ECG Interpretation

made Incredibly Easy!®

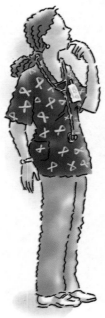

Sixth Edition

Clinical Editor

Jessica Shank Coviello, DNP, APRN, ANP-BC
Associate Professor
Director of the Doctor of Nursing Practice Program
Yale University School of Nursing
West Haven, Connecticut

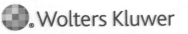. Wolters Kluwer

Philadelphia • Baltimore • New York • London
Buenos Aires • Hong Kong • Sydney • Tokyo

Executive Editor: Shannon W. Magee
Product Development Editor: Maria M. McAvey
Senior Marketing Manager: Mark Wiragh
Senior Production Project Manager: Cynthia Rudy
Design Coordinator: Elaine Kasmer
Manufacturing Coordinator: Kathleen Brown
Prepress Vendor: Aptara, Inc.

Sixth Edition

9 8 7 6 5 4 3 2 1

Printed in China

Library of Congress Cataloging-in-Publication Data

ECG interpretation made incredibly easy! / [edited by] Jessica Shank Coviello. — 6th edition.
   p. ; cm.
  Includes bibliographical references and index.
  ISBN 978-1-4963-0690-6 (alk. paper)
  I. Coviello, Jessica Shank, editor.
  [DNLM: 1. Electrocardiography—methods—Nurses' Instruction. 2. Arrhythmias, Cardiac—diagnosis—Nurses' Instruction. WG 140]
  RC683.5.E5
  616.1'207547—dc23
              2015018775

LWW.com

Contributors

Nancy Bekken, RN, MS, CCRN
Nurse Educator, Adult Critical Care
Spectrum Health
Grand Rapids, Michigan

Carolynn Spera Bruno, PhD, APRN, MSN, CNS, FNP-C
Assistant Professor of Nursing
Division of Primary Care
Yale School of Nursing
West Haven, Connecticut

Karen Crisfulla, RN, MSN, CCNS, CCRN
Clinical Nurse Specialist
Hospital of the University of Pennsylvania
Philadelphia, Pennsylvania

Maurice H. Espinoza, RN, MSN, CNS, CCRN
University of California Irvine Health
Orange, California

Kathleen M. Hill, MSN, RN, CCNS
Clinical Nurse Specialist
Surgical Intensive Care Unit
Cleveland Clinic
Cleveland, Ohio

Mary L. Johnston, APRN
Nurse Practitioner, Cardiology
Middlesex Cardiology Associates
Middletown, Connecticut

Karen Knight-Frank, RN, MS, CS, CCRN, CCNS
Clinical Nurse Specialist, Critical Care
San Joaquin General Hospital
French Camp, California

Marcella Ann Mikalaitis, RN, MSN, CCRN
Clinical Manager
CVICU (Cardiovascular ICU) and IVU
   (Interventional Unit)
Doylestown, Pennsylvania

Leigh Ann Trujillo, RN, MSN
Director Inpatient Orthopedic Services
IU Health La Porte
La Porte, Indiana

Opal V. Wilson, MA, BSN, RN, PCMH CCE
Patient Centered Medical Home (PCMH)
   Project Manger
Family Medicine & Comprehensive Care
LSU Health Shreveport
Shreveport, Louisiana

Previous edition contributors

Diane M. Allen, RN, MSN, ANP, BC, CLS

Nancy Bekken, RN, MS, CCRN

Karen Crisfulla, RN, MSN, CCNS, CCRN

Maurice H. Espinoza, RN, MSN, CNS, CCRN

Kathleen M. Hill, MSN, RN, CCNS

Cheryl Kabeli, RN, MSN, FNP-BC, CNS-BC

Karen Knight-Frank, RN, MS, CS, CCRN, CCNS

Marcella Ann Mikalaitis, RN, MSN, CCRN

Cheryl Rader, RN, BSN, CCRN-CSC

Leigh Ann Trujillo, RN, MSN

Rebecca Unruh, RN, MSN

Opal V. Wilson, MA, BSN, RN, PCMH CCE

Foreword

If you're like me, you're too busy to wade through a foreword that uses pretentious terms and umpteen dull paragraphs to get to the point. So let's cut right to the chase! Here's why this book is so terrific:

1. It will teach you all the important things you need to know about ECG interpretation. (And it will leave out all the fluff that wastes your time.)
2. It will help you remember what you've learned.
3. It will make you smile as it enhances your knowledge and skills.

Don't believe me? Try these recurring logos on for size:

Ages and stages identifies variations in ECGs related to patient age.

Now I get it offers crystal-clear explanations of complex procedures, such as how to use an automated external defibrillator.

Don't skip this strip identifies arrhythmias that have the most serious consequences.

Mixed signals provides tips on how to solve the most common problems in ECG monitoring and interpretation.

I *can't waste time* highlights key points you need to know about each arrhythmia for quick reviews.

See? I told you! And that's not all. Look for me and my friends in the margins throughout this book. We'll be there to explain key concepts, provide important care reminders, and offer reassurance. Oh, and if you don't mind, we'll be spicing up the pages with a bit of humor along the way, to teach and entertain in a way that no other resource can.

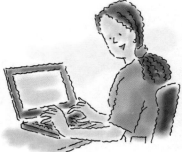

I hope you find this book helpful. Best of luck throughout your career!

Acknowledgments

I would like to thank the wonderful team of nurse contributors who helped revise not only the content, but also several of the illustrations. The caliber of this text would not have been possible without their close attention to detail and their commitment to make this an excellent resource for our colleagues.

Jessica Shank Coviello, DNP, APRN, ANP-BC
Associate Professor
Director of the Doctor of Nursing Practice Program
Yale University School of Nursing

Contents

Part I

ECG fundamentals

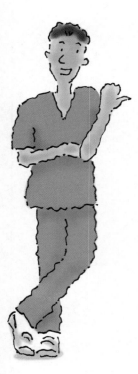

Chapter 1

Cardiac anatomy and physiology

Just the facts

In this chapter, you'll learn:

♦ the location and structure of the heart

♦ the layers of the heart wall

♦ the flow of blood to and through the heart and the structures involved in this flow

♦ phases of the cardiac cycle

♦ properties of cardiac cells

♦ details of cardiac impulse conduction and their relationship to arrhythmias.

A look at cardiac anatomy

Cardiac anatomy includes the location of the heart; the structure of the heart, heart wall, chambers, and valves; and the layout and structure of coronary circulation.

Outside the heart

The heart is a cone-shaped, muscular organ. It's located in the chest, behind the sternum in the mediastinal cavity (or mediastinum), between the lungs, and in front of the spine. The heart lies tilted in this area like an upside-down triangle. The top of the heart, or its base, lies just below the second rib; the bottom of the heart, or its apex, tilts forward and down, toward the left side of the body, and rests on the diaphragm. (See *Location of the pediatric heart*, page 4.)

The heart varies in size depending on the person's body size, but the organ is roughly 5″ (12.5 cm) long and 3½″ (9 cm) wide, or about the size of the person's fist. The heart's weight, typically 9 to 12 oz (255 to 340 g), varies depending on the person's size, age, sex,

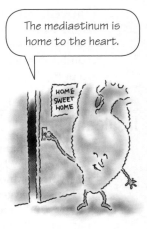

The mediastinum is home to the heart.

and athletic conditioning. An athlete's heart usually weighs more than that of the average person, and an elderly person's heart weighs less. (See *The older adult heart.*) There are differences in male and female cardiovascular anatomy and physiology. A smaller heart and coronary vessels are seen in females versus males. Varying levels of estrogen may be reasons for gender variants in cardiac disease.

Layer upon layer

The heart's wall is made up of three layers: the epicardium, myocardium, and endocardium. (See *Layers of the heart wall.*) The epicardium, the outer layer (and the visceral layer of the serous pericardium), is made up of squamous epithelial cells overlying connective tissue. The myocardium, the middle layer, makes up the largest portion of the heart's wall. This layer of muscle tissue contracts with each heartbeat. The endocardium, the heart's innermost layer, contains endothelial tissue with small blood vessels and bundles of smooth muscle.

A layer of connective tissue called the *pericardium* surrounds the heart and acts as a tough, protective sac. It consists of the fibrous pericardium and the serous pericardium. The fibrous pericardium, composed of tough, white, fibrous tissue, fits loosely around the heart protecting it. The fibrous pericardium attaches to the great vessels, diaphragm, and sternum. The serous pericardium, the thin, smooth, inner portion, has two layers:
- the parietal layer, which lines the inside of the fibrous pericardium
- the visceral layer, which adheres to the surface of the heart

Between the layers

The pericardial space separates the visceral and parietal layers and contains 10 to 20 mL of thin, clear pericardial fluid that lubricates the two surfaces and cushions the heart. Excess pericardial fluid, a condition called *pericardial effusion,* compromises the heart's ability to pump blood.

Inside the heart

The heart contains four chambers—two atria and two ventricles. (See *Inside a normal heart,* page 6.) The right and left atria serve as volume reservoirs for blood being sent into the ventricles. The right atrium receives deoxygenated blood returning from the body through the inferior and superior vena cava and from the heart through the coronary sinus. The left atrium receives oxygenated blood from the lungs through the four pulmonary veins. The interatrial septum divides the chambers and helps them contract. Contraction of the atria forces blood into the ventricles below. Although much emphasis is placed

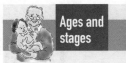

Ages and stages

Location of the pediatric heart

The heart of an infant is positioned more horizontally in the chest cavity than that of the adult. As a result, the apex is at the fourth left intercostal space. Until age 4, the apical impulse is to the left of the midclavicular line. By age 7, the heart is located in the same position as the adult heart.

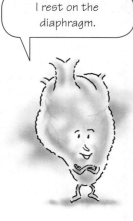

I rest on the diaphragm.

Layers of the heart wall

This cross section of the heart wall shows its various layers.

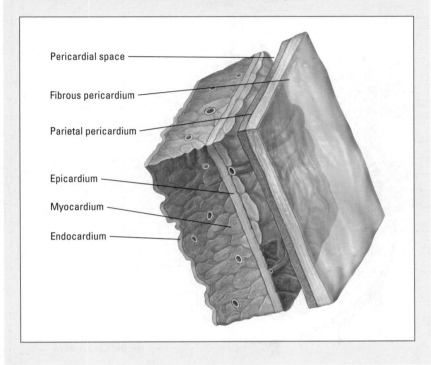

- Pericardial space
- Fibrous pericardium
- Parietal pericardium
- Epicardium
- Myocardium
- Endocardium

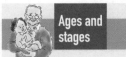

Ages and stages

The older adult heart

As a person ages, his heart usually becomes slightly smaller and loses its contractile strength and efficiency (although exceptions occur in people with hypertension or heart disease). By age 70, cardiac output at rest has diminished by 30% to 35% in many people.

Irritable with age

As the myocardium of the aging heart becomes more irritable, extra systoles may occur, along with sinus arrhythmias and sinus bradycardias. In addition, increased fibrous tissue infiltrates the sinoatrial node and internodal atrial tracts, which may cause atrial fibrillation and flutter.

on left heart function, the right ventricle acts as a key contributor to hemodynamic stability.

Pump up the volume

The right and left ventricles serve as the pumping chambers of the heart. The right ventricle receives blood from the right atrium and pumps it through the pulmonary arteries to the lungs, where it picks up oxygen and drops off carbon dioxide. The left ventricle receives oxygenated blood from the left atrium and pumps it through the aorta and then out to the rest of the body. The interventricular septum separates the ventricles and also helps them to pump.

The thickness of a chamber's walls depends on the amount of high-pressure work the chamber does. Because the atria collect blood for the ventricles and don't pump it far, their walls are considerably thinner than the walls of the ventricles. Likewise, the left ventricle has a much thicker wall than the right ventricle because the left ventricle pumps blood against the higher pressures in the body's

Inside a normal heart

This illustration shows the anatomy of a normal heart.

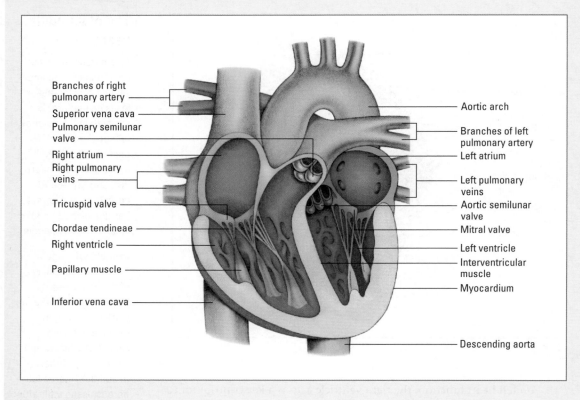

Branches of right pulmonary artery

Superior vena cava

Pulmonary semilunar valve

Right atrium

Right pulmonary veins

Tricuspid valve

Chordae tendineae

Right ventricle

Papillary muscle

Inferior vena cava

Aortic arch

Branches of left pulmonary artery

Left atrium

Left pulmonary veins

Aortic semilunar valve

Mitral valve

Left ventricle

Interventricular muscle

Myocardium

Descending aorta

arterial circulation, whereas the right ventricle pumps blood against the lower pressures in the lungs.

One-way valves

The heart contains four valves—two atrioventricular (AV) valves (tricuspid and mitral) and two semilunar valves (aortic and pulmonic). The valves open and close in response to changes in pressure within the chambers they connect. They serve as one-way doors that keep blood flowing through the heart in a forward direction.

When the valves close, they prevent backflow, or *regurgitation,* of blood from one chamber to another. The closing of the valves creates the heart sounds that are heard through a stethoscope.

The two AV valves, located between the atria and ventricles, are called the *tricuspid* and *mitral valves.* The tricuspid valve is located between the right atrium and the right ventricle. The mitral valve is located between the left atrium and the left ventricle.

Cardiac cords

The mitral valve has two cusps, or *leaflets,* and the tricuspid valve has three. The cusps are anchored to the papillary muscles in the heart wall by fibers called *chordae tendineae.* These cords work together to prevent the cusps from bulging backward into the atria during ventricular contraction. If damage occurs, blood can flow backward into a chamber, resulting in a heart murmur.

Under pressure

The semilunar valves are the pulmonic valve and the aortic valve. These valves are called semilunar because the cusps resemble three half-moons. Because of the high pressures exerted on the valves, their structure is much simpler than that of the AV valves.

They open due to pressure within the ventricles and close due to the back pressure of blood in the pulmonary arteries and aorta, which pushes the cusps closed. The pulmonic valve, located where the pulmonary artery meets the right ventricle, permits blood to flow from the right ventricle to the pulmonary artery and prevents blood backflow into that ventricle. The aortic valve, located where the left ventricle meets the aorta, allows blood to flow from the left ventricle to the aorta and prevents blood backflow into the left ventricle.

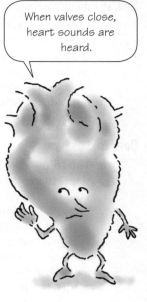

When valves close, heart sounds are heard.

Blood flow through the heart

Understanding how blood flows through the heart is critical to understanding the heart's overall functions and how changes in electrical activity affect peripheral blood flow. Deoxygenated blood from the body returns to the heart through the inferior and superior vena cava and empties into the right atrium. From there, blood flows through the tricuspid valve into the right ventricle.

Circuit city

The right ventricle pumps blood through the pulmonic valve into the pulmonary arteries and then into the lungs. From the lungs, blood flows through the pulmonary veins and empties into the left atrium, which completes a circuit called *pulmonary circulation.*

When pressure rises to a critical point in the left atrium, the mitral valve opens and blood flows into the left ventricle. The left ventricle then contracts and pumps blood through the aortic valve into the aorta, and then throughout the body. Blood returns to the right atrium through the veins, completing a circuit called *systemic circulation.*

Getting into circulation

Like the brain and all other organs, the heart needs an adequate supply of blood to survive. The coronary arteries, which lie on the surface of the heart, supply the heart muscle with blood and oxygen. Understanding coronary blood flow can help you provide better care for a patient with a myocardial infarction (MI) because you'll be able to predict which areas of the heart would be affected by a blockage in a particular coronary artery.

Open that ostium

The coronary ostium, an opening in the aorta that feeds blood to the coronary arteries, is located near the aortic valve. During systole, when the left ventricle is pumping blood through the aorta and the aortic valve is open, the coronary ostium is partially covered. During diastole, when the left ventricle is filling with blood, the aortic valve is closed and the coronary ostium is open, enabling blood to fill the coronary arteries.

With a shortened diastole, which occurs during periods of tachycardia, less blood flows through the ostium into the coronary arteries. Tachycardia also impedes coronary blood flow because contraction of the ventricles squeezes the arteries and lessens blood flow through them.

That's right, coronary

The right coronary artery, as well as the left coronary artery (also known as the *left main artery*), originates as a single branch off the ascending aorta from the area known as the *sinuses of Valsalva*. The right coronary artery supplies blood to the right atrium, the right ventricle, and part of the inferior and posterior surfaces of the left ventricle. In about 50% of the population, the artery also supplies blood to the sinoatrial (SA) node. The bundle of His and the AV node also receive their blood supply from the right coronary artery.

What's left, coronary?

The left coronary artery runs along the surface of the left atrium, where it splits into two major branches, the left anterior descending and the left circumflex arteries. The left anterior descending artery runs down the surface of the left ventricle toward the apex and supplies blood to the anterior wall of the left ventricle, the interventricular septum, the right bundle branch, and the left anterior fasciculus of the left bundle branch. The branches of the left anterior descending artery—the septal perforators and the diagonal arteries—help supply blood to the walls of both ventricles.

> Knowing about coronary blood flow can help me predict which areas of the heart would be affected by a blockage in a particular coronary artery.

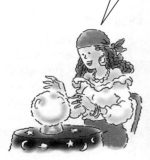

Circling circumflex

The circumflex artery supplies oxygenated blood to the lateral walls of the left ventricle, the left atrium and, in about half of the population, the SA node. In addition, the circumflex artery supplies blood to the left posterior fasciculus of the left bundle branch. This artery circles the left ventricle and provides blood to the ventricle's posterior portion.

Circulation, guaranteed

When two or more arteries supply the same region, they usually connect through anastomoses, junctions that provide alternative routes of blood flow. This network of smaller arteries, called *collateral circulation*, provides blood to capillaries that directly feed the heart muscle. Collateral circulation commonly becomes so strong that even if major coronary arteries become clogged with plaque, collateral circulation can continue to supply blood to the heart.

Veins in the heart

The heart has veins just like other parts of the body. Cardiac veins collect deoxygenated blood from the capillaries of the myocardium. The cardiac veins join to form an enlarged vessel called the *coronary sinus,* which returns blood to the right atrium, where it continues through the circulation.

A look at cardiac physiology

This discussion of cardiac physiology includes descriptions of the cardiac cycle, how the cardiac muscle is innervated (distribution/supply of nerves), how the depolarization–repolarization cycle operates, how impulses are conducted, and how abnormal impulses work. (See *Events of the cardiac cycle,* page 10.)

Cardiac cycle dynamics

During one heartbeat, ventricular diastole (relaxation) and ventricular systole (contraction) occur.

During diastole, the ventricles relax, the atria contract, and blood is forced through the open tricuspid and mitral valves. The aortic and pulmonic valves are closed.

During systole, the atria relax and fill with blood. The mitral and tricuspid valves are closed. Ventricular pressure rises, which forces open the aortic and pulmonic valves. Then the ventricles contract, and blood flows through the circulatory system.

Events of the cardiac cycle

The cardiac cycle consists of the following five events:

• *Isovolumetric ventricular contraction:* In response to ventricular depolarization, tension in the ventricles increases. The rise in pressure within the ventricles leads to closure of the mitral and tricuspid valves. The pulmonic and aortic valves stay closed during the entire phase.

• *Ventricular ejection:* When ventricular pressure exceeds aortic and pulmonary arterial pressure, the aortic and pulmonic valves open and the ventricles eject blood.

• *Isovolumetric relaxation:* When ventricular pressure falls below pressure in the aorta and pulmonary artery, the aortic and pulmonic valves close. All valves are closed during this phase. Atrial diastole occurs as blood fills the atria.

• *Ventricular filling:* Atrial pressure exceeds ventricular pressure, which causes the mitral and tricuspid valves to open. Blood then flows passively into the ventricles. About 70% of ventricular filling takes place during this phase.

• *Atrial systole:* Known as the *atrial kick,* atrial systole (coinciding with late ventricular diastole) supplies the ventricles with the remaining 30% of the blood for each heartbeat.

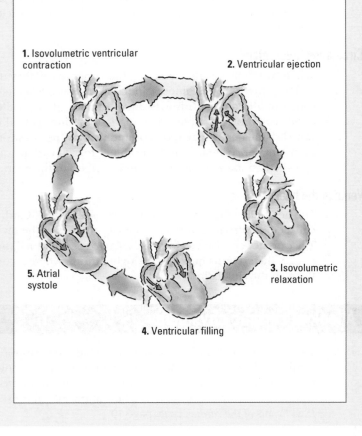

1. Isovolumetric ventricular contraction

2. Ventricular ejection

3. Isovolumetric relaxation

4. Ventricular filling

5. Atrial systole

Atrial kick

The atrial contraction, or atrial kick, contributes about 30% of the cardiac output—the amount of blood pumped by the ventricles in 1 minute. (See *Quick facts about circulation.*) Certain arrhythmias, such as atrial fibrillation, can cause a loss of atrial kick and a subsequent drop in cardiac output. Tachycardia also affects cardiac output by shortening diastole and allowing less time for the ventricles to fill. Less filling time means less blood will be ejected during ventricular systole and less will be sent through the circulation.

A balancing act

The cardiac cycle produces cardiac output, which is the amount of blood the heart pumps in 1 minute. It's measured by multiplying heart rate times stroke volume. (See *Understanding preload, afterload, and contractility,* page 12.) The term stroke volume refers to the amount of blood ejected with each ventricular contraction.

Normal cardiac output is 4 to 8 L/min, depending on body size. The heart pumps only as much blood as the body requires. Three factors affect stroke volume—preload, afterload, and myocardial contractility. A balance of these three factors produces optimal cardiac output.

Preload

Preload is the stretching of muscle fibers in the ventricles and is determined by the pressure and amount of blood remaining in the left ventricle at the end of diastole.

Afterload

Afterload is the amount of pressure the left ventricle must work against to pump blood into the circulation. The greater this resistance, the more the heart works to pump out blood.

Contractility

Contractility is the ability of muscle cells to contract after depolarization. This ability depends on how much the muscle fibers are stretched at the end of diastole. Over stretching or under stretching these fibers alters contractility and the amount of blood pumped out of the ventricles. To better understand this concept, imagine you are trying to shoot a rubber band across the room. If you don't stretch the rubber band enough, it won't go far. If you stretch it too much, it will snap. However, if you stretch it just the right amount, it will go as far as you want it to.

> ### Quick facts about circulation
>
> - It would take about 25 capillaries laid end-to-end to fill 1" (2.5 cm).
> - The body contains about 10 billion capillaries.
> - On average, it takes a red blood cell less than 1 minute to travel from the heart to the capillaries and back again.

Contractility is the heart's ability to stretch—like a balloon!

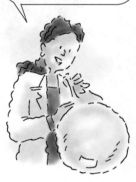

Nerve supply to the heart

The heart is supplied by the two branches of the autonomic nervous system—the sympathetic, or *adrenergic,* and the parasympathetic, or *cholinergic.*

The sympathetic nervous system is basically the heart's accelerator. Two sets of chemicals—norepinephrine and epinephrine—are highly influenced by this system. These chemicals increase heart rate, automaticity, AV conduction, and contractility.

Understanding preload, afterload, and contractility

To better understand preload, afterload, and contractility, think of the heart as a balloon.

Preload

Preload is the passive stretching of muscle fibers in the ventricles. This stretching results from blood volume in the ventricles at end-diastole. According to Starling's law, the more the heart muscles stretch during diastole, the more forcefully they contract during systole. Think of preload as the balloon stretching as air is blown into it. The more air the greater the stretch.

Contractility

Contractility refers to the inherent ability of the myocardium to contract normally. Contractility is influenced by preload. The greater the stretch the more forceful the contraction—or, the more air in the balloon, the greater the stretch and the farther the balloon will fly when air is allowed to expel.

Afterload

Afterload refers to the pressure that the ventricular muscles must generate to overcome the higher pressure in the aorta to get the blood out of the heart. *Resistance* is the knot on the end of the balloon, which the balloon has to work against to get the air out.

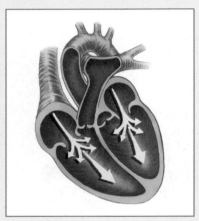

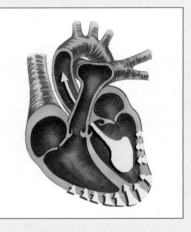

Braking the heart

The parasympathetic nervous system, on the other hand, serves as the heart's brakes. One of this system's nerves, the vagus nerve, carries impulses that slow heart rate and the conduction of impulses through the AV node and ventricles. Stimulating this system releases the chemical acetylcholine, slowing the heart rate.

The vagus nerve is stimulated by baroreceptors, specialized nerve cells in the aorta, and the internal carotid arteries. Conditions that stimulate the baroreceptors also stimulate the vagus nerve.

For example, a stretching of the baroreceptors, which can occur during periods of hypertension or when applying pressure to the carotid artery, stimulates the receptors. In a maneuver called carotid sinus massage, baroreceptors in the carotid arteries are purposely activated in an effort to slow a rapid heart rate.

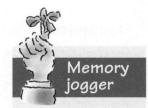

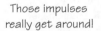

Memory jogger

To help you remember the difference between depolarization and repolarization, think of the **R** in repolarization as standing for **REST.** Remember that repolarization is the resting phase of the cardiac cycle.

Transmission of electrical impulses

The heart can't pump unless an electrical stimulus occurs first. Generation and transmission of electrical impulses depend on four characteristics of cardiac cells:

- *Automaticity* refers to a cell's ability to spontaneously initiate an impulse. Pacemaker cells possess this ability.
- *Excitability* results from ion shifts across the cell membrane and indicates how well a cell responds to an electrical stimulus.
- *Conductivity* is the ability of a cell to transmit an electrical impulse to another cardiac cell.
- *Contractility* refers to how well the cell contracts after receiving a stimulus.

"De"-cycle and "re"-cycle

As impulses are transmitted, cardiac cells undergo cycles of depolarization and repolarization. (See *Depolarization–repolarization cycle,* page 14.) Cardiac cells at rest are considered polarized, meaning that no electrical activity takes place. Cell membranes separate different concentrations of ions, such as sodium and potassium, and create a more negative charge inside the cell. This is called the resting potential. After a stimulus occurs, ions cross the cell membrane and cause an action potential, or cell depolarization.

When a cell is fully depolarized, it attempts to return to its resting state in a process called repolarization. Electrical charges in the cell reverse and return to normal.

A cycle of depolarization–repolarization consists of five phases—0 through 4. The action potential is represented by a curve that shows voltage changes during the five phases. (See *Action potential curve,* page 15.)

Those impulses really get around!

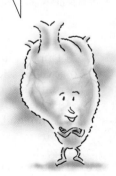

Many phases of the curve

During phase 0, the cell receives an impulse from a neighboring cell and is depolarized. Phase 1 is marked by early, rapid repolarization. Phase 2, the plateau phase, is a period of slow repolarization.

Depolarization–repolarization cycle

The depolarization–repolarization cycle consists of the following phases:

Phase 0:
Rapid depolarization
- Sodium (Na$^+$) moves rapidly into cell.
- Calcium (Ca^{++}) moves slowly into cell.

CELL

CELL
MEMBRANE

Na+
Ca++

Phase 1:
Early repolarization
- Sodium channels close.

Na+

Phase 2:
Plateau phase
- Calcium continues to flow in.
- Potassium (K$^+$) continues to flow out.

Ca++
K+

Phase 3:
Rapid repolarization
- Calcium channels close.
- Potassium flows out rapidly.
- Active transport via the sodium–potassium pump begins restoring potassium to the inside of the cell and sodium to the outside of the cell.

Ca++
K+
Sodium-
potassium
pump
K+
Na+

Phase 4:
Resting phase
- Cell membrane is impermeable to sodium.
- Potassium moves out of the cell.

Na+
K+

During phases 1 and 2 and at the beginning of phase 3, the cardiac cell is said to be in its absolute refractory period. During that period, no stimulus, no matter how strong, can excite the cell.

Phase 3, the rapid repolarization phase, occurs as the cell returns to its original state. During the last half of this phase, when the cell is in its relative refractory period, a very strong stimulus can depolarize it.

Phase 4 is the resting phase of the action potential. By the end of phase 4, the cell is ready for another stimulus.

All that electrical activity is represented on an electrocardiogram (ECG). Keep in mind that the ECG represents electrical activity only, not actual pumping of the heart.

Action potential curve

An action potential curve shows the electrical changes in a myocardial cell during the depolarization–repolarization cycle. This graph shows the changes in a non-pacemaker cell.

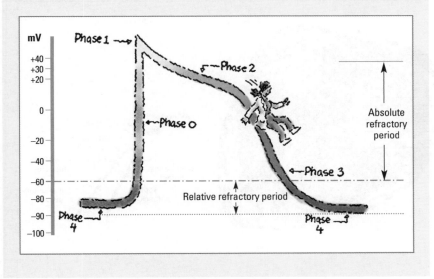

Pathway through the heart

After depolarization and repolarization occur, the resulting electrical impulse travels through the heart along a pathway called the *conduction system*. (See *The cardiac conduction system*, page 16.)

Impulses travel out from the SA node and through the internodal tracts and Bachmann's bundle to the AV node. From there, they travel through the bundle of His, the bundle branches, and lastly to the Purkinje fibers.

Setting the pace

The SA node is located in the upper right corner of the right atrium, where the superior vena cava joins the atrial tissue mass. It's the heart's main pacemaker, generating impulses 60 to 100 times per minute. When initiated, the impulses follow a specific path through the heart. They usually can't flow backward because the cells can't respond to a stimulus immediately after depolarization.

The cardiac conduction system

Specialized fibers propagate electrical impulses throughout the heart's cells, causing the heart to contract. This illustration shows the elements of the cardiac conduction system.

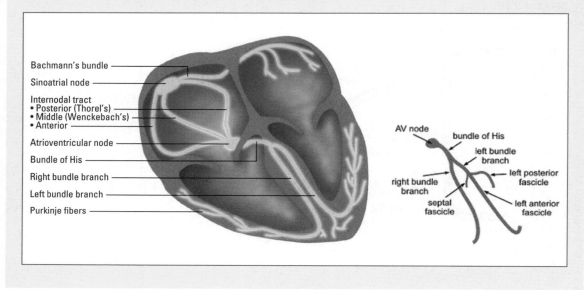

Bachmann's bundle of nerves

Impulses from the SA node next travel through Bachmann's bundle, tracts of tissue extending from the SA node to the left atrium. Impulses are thought to be transmitted throughout the right atrium through the anterior, middle, and posterior internodal tracts. Whether those tracts actually exist, however, is unclear. Impulse transmission through the right and left atria occurs so rapidly that the atria contract almost simultaneously.

AV: The slow node

The AV node, located in the inferior right atrium near the ostium of the coronary sinus, is responsible for delaying the impulses that reach it. Although the nodal tissue itself has no pacemaker cells, the tissue surrounding it (called *junctional tissue*) contains pacemaker cells that can fire at a rate of 40 to 60 times per minute.

The AV node's main function is to delay impulses by 0.04 second to keep the ventricles from contracting too quickly. This delay allows the ventricles to complete their filling phase as the atria contract. It also allows the cardiac muscle to stretch to its fullest for peak cardiac output.

Branch splitting

The bundle of His, a tract of tissue extending into the ventricles next to the interventricular septum, resumes the rapid conduction of the impulse through the ventricles. The bundle eventually divides into the right and left bundle branches.

The right bundle branch extends down the right side of the interventricular septum and through the right ventricle. The left bundle branch extends down the left side of the interventricular septum and through the left ventricle.

The left bundle branch then splits into two branches, or fasciculi: the left anterior fasciculus, which extends through the anterior portion of the left ventricle, and the left posterior fasciculus, which runs through the lateral and posterior portions of the left ventricle. Impulses travel much faster down the left bundle branch (which feeds the larger, thicker-walled left ventricle) than the right bundle branch (which feeds the smaller, thinner-walled right ventricle).

The difference in the conduction speed allows both ventricles to contract simultaneously. The entire network of specialized nervous tissue that extends through the ventricles is known as the *His-Purkinje system*.

Those perky Purkinje fibers

Purkinje fibers extend from the bundle branches into the endocardium, deep into the myocardial tissue. These fibers conduct impulses rapidly through the muscle to assist in its depolarization and contraction.

Purkinje fibers can also serve as a pacemaker and are able to discharge impulses at a rate of 20 to 40 times per minute, sometimes even more slowly. (See *Pacemakers of the heart*, page 18.) Purkinje fibers usually aren't activated as a pacemaker unless conduction through the bundle of His becomes blocked or a higher pacemaker (SA or AV node) doesn't generate an impulse. (See *Pediatric pacemaker rates*, page 18.)

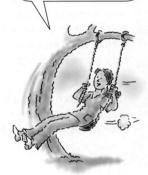

The bundle of His eventually divides into the right and left bundle branches. This branch works just fine for me!

Pacemakers of the heart

Pacemaker cells in lower areas, such as the junctional tissue and the Purkinje fibers, normally remain dormant because they receive impulses from the sinoatrial (SA) node. They initiate an impulse only when they don't receive one from above, such as when the SA node is damaged from a myocardial infarction.

Firing rates

This illustration shows intrinsic firing rates of pacemaker cells located in three critical areas of the heart.

SA node,
60 to 100/minute

Atrioventricular junction,
40 to 60/minute

Purkinje fibers,
20 to 40/minute

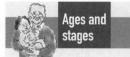

Ages and stages

Pediatric pacemaker rates

In children younger than age 3, the atrioventricular node may discharge impulses at a rate of 50 to 80 times per minute; the Purkinje fibers may discharge at a rate of 40 to 50 times per minute.

Abnormal impulses

Now that you understand how the heart generates a normal impulse, let's look at some causes of abnormal impulse conduction, including automaticity, backward conduction of impulses, re-entry abnormalities, and ectopy.

When the heart goes on "manual"

Automaticity is a special characteristic of pacemaker cells that generates impulses automatically, without being stimulated to do so. If a cell's automaticity is increased or decreased, an arrhythmia can occur. Tachycardia, for example, is commonly caused by an increase in the automaticity of pacemaker cells below the SA node. Likewise, a decrease in automaticity of cells in the SA node can cause the development of bradycardia or an escape rhythm (a compensatory beat generated by a lower pacemaker site).

Out of synch

Impulses that begin below the AV node can be transmitted backward toward the atria. This backward, or retrograde, conduction usually takes longer than normal conduction and can cause the atria and ventricles to beat out of synch.

Coming back for more

Sometimes impulses cause depolarization twice in a row at a faster-than-normal rate. Such events are referred to as *re-entry events*. In re-entry, impulses are delayed long enough that cells have time to repolarize. In these cases, the active impulse re-enters the same area and produces another impulse.

Repeating itself

An injured pacemaker (or nonpacemaker) cell may partially depolarize, rather than fully depolarizing. Partial depolarization can lead to spontaneous or secondary depolarization, which involves repetitive ectopic firings called *triggered activity*.

The resultant depolarization is called *afterdepolarization*. Early afterdepolarization occurs before the cell is fully repolarized and can be caused by hypokalemia, slow pacing rates, or drug toxicity. If it occurs after the cell has been fully repolarized, it's called *delayed afterdepolarization*. These problems can be caused by digoxin toxicity, hypercalcemia, or increased catecholamine release. Atrial or ventricular tachycardias may result. You'll learn more about these and other arrhythmias in later chapters.

That's a wrap!

Cardiac anatomy and physiology review

The heart's valves
- *Tricuspid*—AV valve between the right atrium and right ventricle
- *Mitral*—AV valve between the left atrium and left ventricle
- *Aortic*—semilunar valve between the left ventricle and the aorta
- *Pulmonic*—semilunar valve between the right ventricle and the pulmonary artery

Blood flow
- Deoxygenated blood from the body returns to the right atrium and then flows to the right ventricle.
- The right ventricle pumps blood into the lungs where it's oxygenated. Then the blood returns to the left atrium and flows to the left ventricle.
- Oxygenated blood is pumped to the aorta and the body by the left ventricle.

Coronary arteries and veins
- *Right coronary artery*—supplies blood to the right atrium and ventricle and part of the left ventricle
- *Left anterior descending artery*—supplies blood to the anterior wall of the left ventricle, interventricular septum, right bundle branch, and left anterior fasciculus of the left bundle branch
- *Circumflex artery*—supplies blood to the lateral walls of the left ventricle, left atrium, and left posterior fasciculus of the left bundle branch
- *Cardiac veins*—collect blood from the capillaries of the myocardium
- *Coronary sinus*—returns blood to the right atrium

Cardiac cycle dynamics
- *Atrial kick*—atrial contraction, contributing about 30% of the cardiac output

(continued)

Cardiac anatomy and physiology review *(Continued)*

- *Cardiac output*—the amount of blood the heart pumps in 1 minute, calculated by multiplying heart rate times stroke volume
- *Stroke volume*—the amount of blood ejected with each ventricular contraction (it's affected by preload, afterload, and contractility)
- *Preload*—the passive stretching exerted by blood on the ventricular muscle at the end of diastole
- *Afterload*—the amount of pressure the left ventricle must work against to pump blood into the aorta
- *Contractility*—the ability of the heart muscle cells to contract after depolarization

Innervation of the heart

Two branches of the autonomic nervous system supply the heart:
- *Sympathetic nervous system*—increases heart rate, automaticity, AV conduction, and contractility through release of norepinephrine and epinephrine
- *Parasympathetic nervous system*—vagus nerve stimulation reduces heart rate and AV conduction through release of acetylcholine

Transmission of electrical impulses

Generation and transmission of electrical impulses depend on these cell characteristics:
- *Automaticity*—a cell's ability to spontaneously initiate an impulse, such as found in pacemaker cells
- *Excitability*—how well a cell responds to an electrical stimulus
- *Conductivity*—the ability of a cell to transmit an electrical impulse to another cardiac cell

- *Contractility*—how well the cell contracts after receiving a stimulus

Depolarization–repolarization cycle

Cardiac cells undergo the following cycles of depolarization and repolarization as impulses are transmitted:
- *Phase 0: Rapid depolarization*—the cell receives an impulse from a nearby cell and is depolarized
- *Phase 1: Early repolarization*—early rapid repolarization occurs
- *Phase 2: Plateau phase*—a period of slow repolarization occurs
- *Phase 3: Rapid repolarization*—the cell returns to its original state
- *Phase 4: Resting phase*—the cell rests and readies itself for another stimulus

Cardiac conduction

- The electrical impulse begins in the SA node and travels through the internodal tracts and Bachmann's bundle to the AV node
- From the AV node, the impulse travels down the bundle of His, along the bundle branches, and through the Purkinje fibers

Intrinsic firing rates

- *SA node*—60 to 100/min
- *AV junction*—40 to 60/min
- *Purkinje fibers*—20 to 40/min

Abnormal impulses

- *Automaticity*—the ability of a cardiac cell to initiate an impulse on its own
- *Retrograde conduction*—impulses that are transmitted backward toward the atria
- *Re-entry*—when an impulse follows a circular, rather than the normal, conduction path

Quick quiz

1. The term *automaticity* refers to the ability of a cell to:
   A. initiate an impulse on its own.
   B. send impulses in all directions.
   C. block impulses formed in areas other than the SA node.
   D. generate an impulse when stimulated.

Answer: A. Automaticity, the ability of a cell to initiate an impulse on its own, is a unique characteristic of cardiac cells.

2. Parasympathetic stimulation of the heart results in:
   A. increased heart rate and decreased contractility.
   B. increased heart rate and faster AV conduction.
   C. decreased heart rate and slower AV conduction.
   D. decreased heart rate and increased contractility.

Answer: C. Parasympathetic stimulation of the vagus nerve causes a decrease in heart rate and slowed AV conduction.

3. The normal pacemaker of the heart is the:
   A. SA node.
   B. AV node.
   C. bundle of His.
   D. Purkinje fibers.

Answer: A. The SA node is the normal pacemaker of the heart, firing at an intrinsic rate of 60 to 100 times per minute.

4. The impulse delay produced by the AV node allows the atria to:
   A. repolarize simultaneously.
   B. contract before the ventricles.
   C. send impulses to the bundle of His.
   D. complete their filling.

Answer: B. The 0.04-second delay allows the atria to contract and the ventricles to completely fill, which optimizes cardiac output.

5. The coronary arteries fill with blood during:
   A. atrial systole.
   B. atrial diastole.
   C. ventricular systole.
   D. ventricular diastole.

Answer: D. The coronary arteries fill with blood when the ventricles are in diastole and filling with blood. The aortic valve is closed at that time, so it no longer blocks blood flow through the coronary ostium into the coronary arteries.

6. When stimulated, baroreceptors cause the heart rate to:
   A. increase.
   B. decrease.
   C. stay the same.
   D. become irregular.

Answer: B. Baroreceptors, when stimulated, cause the heart rate to decrease.

7. The two valves called the *semilunar valves* are the:
   A. pulmonic and tricuspid valves.
   B. pulmonic and aortic valves.
   C. aortic and mitral valves.
   D. aortic and tricuspid valves.

Answer: B. The pulmonic and aortic valves are semilunar.

8. Passive stretching exerted by blood on the ventricular muscle at the end of diastole is referred to as:
   A. preload.
   B. afterload.
   C. the atrial kick.
   D. cardiac output.

Answer: A. Preload is the passive stretching exerted by blood on the ventricular muscle at the end of diastole. It increases with an increase in venous return to the heart.

9. A patient admitted with an acute MI has a heart rate of 36 beats/minute. Based on this finding, which area of the heart is most likely serving as the pacemaker?
   A. SA node
   B. AV node
   C. Bachmann's bundle
   D. Purkinje fibers

Answer: D. If the SA node (which fires at a rate of 60 to 100 times per minute) and the AV node (which takes over firing at 40 to 60 times per minute) are damaged, the Purkinje fibers take over firing at a rate of 20 to 40 times per minute.

Scoring

★★★ If you answered all nine questions correctly, hooray! You're a happenin', heart-smart hipster.

★★ If you answered six to eight questions correctly, way to go! You're clearly heart smart.

★ If you answered fewer than six questions correctly, take heart. Just review this chapter and you'll be up to speed.

Recommended references

Buddiga, P. (2014). *Cardiovascular system anatomy.* Medscape Reference. Retrieved November 20, 2014 from http://emedicine.medscape.com/article/1948510-overview

Ellis, K. (2012). *EKG plain and simple* (3rd ed.). Pearson. Retrieved from http://online.statref.com/Document.aspx?FxId=195&SessionId=E66894SWQOSRWRB

Mohrman, D. E., & Hellen, L. (2014). Overview of the cardiovascular system. In D. H. Mohrman (Ed.), *Cardiovascular physiology* (8th ed., Ch. 1). New York, NY: McGraw Hill. Retrieved November 13, 2014, from http://accessmedicine.mhmedical.com/content.aspx?bookid=843&sectionid=48779649

Rigolin, V. H., Robiolio, P. A., Wilson, J. S., Harrison, J. K., & Bashore, T. M. (1995). The forgotten chamber: the importance of the right ventricle. *Catheterization and Cardiovascular Diagnosis, 35*(1), 18–28.

Wingate, S. (1997). Cardiovascular anatomy and physiology in the female. *Critical Care Nursing Clinics of North America, 9*(4), 447–452.

Zamorano, J. L., González-Gómez, A., & Lancellotti, P. (2014). Mitral valve anatomy: implications for transcatheter mitral valve interventions. *EuroIntervention,* 1–6. Europepmc.org/abstract/med/25256321

Chapter 2

Obtaining a rhythm strip

Just the facts

In this chapter, you'll learn:

◆ the importance of ECGs in providing effective patient care

◆ the functions of leads and planes

◆ types of ECG monitoring systems

◆ proper techniques for applying electrodes, selecting leads, and obtaining rhythm strips

◆ solutions for cardiac-monitoring problems.

A look at ECG recordings

The heart's electrical activity produces currents that radiate through the surrounding tissue to the skin. When electrodes are attached to the skin, they sense those electrical currents and transmit them to an ECG monitor. The currents are then transformed into waveforms that represent the heart's depolarization–repolarization cycle.

You might remember that myocardial depolarization occurs when a wave of stimulation passes through the heart and stimulates the heart muscle to contract. Repolarization is the return to the resting state and results in relaxation.

An ECG shows the precise sequence of electrical events occurring in the cardiac cells throughout that process. It allows the nurse to monitor phases of myocardial contraction and to identify rhythm and conduction disturbances. A series of ECGs can be used as a baseline comparison to assess cardiac function.

An ECG shows the sequence of cardiac events.

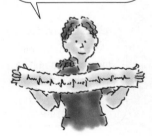

Leads and planes

To understand electrocardiography, you need to understand leads and planes. Electrodes placed on the skin measure the direction of electrical current discharged by the heart. That current is then transformed into waveforms.

An ECG records information about those waveforms from different views or perspectives. Those perspectives are called *leads* and *planes*.

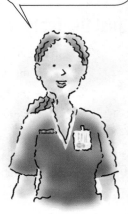

Leads and planes offer different views of the heart's electrical activity

Take the lead

A lead provides a view of the heart's electrical activity between one positive pole and one negative pole. Between the two poles lies an imaginary line representing the lead's axis, a term that refers to the direction of the current moving through the heart.

The direction of the current affects the direction in which the waveform points on an ECG. (See *Current direction and wave deflection*.) When no electrical activity occurs or the activity is too weak to measure, the waveform looks like a straight line, called an isoelectric waveform.

Current direction and wave deflection

This illustration shows possible directions of electrical current, or depolarization, on a lead. The direction of the electrical current determines the upward or downward deflection of an electrocardiogram waveform.

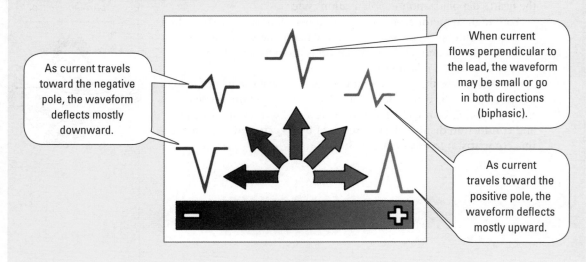

As current travels toward the negative pole, the waveform deflects mostly downward.

When current flows perpendicular to the lead, the waveform may be small or go in both directions (biphasic).

As current travels toward the positive pole, the waveform deflects mostly upward.

Plane and simple

The term *plane* refers to a cross-sectional perspective of the heart's electrical activity. The frontal plane, a vertical cut through the middle of the heart, provides an anterior-to-posterior view of electrical activity. The horizontal plane, a transverse cut through the middle of the heart, provides either a superior or an inferior view.

Types of ECGs

The two types of ECG recordings are the 12-lead ECG and a rhythm strip. Both types give valuable information about heart function.

A dozen views

A 12-lead ECG records information from 12 different views of the heart and provides a complete picture of electrical activity. These 12 views are obtained by placing electrodes on the patient's limbs and chest. The limb leads and the chest, or precordial leads reflect information from the different planes of the heart.

Different leads provide different information. The six limb leads—I, II, III, augmented vector right (aV_R), augmented vector left (aV_L), and augmented vector foot (aV_F)—provide information about the heart's frontal (vertical) plane. Leads I, II, and III require a negative and positive electrode for monitoring, which makes those leads bipolar. The augmented leads record information from one lead and are called *unipolar*.

The six precordial or V leads—V_1, V_2, V_3, V_4, V_5, and V_6—provide information about the heart's horizontal plane. Like the augmented leads, the precordial leads are also unipolar, requiring only a single electrode. The opposing pole of those leads is the center of the heart as calculated by the ECG.

Just one view

A rhythm strip, which can be used to monitor cardiac status, provides information about the heart's electrical activity from one or more leads simultaneously. Chest electrodes pick up the heart's electrical activity for display on the monitor. The monitor also displays heart rate and other measurements and allows for printing strips of cardiac rhythms.

Commonly monitored leads include the bipolar leads I, II, III, V_1, V_6, MCL_1, and MCL_6. The initials MCL stand for modified chest lead. These leads are similar to the unipolar leads V_1 and V_6 of the 12-lead ECG. MCL_1 and MCL_6, however, are bipolar leads.

Monitoring ECGs

The type of ECG monitoring system you'll use—hardwire monitoring or telemetry—depends on the patient's condition and where you work. Let's look at each system.

Hardwire basics

With hardwire monitoring, the electrodes are connected directly to the cardiac monitor. Most hardwire monitors are mounted permanently on a shelf or wall near the patient's bed. Some monitors are mounted on an I.V. pole for portability, and some may include a defibrillator.

The monitor provides a continuous cardiac rhythm display and transmits the ECG tracing to a console at the nurses' station. Both the monitor and the console have alarms and can print rhythm strips. Hardwire monitors can also track pulse oximetry, blood pressure, hemodynamic measurements, and other parameters through various attachments to the patient.

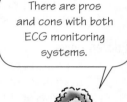

There are pros and cons with both ECG monitoring systems.

Some drawbacks

Hardwire monitoring is generally used in intensive care units and emergency departments because it permits continuous observation of one or more patients from more than one area in the unit. However, this type of monitoring does have drawbacks, among them:

- limited patient mobility because the patient is tethered to a monitor by a cable
- patient discomfort because the electrodes and cables are attached to the chest
- possibility of lead disconnection and loss of cardiac monitoring when the patient moves.

Portable points

Telemetry monitoring is generally used in step-down units and medical-surgical units where patients are permitted more activity. With telemetry monitoring, the patient carries a small, battery-powered transmitter that sends electrical signals to another location where the signals are displayed on a monitor screen. This type of ECG monitoring frees the patient from cumbersome wires and cables associated with hardwire monitoring.

Telemetry monitoring still requires skin electrodes to be placed on the patient's chest. Each electrode is connected by a thin wire to a small transmitter box carried in a pocket or pouch. It's especially useful for detecting arrhythmias that occur with activity or stressful situations. Most systems, however, can monitor heart rate and rhythm only.

All about leads

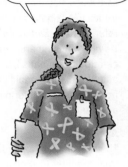

Adjust the leads according to the patient's condition.

Electrode placement is different for each lead, and different leads provide different views of the heart. A lead may be chosen to highlight a particular part of the ECG complex or the electrical events of a specific cardiac cycle.

Although leads II, V_1, and V_6 are among the most commonly used leads for monitoring, you should adjust the leads according to the patient's condition. If your monitoring system has the capability, you may also monitor the patient in more than one lead.

Going to ground

All bipolar leads have a third electrode, known as the *ground*, which is placed on the chest to prevent electrical interference from appearing on the ECG recording.

Heeeere's lead I

Lead I provides a view of the heart that shows current moving from right to left. Because current flows from negative to positive, the positive electrode for this lead is placed on the left arm or on the left side of the chest; the negative electrode is placed on the right arm. Lead I produces a positive deflection on ECG tracings and is helpful in monitoring atrial rhythms and hemiblocks.

Introducing lead II

Lead II produces a positive deflection. Place the positive electrode on the patient's left leg and the negative electrode on the right arm. For continuous monitoring, place the electrodes on the torso for convenience, with the positive electrode below the lowest palpable rib at the left midclavicular line and the negative electrode below the right clavicle. The current travels down and to the left in this lead. Lead II tends to produce a positive, high-voltage deflection, resulting in tall P, R, and T waves. This lead is commonly used for routine monitoring and is useful for detecting sinus node and atrial arrhythmias.

Next up, lead III

Lead III produces a positive deflection. The positive electrode is placed on the left leg; the negative electrode, on the left arm. Along with lead II, this lead is useful for detecting changes associated with an inferior wall myocardial infarction.

The axes of the three bipolar limb leads—I, II, and III—form a triangle around the heart and provide a frontal plane view of the heart. (See *Einthoven's triangle*, page 30.)

Einthoven's triangle

When setting up standard limb leads, you'll place electrodes in positions commonly referred to as *Einthoven's triangle,* shown here. The electrodes for leads I, II, and III are about equidistant from the heart and form an equilateral triangle.

Axes

The axis of lead I extends from shoulder to shoulder, with the right-arm electrode being the negative electrode and the left-arm electrode positive.

The axis of lead II runs from the negative right-arm electrode to the positive left-leg electrode. The axis of lead III extends from the negative left-arm electrode to the positive left-leg electrode.

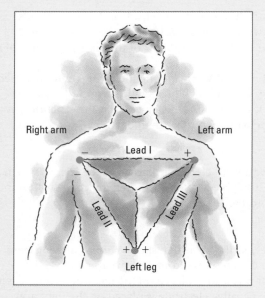

Right arm   Left arm

Lead I

Lead II   Lead III

Left leg

The "a" leads

Leads aV_R, aV_L, and aV_F are called *augmented leads* because the small waveforms that normally would appear from these unipolar leads are enhanced by the ECG. (See *Augmented leads.*) The "a" stands for "augmented," and "R, L, and F" stand for the positive electrode position of the lead.

In lead aV_R, the positive electrode is placed on the right arm (hence, the R) and produces a negative deflection because the heart's electrical activity moves away from the lead. In lead aV_L, the positive electrode is on the left arm and produces a positive deflection on the ECG. In lead aV_F, the positive electrode is on the left leg (despite the name aV_F where the F is referring to "foot") and produces a positive deflection. These three limb leads also provide a view of the heart's frontal plane.

The preeminent precordials

The six unipolar precordial leads are placed in sequence across the chest and provide a view of the heart's horizontal plane. (See *Precordial views,* page 32.) These leads include:

> Placed in sequence across the chest, precordial leads V_1 through V_6 provide a view of the heart's horizontal plane.

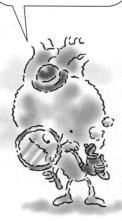

Augmented leads

Leads aV$_R$, aV$_L$, and aV$_F$ are called *augmented leads*. They measure electrical activity between one limb and a single electrode. Lead aV$_R$ provides no specific view of the heart. Lead aV$_L$ shows electrical activity coming from the heart's lateral wall. Lead aV$_F$ shows electrical activity coming from the heart's inferior wall.

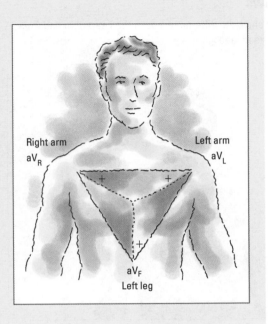

Augmented leads diagram labels

Right arm aV$_R$

Left arm aV$_L$

aV$_F$

Left leg

- *Lead V$_1$*—The precordial lead V$_1$ electrode is placed on the right side of the sternum at the fourth intercostal rib space. This lead corresponds to the modified chest lead MCL$_1$ and shows the P wave, QRS complex, and ST segment particularly well. It helps to distinguish between right and left ventricular ectopic beats that result from myocardial irritation or other cardiac stimulation outside the normal conduction system. Lead V$_1$ is also useful in monitoring ventricular arrhythmias, ST-segment changes, and bundle-branch blocks.
- *Lead V$_2$*—Lead V$_2$ is placed at the left of the sternum at the fourth intercostal rib space.
- *Lead V$_3$*—Lead V$_3$ goes between V$_2$ and V$_4$. Leads V$_1$, V$_2$, and V$_3$ are biphasic, with both positive and negative deflections. Leads V$_2$ and V$_3$ can be used to detect ST-segment elevation.
- *Lead V$_4$*—Lead V$_4$ is placed at the fifth intercostal space at the mid-clavicular line and produces a biphasic waveform.
- *Lead V$_5$*—Lead V$_5$ is placed at the fifth intercostal space at the anterior axillary line. It produces a positive deflection on the ECG and, along with V$_4$, can show changes in the ST segment or T wave.
- *Lead V$_6$*—Lead V$_6$, the last of the precordial leads, is placed level with V$_4$ at the midaxillary line. This lead produces a positive deflection on the ECG.

Precordial views

These illustrations show the different views of the heart obtained from each precordial (chest) lead.

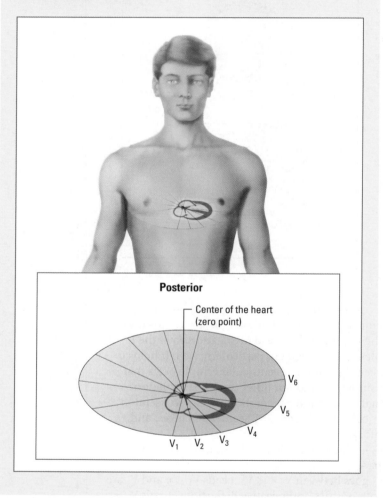

The modest modified lead

MCL$_1$ is similar to lead V$_1$ on the 12-lead ECG and is created by placing the negative electrode on the left upper chest, the positive electrode on the right side of the sternum at the fourth intercostal space, and the ground electrode usually on the right upper chest below the clavicle.

When the positive electrode is on the right side of the heart and the electrical current travels toward the left ventricle, the waveform has a negative deflection. As a result, ectopic or abnormal beats deflect in a positive direction.

You can use this lead to monitor premature ventricular contractions and to distinguish different types of tachycardia, such as ventricular tachycardia and supraventricular tachycardia. Lead MCL_1 can also be used to assess bundle-branch defects and P-wave changes and to confirm pacemaker wire placement.

A positive option

MCL_6 may be used as an alternative to MCL_1. Like MCL_1 it monitors ventricular conduction changes. The positive lead in MCL_6 is placed in the same location as its equivalent, lead V_6. The positive electrode is placed at the fifth intercostal space at the midaxillary line, the negative electrode below the left shoulder, and the ground below the right shoulder.

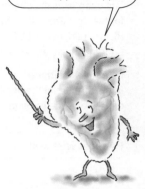

A five-leadwire system allows you to monitor any six modified chest leads and the standard limb leads. Yippee, Skippy!

Electrode basics

A three- or five-electrode (or *leadwire*) system may be used for cardiac monitoring. (See *Leadwire systems,* page 34.) Both systems use a ground electrode to prevent accidental electrical shock to the patient.

A three-electrode system has one positive electrode, one negative electrode, and a ground.

The popular five-electrode system uses an exploratory chest lead to monitor any six modified chest leads as well as the standard limb leads. (See *Using a five-leadwire system,* page 35.) This system uses standardized chest placement. Wires that attach to the electrodes are usually color-coded to help you to place them correctly on the patient's chest.

One newer application of bedside cardiac monitoring is a reduced lead continuous 12-lead ECG system (EASI* system), which uses an advanced algorithm and only five electrodes uniquely placed on the torso to derive a 12-lead ECG. The system allows all 12 leads to be simultaneously displayed and recorded. (See *Understanding the EASI* system,* page 36.)

How to apply electrodes

Before you attach electrodes to your patient, make sure they know you're monitoring their heart rate and rhythm, not controlling them. Tell them not to become upset if they hear an alarm during the procedure; it probably just means a leadwire has come loose.

Explain the electrode placement procedure to the patient, provide privacy, and wash your hands. Expose the patient's chest and select *(Text continues on page 36.)*

Leadwire systems

This chart shows the correct electrode positions for some of the leads you'll use most often—the five-leadwire, three-leadwire, and telemetry systems. The chart uses the abbreviations RA for the right arm, LA for the left arm, RL for the right leg, LL for the left leg, C for the chest, and G for the ground.

Electrode positions

In the three- and the five-leadwire systems, electrode positions for one lead may be identical to those for another lead. When that happens, change the lead selector switch to the setting that corresponds to the lead you want. In some cases, you'll need to reposition the electrodes.

Telemetry

In a telemetry monitoring system, you can create the same leads as the other systems with just two electrodes and a ground wire.

> *These are the electrode positions you'll use most often.*

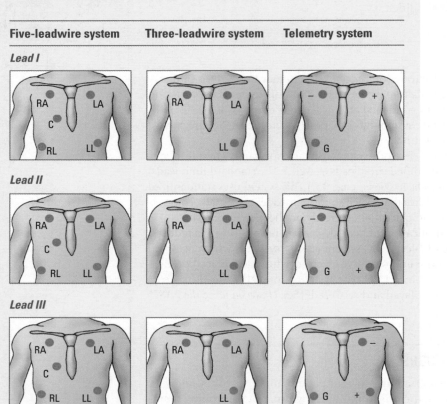

Five-leadwire system	Three-leadwire system	Telemetry system

Lead I

Lead II

Lead III

Leadwire systems *(Continued)*

Five-leadwire system	**Three-leadwire system**	**Telemetry system**

Lead MCL₁

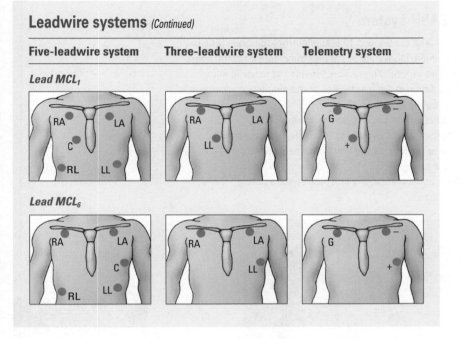

Lead MCL₆

Using a five-leadwire system

This illustration shows the correct placement of the leadwires for a five-leadwire system. The chest electrode shown is located in the V$_1$ position, but you can place it in any of the chest-lead positions. The electrodes are color-coded as follows.

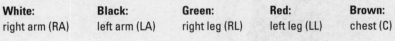

White:	**Black:**	**Green:**	**Red:**	**Brown:**
right arm (RA)	left arm (LA)	right leg (RL)	left leg (LL)	chest (C)

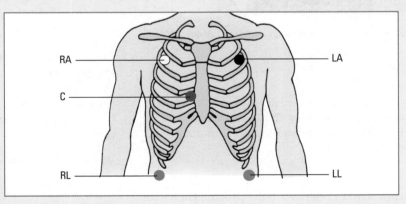

Understanding the EASI* system

The five-lead EASI* (reduced lead continuous 12-lead electrocardiogram [ECG]) configuration gives a three-dimensional view of the electrical activity of the heart from the frontal, horizontal, and sagittal planes. This provides 12 leads of information. A mathematical calculation in the electronics of the monitoring system is applied to the information, creating a derived 12-lead ECG.

Placement of the electrodes for the EASI* system includes:

- *E lead:* lower part of the sternum at the level of the fifth intercostal space
- *A lead:* left midaxillary line at the level of the fifth intercostal space
- *S lead:* upper part of the sternum
- *I lead:* right midaxillary line at the level of the fifth intercostal space
- *Ground:* anywhere on the torso.

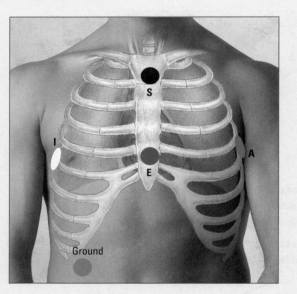

*EASI is a product of Philips Medical Systems, a Division of Philips Healthcare, Andover, MA, 01810-1099.

electrode sites for the chosen lead. Choose sites over soft tissues or close to bone, not over bony prominences, thick muscles, or skin folds. Those areas can produce ECG artifacts—waveforms not produced by the heart's electrical activity.

Prepare the skin

Next, prepare the patient's skin. To begin, wash the patient's chest with soap and water and then dry it thoroughly. Because hair may interfere with electrical contact, clip dense hair with clippers or scissors. Then

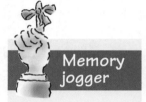

Memory jogger

To help you remember where to place electrodes in a five-electrode configuration, think of the phrase "White to the upper right." Then think of snow over trees (white electrode above green electrode) and smoke over fire (black electrode above red electrode). And of course, chocolate (brown electrode) lies close to the heart.

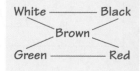

use the special rough patch on the back of the electrode, a dry wash-cloth, or a gauze pad to briskly rub each site until the skin reddens. Make sure that you don't damage or break the skin. Brisk scrubbing helps to remove dead skin cells and improves electrical contact.

If the patient has oily skin, clean each site with an alcohol pad and let it air-dry. This ensures proper adhesion and prevents the alcohol from becoming trapped beneath the electrode, which can irritate the skin and cause skin breakdown.

Stick it to me

To apply the electrodes, remove the backing and make sure each pre-gelled electrode is still moist. If an electrode has become dry, discard it and select another. A dry electrode decreases electrical contact and interferes with waveforms.

Apply one electrode to each prepared site using this method:
- Press one side of the electrode against the patient's skin, pull gently, and then press the opposite side of the electrode against the skin.
- Using two fingers, press the adhesive edge around the outside of the electrode to the patient's chest. This fixes the gel and stabilizes the electrode.
- Repeat this procedure for each electrode.
- Every 24 hours, remove the electrodes, assess the patient's skin, and put new electrodes in place.

Clip, clip, snap, snap

You'll also need to attach leadwires or cable connections to the monitor and attach leadwires to the electrodes. Leadwires may clip on or, more commonly, snap on. (See *Clip-on and snap-on leadwires.*) If you're using the snap-on type, attach the electrode to the leadwire just before applying it to the patient's chest. Keep in mind that you may lose electrode contact if you press down to apply the leadwire.

When you use a clip-on leadwire, apply it after the electrode has been secured to the patient's skin. That way, applying the clip won't interfere with the electrode's contact with the skin.

Observing the cardiac rhythm

After the electrodes are in proper position, the monitor is on, and the necessary cables are attached, observe the screen. You should see the patient's ECG waveform. Although some monitoring systems allow you to make adjustments by touching the screen, most require you to manipulate buttons. If the waveform appears too large or too small, change the size by adjusting the gain control. If the waveform appears too high or too low on the screen, adjust the position.

Clip-on and snap-on leadwires

Several kinds of leadwires are available for monitoring. A clip-on leadwire should be attached to the electrode *after* it has been placed on the patient's chest. A snap-on leadwire should be attached to the electrode just *before* it has been placed on the patient's chest. Doing so prevents patient discomfort and disturbance of the contact between the electrode and the skin.

Clip-on leadwire

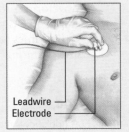

Leadwire
Electrode

Snap-on leadwire

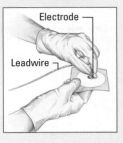

Electrode

Leadwire

Verify that the monitor detects each heartbeat by comparing the patient's apical rate with the rate displayed on the monitor. Set the upper and lower limits of the heart rate according to your facility's policy and the patient's condition. Heart rate alarms are generally set 10 to 20 beats per minute higher and lower than the patient's heart rate.

Monitors with arrhythmia detectors generate a rhythm strip automatically whenever the alarm goes off. You can obtain other views of your patient's cardiac rhythm by selecting different leads. You can select leads with the lead selector button or switch.

Printing it out

To get a printout of the patient's cardiac rhythm, press the record control on the monitor. The ECG strip will be printed at the central console. Some systems print the rhythm from a recorder box on the monitor itself.

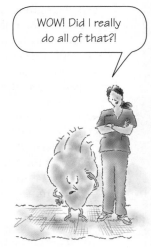

WOW! Did I really do all of that?!

Most monitor recording systems print the date, time, and the patient's name and identification number; however, if the monitor you're using can't do this, label the rhythm strip with the date, time, patient's name, identification number, and rhythm interpretation. Add any appropriate clinical information to the ECG strip, such as any medication administered, presence of chest pain, or patient activity at the time of the recording. Be sure to place the rhythm strip in the appropriate section of the patient's medical record.

It's all on paper

Waveforms produced by the heart's electrical current are recorded on graphed ECG paper by a stylus. ECG paper consists of horizontal and vertical lines forming a grid. A piece of ECG paper is called an *ECG strip* or *tracing*. (See *ECG grid*.)

ECG grid

This ECG grid shows the horizontal axis and vertical axis and their respective measurement values.

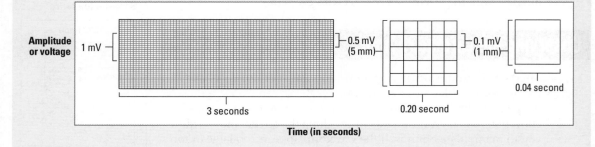

The horizontal axis of the ECG strip represents time. Each small block equals 0.04 second, and five small blocks form a large block, which equals 0.2 second. This time increment is determined by multiplying 0.04 second (for one small block) by 5, the number of small blocks that compose a large block. Five large blocks equal 1 second (5 × 0.2). When measuring or calculating a patient's heart rate, a 6-second strip consisting of 30 large blocks is usually used.

The ECG strip's vertical axis measures amplitude in millimeters (mm) or electrical voltage in millivolts (mV). Each small block represents 1 mm or 0.1 mV; each large block, 5 mm or 0.5 mV. To determine the amplitude of a wave, segment, or interval, count the number of small blocks from the baseline to the highest or lowest point of the wave, segment, or interval.

Monitor problems

For optimal cardiac monitoring, you need to recognize problems that can interfere with obtaining a reliable ECG recording. (See *Troubleshooting monitor problems*, pages 40 and 41.) Causes of interference include artifact from patient movement and poorly placed or poorly functioning equipment.

Artifact

Artifact, also called *waveform interference*, may be seen with excessive movement (somatic tremor). The baseline of the ECG appears wavy, bumpy, or tremulous. Dry electrodes may also cause this problem due to poor contact.

Interference

Electrical interference, also called *60-cycle interference*, is caused by electrical power leakage. It may also occur due to interference from other room equipment or improperly grounded equipment. As a result, the lost current pulses at a rate of 60 cycles per second. This interference appears on the ECG as a baseline that's thick and unreadable.

Wandering baseline

A wandering baseline undulates, meaning that all waveforms are present but the baseline isn't stationary. Movement of the chest wall during respiration, poor electrode placement, or poor electrode contact usually causes this problem.

Faulty equipment

Faulty equipment, such as broken leadwires and cables, can also cause monitoring problems. Excessively worn equipment can cause

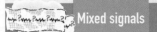

Mixed signals

Troubleshooting monitor problems

This chart shows several ECG monitoring problems, along with their causes and possible solutions.

What you see	What might cause it	What to do about it
Artifact (waveform interference) 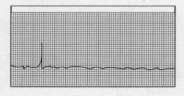	• Patient experiencing seizures, chills, or anxiety	• If the patient is having a seizure, notify the practitioner and intervene as ordered. • Keep the patient warm and encourage him to relax.
	• Dirty or corroded connections • Improper electrode application	• Replace dirty or corroded wires. • Check the electrodes and reapply them if needed. Clean the patient's skin well because skin oils and dead skin cells inhibit conduction. • Check the electrode gel. If the gel is dry, apply new electrodes.
	• Short circuit in leadwires or cable • Electrical interference from other equipment in the room	• Replace broken equipment. • Make sure all electrical equipment are attached to a common ground. Check all three-pronged plugs to ensure that none of the prongs are loose. Notify the biomedical department.
	• Static electricity interference from inadequate room humidity	• Regulate room humidity to 40% if possible.
False high-rate alarm 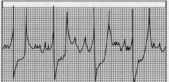	• Gain setting too high, particularly with MCL₁ setting	• Reset gain.
Weak signals 	• Improper electrode application • QRS complex too small to register • Wire or cable failure	• Reapply the electrodes. • Reset gain so that the height of the complex is greater than 1 mV. • Try monitoring the patient on another lead. • Replace any faulty wires or cables.

Troubleshooting monitor problems *(Continued)*

What you see	What might cause it	What to do about it
Wandering baseline 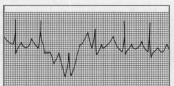	• Patient restless • Chest wall movement during respiration • Improper electrode application; electrode positioned over bone	• Encourage the patient to relax. • Make sure that tension on the cable isn't pulling the electrode away from the patient's body. • Reposition improperly placed electrodes.
Fuzzy baseline (electrical interference) 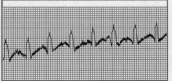	• Electrical interference from other electrical equipment in the room • Improper grounding of the patient's bed • Electrode malfunction	• Ensure that all electrical equipment is attached to a common ground. • Check all three-pronged plugs to make sure none of the prongs are loose. • Ensure that the bed ground is attached to the room's common ground. • Replace the electrodes.
Baseline (no waveform) 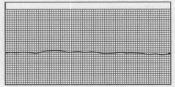	• Improper electrode placement (perpendicular to axis of heart) • Electrode disconnected • Dry electrode gel • Wire or cable failure	• Reposition improperly placed electrodes • Check if electrodes are disconnected. Reapply them as necessary. • Check electrode gel. If the gel is dry, apply new electrodes. • Replace faulty wires or cables.

improper grounding, putting the patient at risk for accidental shock.

Be aware that some types of artifact resemble arrhythmias and the monitor will interpret them as such. For example, the monitor may sense a small movement, such as the patient brushing his teeth, as a potentially lethal ventricular tachycardia. So remember to treat the patient, not the monitor. The more familiar you become with your unit's monitoring system—and with your patient—the more quickly you can recognize and interpret problems and act appropriately.

Worn equipment can cause problems—including a possible shock for the patient.

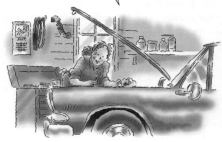

That's a wrap!

Obtaining a rhythm strip review

Leads and planes
- A *lead* provides a view of the heart's electrical activity between a positive and negative pole.
  - When electrical current travels toward the negative pole, the waveform deflects mostly downward.
  - When the current flows toward the positive pole, the waveform deflects mostly upward.
- A *plane* refers to a cross-section view of the electrical activity of the heart.
  - Frontal plane, a vertical cut through the middle of the heart, provides an anterior–posterior view.
  - Horizontal plane, a transverse cut through the middle of the heart, provides a superior or inferior view.

Types of ECGs
- *12-lead ECG* records electrical activity from 12 views of the heart.
- *Single-lead or dual-lead monitoring* provides continuous cardiac monitoring.

12-lead ECG
- Six limb leads provide information about the heart's frontal (vertical) plane.
- Bipolar (leads I, II, and III) require a negative and positive electrode for monitoring.
- Unipolar (leads aV_R, aV_L, and aV_F) record information from one lead and require only one electrode.
- The six precordial leads (leads V_1 through V_6) provide information about the heart's horizontal plane.

Leads I, II, and III
- Leads I, II, and III typically produce positive deflection on ECG tracings.
- Lead I helps monitor atrial arrhythmias and hemiblocks.
- Lead II commonly aids in routine monitoring and detecting of sinus node and atrial arrhythmias.
- Lead III helps detect changes associated with inferior wall myocardial infarction.

Precordial leads
- Lead V_1
  - Biphasic
  - Distinguishes between right and left ventricular ectopic beats
  - Monitors ventricular arrhythmias, ST-segment changes, and bundle-branch blocks
- Leads V_2 and V_3
  - Biphasic
  - Monitors ST-segment elevation
- Lead V_4
  - Produces a biphasic waveform
  - Monitors ST-segment and T-wave changes
- Lead V_5
  - Produces a positive deflection on the ECG
  - Monitors ST-segment or T-wave changes (when used with lead V_4)
- Lead V_6
  - Produces a positive deflection on the ECG
  - Detects bundle-branch blocks

Obtaining a rhythm strip review *(Continued)*

Modified leads
- Lead MCL$_1$
  - Similar to V$_1$
  - Assesses QRS-complex arrhythmias, P-wave changes, and bundle-branch defects
  - Monitors premature ventricular contractions
  - Distinguishes different types of tachycardia
- Lead MCL$_6$
  - Similar to V$_6$
  - Monitors ventricular conduction changes

Electrode configurations
- Three-electrode system uses one positive electrode, one negative electrode, and a ground.
- *Five-electrode system* uses an exploratory chest lead to monitor modified chest or standard limb leads.

ECG strip
- 1 small horizontal block = 0.04 second
- 5 small horizontal blocks = 1 large block = 0.2 second
- 5 large horizontal blocks = 1 second
- Normal 6 second strip = 30 large horizontal blocks
- 1 small vertical block = 0.1 mV
- 1 large vertical block = 0.5 mV
- Amplitude (mV) = number of small blocks from baseline to highest or lowest point

Monitoring problems
- *Artifact*—excessive movement or dry electrode that causes baseline to appear wavy, bumpy, or tremulous
- *Interference*—electrical power leakage, interference from other equipment, or improper equipment grounding that produces a thick, unreadable baseline
- *Wandering baseline*—chest wall movement, poor electrode placement, or poor electrode contact that causes an undulating baseline
- *Faulty equipment*—faulty and worn equipment that causes monitoring problems and places the patient at risk for shock

Quick quiz

1. On ECG graph paper, the horizontal axis measures:
   A. time.
   B. speed.
   C. voltage.
   D. amplitude.

   Answer: A. The horizontal axis measures time and is recorded in increments of 0.04 second for each small box.

2.   On ECG graph paper, the vertical axis measures:
   A.   time.
   B.   speed.
   C.   voltage.
   D.   amplitude.

Answer: C. The vertical axis measures voltage by the height of a waveform.

3.   A biphasic deflection will occur on an ECG if the electrical current is traveling in a direction:
   A.   posterior to the positive electrode.
   B.   perpendicular to the positive electrode.
   C.   superior to the positive electrode.
   D.   anterior to the positive electrode.

Answer: B. A current traveling in a route perpendicular to the positive electrode will generate a biphasic wave, partially above and below the isoelectric line.

4.   If a lead comes off the patient's chest, the waveform:
   A.   will appear much larger on the monitor.
   B.   will appear much smaller on the monitor.
   C.   will appear to wander on the monitor.
   D.   won't be seen at all on the monitor.

Answer: D. Leadwire disconnection will stop the monitoring process, and the waveform won't be seen on the monitor.

5.   To monitor lead II, you would place the:
   A.   positive electrode below the lowest palpable rib at the left midclavicular line and the negative electrode below the right clavicle.
   B.   positive electrode below the right clavicle at the midline and the negative electrode below the left clavicle at the midline.
   C.   positive electrode below the left clavicle and the negative electrode below the right clavicle at the midclavicular line.
   D.   positive electrode below the lowest palpable rib at the right midclavicular line and the negative electrode below the left clavicle.

Answer: A. This electrode position is the proper one for monitoring in lead II.

Scoring

☆☆☆   If you answered all five questions correctly, superb! We're ready to go out on a limb lead for you.

   ☆☆   If you answered four questions correctly, great! We hardly need to monitor your progress.

     ☆   If you answered fewer than four questions correctly, keep at it! A review of the chapter can get your current flowing in the right direction.

Recommended references

Brown, D. F. M., & Martindale, J. L. (2012). *Rapid interpretation of ECG's in emergency medicine.* Philadelphia, PA: Wolters Kluwer.

García-Niebla, J. (2009). Comparison of P-wave patterns derived from correct and incorrect placement of V1-V2 electrodes. *Journal of Cardiovascular Nursing, 24*(2), 156–161.

Katritsis, D. G., Gersch, B. J., & Camm. A. J. (2013). *Clinical cardiology: Current practice guidelines.* Oxford, United Kingdom: Oxford University Press.

Lynn-McHale Wiegand, D. J. (Ed.). (2010). *AACN procedure manual for critical care* (6th ed.). Philadelphia, PA: Saunders | Elsevier.

McLaughlin, M. A. (clinical ed.). (2014). *Cardiovascular care made incredibly easy* (3rd ed.). Philadelphia, PA: Wolters Kluwer.

Rosen, A. V., Koppikan, S., Shaw, C., & Baranchuk, A. (2014). Common ECG lead placement errors. Part II: Pericardial misplacements. *International Journal of Medical Students, 2*(3), 99–103.

Chapter 3

Interpreting a rhythm strip

Just the facts

In this chapter, you'll learn:

◆ the components of an ECG complex and their significance and variations

◆ techniques for calculating the rate and rhythm of an ECG recording

◆ the step-by-step approach to ECG interpretation

◆ properties of normal sinus rhythm.

A look at an ECG complex

An ECG complex represents the electrical events occurring in one cardiac cycle. A complex consists of five waveforms labeled with the letters P, Q, R, S, and T. The middle three letters—Q, R, and S—are referred to as a unit, the QRS complex. ECG tracings represent the conduction of electrical impulses from the atria to the ventricles. (See *Normal ECG*, page 48.)

The P wave

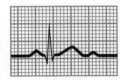

The P wave is the first component of a normal ECG waveform. It represents atrial depolarization—conduction of an electrical impulse through the atria. When evaluating a P wave, look closely at its characteristics, especially its location, amplitude, duration, configuration, and deflection. In a normal ECG, there should be one P wave, which precedes the QRS complex and has the following characteristics:
• location—precedes the QRS complex
• amplitude—<0.25 mV (2.5 mm or 2.5 small squares high)
• duration—<0.12 second (3 small squares in length; each horizontal square equals 0.04 second)
• configuration—usually rounded and upright

- deflection—positive or upright in leads I, II, aV_F, and V_2 to V_6; usually positive but variable in leads III and aV_L; negative or inverted in lead aV_R; biphasic or variable in lead V_1.

  If the deflection and configuration of a P wave are normal—for example, if the P wave is upright in lead II and is rounded and smooth—and if one P wave precedes each QRS complex, you can assume that this electrical impulse originated in the sinoatrial (SA) node of the right atrium. Electrical activity of the myocardium precedes muscular contraction. Therefore, the atria contract partway through the P wave and is not recorded on the ECG. Remember, the ECG records electrical activity only, not mechanical activity or contraction.

Normal ECG

This strip shows the components of a normal ECG waveform.

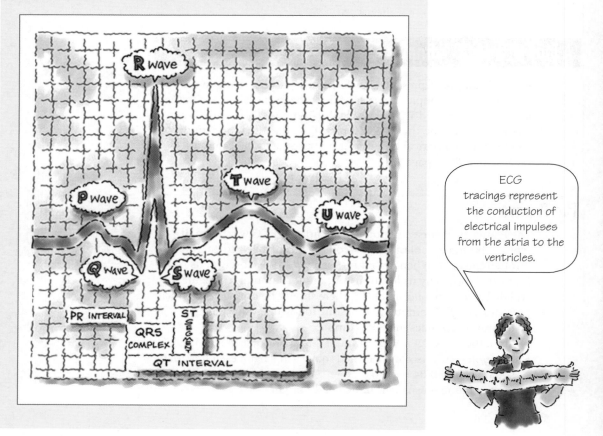

ECG tracings represent the conduction of electrical impulses from the atria to the ventricles.

The odd Ps

The configuration and amplitude of the P wave are important to note. When a P wave has an amplitude of >2.5 mm in lead II or >1.5 mm in V_1, right atrial enlargement may be indicated. A prolonged P wave, such as ≥0.12 second, in the frontal plan (such as lead II), can suggest left atrial enlargement. Other conditions associated with peaked, notched, or enlarged P waves include chronic obstructive pulmonary disease, pulmonary emboli, valvular disease, or heart failure.

Recall that the SA node, pacemaker of the heart, generates electrical impulses that are relayed to the atrioventricular (AV) node located in the posterioinferior region of the interatrial septum and travel to the ventricles, lower chambers of the heart. Inverted P waves may signify retrograde atrial depolarization or reverse conduction from the AV junction toward the atria. If the P wave has flipped on a repeat ECG, an upright sinus P wave becomes inverted, consider retrograde or reverse conduction as possible conditions.

Varying P waves indicate that the impulse may be generated from different sites, as with a wandering pacemaker rhythm, irritable atrial tissue, or damage near the SA node. Absent P waves may signify conduction by a route other than the SA node, as with a junctional rhythm, atrial flutter or fibrillation. In some cases, absent P waves may be caused by hyperkalemia. A flattened baseline with absent or numerous erratic P waves may indicate rapid atrial contraction caused by rhythm disturbances, such as atrial flutter or fibrillation. In atrial flutter, although P waves are not distinct, a saw-toothed flutter wave(s) is apparent on the ECG.

The PR interval

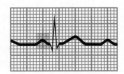

The PR interval is measured on the horizontal axis of the ECG from the beginning of the P wave to the beginning of the adjacent QRS interval. The PR interval tracks the atrial impulse from the atria through the AV node, bundle of His, and right and left bundle branches. When evaluating a PR interval, note duration. Changes in the PR interval indicate an altered impulse formation or a conduction delay, as seen in AV block. While the amplitude, configuration, and deflection of the PR interval are not measured, it is important to note the following characteristics:
- location—from the beginning of the P wave to the beginning of the QRS complex
- duration—0.12 to 0.20 second (3 to 5 small squares in length; each horizontal square equals 0.04 second)

These characteristics are different for pediatric patients. (See *Pediatric rates and intervals,* page 50.)

Pediatric rates and intervals

The hearts of infants and children beat faster than those of adults because children have smaller ventricular size and higher metabolic needs. The fast heart rate and small heart size produces short PR intervals and QRS intervals.

Age	Heart rate (beats/minute)	PR interval (in seconds)	QRS interval (in seconds)
0–7 days	95–160	0.08–0.12	0.05
1–3 weeks	105–180	0.08–0.12	0.05
1–6 months	110–180	0.08–0.13	0.05
6–12 months	110–170	0.10–0.14	0.05
1–3 years	90–150	0.10–0.14	0.06
4–5 years	65–135	0.11–0.15	0.07
6–8 years	60–130	0.12–0.16	0.07
9–11 years	60–110	0.12–0.17	0.07
12–16 years	60–110	0.12–0.17	0.07

The short and long of it

Short PR intervals (less than 0.12 second) indicate that the impulse originated somewhere other than the SA node. This variation is associated with junctional arrhythmias and pre-excitation syndromes. Prolonged PR intervals (greater than 0.20 second), slowing through the atria or AV junction, which may represent a conduction delay due to digoxin toxicity, heart block, or myocardial ischemia/infarction associated with heart injury or damaged heart tissue.

The QRS complex

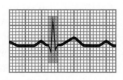

The QRS complex that follows the P wave represents ventricular depolarization and contraction and is also known as ventricular systole. At this time, the atria repolarize and relax. The impulse is transmitted from the AV node to the bundle of His and Purkinje fibers located in the ventricular walls. Ventricular contraction proceeds from the apex of the heart to its base and results in blood being ejected from the ventricles through the semilunar valves (aortic and pulmonary) into the arterial system perfusing the body with oxygenated blood and creating a pulse.

Not necessarily mechanical

The ECG waveform represents only electrical activity of the heart. Remember that mechanical contraction of heart and its contents follows electrical conduction, but is not a guarantee of successful perfusion. When monitoring the cardiac rhythm, it is important to remember that proper assessment of the patient includes other clinical indicators to determine health and stability. Muscular contraction of the heart can be weak and ineffective in perfusing the body, as may occur with premature ventricular contractions; or pulse may be absent, as with pulseless electrical activity. Always check the patient's physiological status (including pulse, blood pressure, mentation) when performing ECG monitoring.

It's all normal

Pay special attention to the duration and configuration when evaluating a QRS complex. A normal complex has the following characteristics:
- location—follows the PR interval
- amplitude—5 to 30 mV (1 mm or 6 small squares high) but differs for each lead used
- duration—0.06 to 0.12 second (1.5 to 3 small squares in length; each horizontal square equals 0.04 second); or roughly half of the PR interval. Duration is measured from the beginning of the Q wave to the end of the S wave or from the beginning of the R wave if the Q wave is absent.
- configuration—consists of the Q wave (the first negative deflection after the P wave), the R wave (the first positive deflection after the P wave or the Q wave), and the S wave (the first negative deflection after the R wave). All three waves may not always be evident on the ECG. The ventricles depolarize quickly, minimizing contact time between the stylus and the ECG paper, so the QRS complex typically appears thinner than other ECG components. QRS complexes may also appear differently in each lead. (See *QRS waveform variety*, page 52.)
- deflection—positive in leads I, II, III, aV_L, aV_F, and V_4 to V_6 and negative in leads aV_R and V_1 to V_3.

Crucial I.D.

Remember that the QRS complex represents intraventricular conduction time. That's why identifying and correctly interpreting it is so crucial. If no P wave appears before the QRS complex, one consideration is that the impulse may have originated in the ventricles, indicating a ventricular arrhythmia. (See *Older adult ECGs*.)

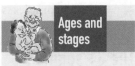
Ages and stages

Older adult ECGs

Always keep the patient's age in mind when interpreting the ECG. ECG changes in the older adult include increased PR, QRS, and QT intervals, decreased amplitude of the QRS complex, and a shift of the QRS axis to the left.

QRS waveform variety

The illustrations below show the various configurations of QRS complexes. When documenting the QRS complex, use uppercase letters to indicate a wave with a normal or high amplitude (greater than 5 mm) and lowercase letters to indicate a wave with a low amplitude (less than 5 mm). In some instances, a second R wave may appear in a QRS complex. This is called R'.

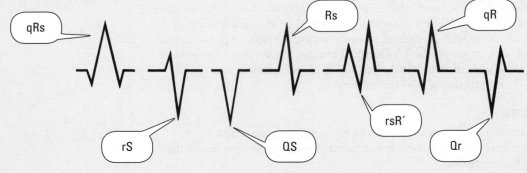

Deep and wide

Deep, wide Q waves may represent myocardial infarction. In this case, the Q-wave amplitude is 25% of the R-wave amplitude, or the duration of the Q wave is 0.04 second. A notched R wave may signify a bundle-branch block. A widened QRS complex (greater than 0.12 second) may signify a ventricular conduction delay. Missing QRS complexes may indicate AV block or ventricular standstill.

The ST segment

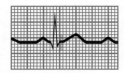

The ST segment represents the end of ventricular depolarization or conduction and the beginning of ventricular repolarization or recovery. The flat, isoelectric portion of the ECG that occurs at the end of the S wave to the beginning of the T wave is known as the ST segment. The point that marks the end of the QRS complex and the beginning of the ST segment is known as the *J point*.

Normal ST

Pay special attention to the deflection of an ST segment. A normal ST segment has the following characteristics:
- location—extends from the S wave to the beginning of the T wave
- deflection—usually isoelectric (neither positive nor negative); may vary from –0.5 to +1 mm in some precordial leads.

Changes in the ST segment

It is critically important to closely monitor the ST segment on a patient's ECG in order to detect myocardial ischemia or infarction and to limit damage.

ST-segment depression

An ST segment is considered depressed when it's 0.5 mm or more below the baseline. A depressed ST segment may indicate myocardial ischemia or digoxin toxicity.

Observe the ST segment for depression, such as upsloping, downsloping, or a horizontal configuration.

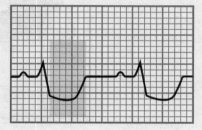

ST-segment elevation

An ST segment is considered elevated when it's 1 mm or more above the baseline. An elevated ST segment may indicate myocardial injury.

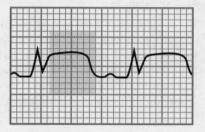

Not so normal ST

A change in the ST segment may indicate myocardial ischemia or infarction. An ST segment may become either elevated or depressed. Observe the ST segment for characteristic patterns of depression changes known as upsloping, downsloping, or horizontal. (See *Changes in the ST segment.*)

The T wave

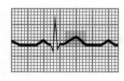

The T wave represents ventricular repolarization or recovery. When evaluating a T wave, look at the amplitude, configuration, and deflection. Normal T waves have the following characteristics (duration isn't measured):

- location—follows the S wave
- amplitude—0.5 mm in leads I, II, and III and up to 10 mm in the precordial leads
- configuration—typically round and smooth
- deflection—usually upright in leads I, II, and V_3 to V_6; inverted in lead aV_R; variable in all other leads.

Why is that T so bumpy?

The T wave may be asymmetrical, the first slope may appear more gradual than the second one. The T wave's peak represents the relative refractory period of ventricular repolarization, a period during which cells are especially vulnerable to extra stimuli. Bumps in a T wave may indicate that a P wave is hidden in it. If a P wave is hidden, atrial depolarization has occurred, the impulse having originated at a site above the ventricles.

Tall, inverted, or pointy Ts

The amplitude of the T wave typically corresponds to the amplitude of the preceding R wave. T waves may appear taller in leads V_3 and V_4. Tall, peaked, or tented T waves indicate myocardial ischemia or hyperkalemia. Inverted T waves in leads I, II, or V_3 through V_6 may represent myocardial ischemia. Heavily notched or pointed T waves in an adult may suggest pericarditis.

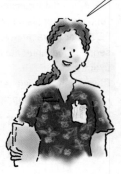

Heavily notched or pointed T waves in an adult may mean pericarditis.

The QT interval

The QT interval measures ventricular depolarization and repolarization. The length of the QT interval varies according to heart rate. The faster the heart rate, the shorter the QT interval. When checking the QT interval, look closely at the duration.

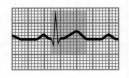

A normal QT interval has the following characteristics (amplitude, configuration, and deflection aren't observed):
- location—extends from the beginning of the QRS complex to the end of the T wave
- duration—varies according to age, sex, and heart rate; usually lasts from 0.36 to 0.44 second; should not be greater than half the distance between consecutive R waves (R to R interval) when the rhythm is regular.

The importance of QT

The QT interval shows the time needed for the ventricular depolarization–repolarization cycle. An abnormality in duration may indicate myocardial problems. Prolonged QT intervals indicate that the relative refractory period is longer. A prolonged QT interval increases the risk of a life-threatening arrhythmia known as *torsades de pointes*.

Drugs that increase the QT interval

This chart lists drugs that have been shown to increase the QT interval, which increases the patient's risk of developing torsades de pointes.

Drug name	Drug class	Drug name	Drug class
Amiodarone (Cordarone) or (Pacerone)	Antiarrhythmic	Haloperidol (Haldol)	Antipsychotic
		Ibutilide (Corvert)	Antiarrhythmic
Amitriptyline (Elavil)	Antidepressant	Ketoconazole (Nizoral)	Antifungal
Chlorpromazine	Antipsychotic/antiemetic	Levofloxacin (Levaquin)	Antibiotic
Clarithromycin (Biaxin)	Antibiotic	Methadone (Methadose or Dolophine)	Opiate agonist
Desipramine (Norpramin)	Antidepressant		
Disopyramide (Norpace)	Antiarrhythmic	Procainamide	Antiarrhythmic
Dofetilide (Tikosyn)	Antiarrhythmic	Quinidine sulphate	Antiarrhythmic
Dolasetron (Anzemet)	Antiemetic	Sertraline (Zoloft)	Antidepressant
Droperidol (Inapsine)	Sedative; antinauseant	Sotalol (Betapace)	Antiarrhythmic
Erythromycin (Erythrocin)	Antibiotic; GI stimulant	Sumatriptan (Imitrex)	Antimigraine
Fluoxetine (Prozac)	Antidepressant	Thioridazine (Mellaril)	Antipsychotic

This variation is also associated with certain medications such as Class IA antiarrhythmics. (See *Drugs that increase the QT interval.*) Prolonged QT syndrome is a congenital conduction-system defect present in certain families. Short QT intervals may result from digoxin toxicity or hypercalcemia.

The U wave

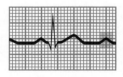

The U wave represents the recovery period of the Purkinje or ventricular conduction fibers. It is seen as a small deflection following the T wave; however, is not present on every rhythm strip. The configuration is the most important characteristic of the U wave.

When present, a normal U wave has the following characteristics (amplitude and duration aren't measured):
- location—follows the T wave
- configuration—typically upright except in aV_R, and rounded
- deflection—upright.

The U wave may not appear on an ECG. A prominent U wave may be due to hypercalcemia, hypokalemia, or digoxin toxicity.

8-step method

Interpreting a rhythm strip is a skill developed through practice. You can use several methods, as long as you employ consistent technique. Rhythm strip analysis requires a sequential and systematic approach, such as the eight steps outlined here.

> What are the keys for reading a rhythm strip?

> A sequential, systematic approach will serve you best.

Step 1: Determine the rhythm

To determine the heart's atrial and ventricular rhythms, use either the paper-and-pencil method or the caliper method. (See *Methods of measuring rhythm.*)

For atrial rhythm, measure the P-P intervals—the intervals between consecutive P waves. These intervals should occur regularly with only small variations associated with respirations. Then compare the P-P intervals in several cycles. Consistently similar P-P intervals indicate regular atrial rhythm; dissimilar P-P intervals indicate irregular atrial rhythm.

To determine the ventricular rhythm, measure the intervals between two consecutive R waves in the QRS com-

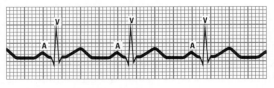

plexes. If an R wave isn't present, use the Q wave of consecutive QRS complexes. The R-R intervals should occur regularly.

Then compare R-R intervals in several cycles. As with atrial rhythms, consistently similar intervals mean a regular rhythm; dissimilar intervals point to an irregular rhythm.

Ask yourself: How irregular is the rhythm? Is it slightly irregular or markedly so? Does the irregularity occur in a pattern (a regularly irregular pattern)? Keep in mind that variations of up to 0.04 second are considered normal.

Methods of measuring rhythm

You can use the paper-and-pencil or caliper method to determine atrial or ventricular rhythm.

Paper-and-pencil method

Place the ECG strip on a flat surface. Then position the straight edge of a piece of paper along 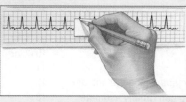 the strip's baseline. Move the paper up slightly so the straight edge is near the peak of the R wave. With a pencil, mark the paper at the R waves of two consecutive QRS complexes, as shown above. This is the R-R interval.

Next, move the paper across the strip, aligning the two marks with succeeding R-R intervals. If the distance for each R-R interval is the same, the ventricular rhythm is regular. If the distance varies, the rhythm is irregular.

Use the same method to measure the distance between the P waves (the P-P interval) and determine whether the atrial rhythm is regular or irregular.

Caliper method

With the ECG on a flat surface, place one point of the caliper on the peak of the first R wave of two consecutive QRS complexes. 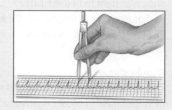 Then adjust the caliper legs so the other point is on the peak of the next R wave, as shown above. This distance is the R-R interval.

Now pivot the first point of the caliper toward the third R wave and note whether it falls on the peak of that wave. Check succeeding R-R intervals in the same way. If the R-R intervals are the same length, the ventricular rhythm is regular. If the length varies, the ventricular rhythm is irregular.

Use the same method to measure the P-P intervals to determine whether the atrial rhythm is regular or irregular.

Step 2: Determine the rate

You can use one of three methods to determine an approximate atrial and ventricular heart rate. Always check a pulse to correlate it with the heart rate on the ECG.

10-times method

The easiest way to calculate heart rate is the 10-times method, especially if the rhythm is irregular. You'll notice that ECG paper is marked in increments of 3 seconds, or 15 large boxes. To figure the atrial rate, obtain a 6-second strip, count the number of P waves, and multiply by 10. Ten 6-second strips represent 1 minute. Calculate ventricular rate the same way, using the R waves.

Calculating heart rate

This table can help make the sequencing method of determining heart rate more precise. After counting the number of boxes between the R waves, use the table shown at right to find the rate.

For example, if you count 20 small blocks or 4 large blocks, the rate would be 75 beats/minute. To calculate the atrial rate, use the same method with P waves instead of R waves.

Rapid estimation

This rapid-rate calculation is also called the *countdown method.* Using the number of large boxes between R waves or P waves as a guide, you can rapidly estimate ventricular or atrial rates by memorizing the sequence "300, 150, 100, 75, 60, 50."

Number of small blocks	Heart rate
5 (1 large block)	300
6	250
7	214
8	187
9	166
10 (2 large blocks)	150
11	136
12	125
13	115
14	107
15 (3 large blocks)	100
16	94
17	88
18	83
19	79
20 (4 large blocks)	75
21	71
22	68
23	65
24	63
25 (5 large blocks)	60
26	58
27	56
28	54
29	52
30 (6 large blocks)	50
31	48
32	47
33	45
34	44
35 (7 large blocks)	43
36	42
37	41
38	39
39	38
40 (8 large blocks)	37

1,500 method

If the heart rhythm is regular, use the 1,500 method—so named because 1,500 small squares represent 1 minute. Count the small squares between identical points on two consecutive P waves and then divide 1,500 by that number to get the atrial rate. To obtain the ventricular rate, use the same method with two consecutive R waves.

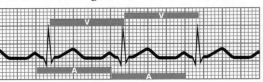

Sequence method

The third method of estimating heart rate is the sequence method, which requires that you memorize a sequence of numbers. (See *Calculating heart rate.*) To get the atrial rate, find a P wave that peaks on a heavy black line and assign the following numbers to the next six heavy black lines: 300, 150, 100, 75, 60, and 50. Then find the next P wave peak and estimate the atrial rate, based on the number assigned to the nearest heavy black line. Estimate the ventricular rate the same way, using the R wave.

Step 3: Evaluate the P wave

When examining a rhythm strip for P waves, ask yourself: Are P waves present? Do they all have normal configurations? Do they all have a similar size, shape, and location on the ECG? Is there one P wave preceding every QRS complex?

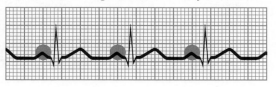

Step 4: Determine the duration of the PR interval

To measure the PR interval, count the small squares between the start of the P wave and the start of the QRS complex; then multiply the number of squares by 0.04 second. Now ask yourself: Is the duration a normal 0.12 to 0.20 second? Is the PR interval constant?

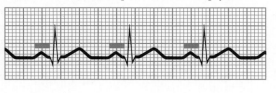

Step 5: Determine the duration of the QRS complex

When determining QRS duration, be sure to measure straight across from the end of the PR interval to the end of the S wave, not just to the peak. Remember, the QRS has no horizontal components. To calculate duration, count the number of small squares between the beginning and end of the QRS complex and multiply this number by 0.04 second. Then ask yourself: Is the duration a normal 0.06 to 0.12 second? Are all QRS complexes the same size and shape? (If not, measure each one and describe it individually.) Does a QRS complex appear after every P wave?

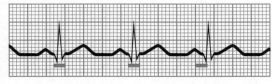

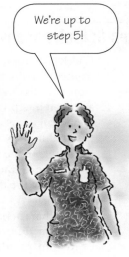

We're up to step 5!

Step 6: Evaluate the T waves

Examine the strip for T waves. Then ask yourself: Are T waves present? Do they all have a normal shape? Do they all have a normal amplitude? Do they all have the same amplitude? Do the T waves have the same deflection as the QRS complexes?

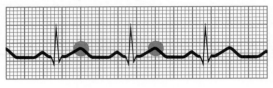

Step 7: Determine the duration of the QT interval

Count the number of small squares between the beginning of the QRS complex and the end of the T wave, where the T wave returns to the baseline. Multiply this number by 0.04 second. Ask yourself: Is the duration a normal 0.36 to 0.44 second? (See *Correcting the QT interval.*)

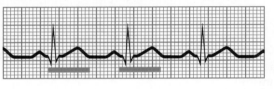

Step 8: Evaluate any other components

Check for ectopic beats and other abnormalities. Also check the ST segment for abnormalities, and look for the presence of a U wave.

Note your findings, and then interpret them by naming the rhythm strip according to one or all of these findings:

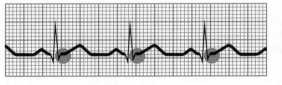

- origin of the rhythm (e.g., sinus node, atria, AV node, or ventricles)
- rate characteristics (e.g., bradycardia or tachycardia)
- rhythm abnormalities (e.g., flutter, fibrillation, heart block, escape rhythm, or other arrhythmias)

Correcting the QT interval

The QT interval is affected by the patient's heart rate. As the heart rate increases, the QT interval decreases; as the heart rate decreases, the QT interval increases. For this reason, evaluating the QT interval based on a standard heart rate of 60 is recommended. This corrected QT interval is known as *QTc*:

The following formula is used to determine the *QTc*

$$\frac{QT\ Interval}{\sqrt{R\text{-}R\ interval\ in\ seconds}}$$

The normal QTc for women is less than 0.45 second and for men is less than 0.43 second. When the QTc is longer than 0.50 second in men or women, torsades de pointes is more likely to develop.

Recognizing normal sinus rhythm

Before you can recognize an arrhythmia, you must first be able to recognize normal sinus rhythm. Normal sinus rhythm records an impulse that starts in the sinus node and progresses to the ventricles through a normal conduction pathway—from the sinus node to the atria and AV node, through the bundle of His, to the bundle branches, and on to the Purkinje fibers. Normal sinus rhythm is the standard against which all other rhythms are compared. (See *Normal sinus rhythm.*)

What makes for normal?

Using the 8-step method previously described, these are the characteristics of normal sinus rhythm:
- Atrial and ventricular rhythms are regular.
- Atrial and ventricular rates fall between 60 and 100 beats/minute, the SA node's normal firing rate, and all impulses are conducted to the ventricles.
- P waves are rounded, smooth, and upright in lead II, signaling that a sinus impulse has reached the atria.

Normal sinus rhythm

Normal sinus rhythm, shown below, represents normal impulse conduction through the heart.

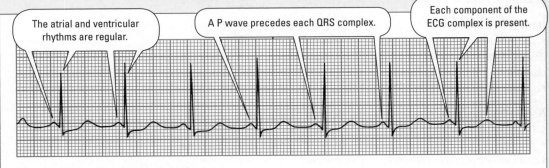

Characteristics of normal sinus rhythm:
- Regular rhythm
- Normal rate
- A P wave for every QRS complex; all P waves similar in size and shape
- All QRS complexes similar in size and shape
- Normal PR and QT intervals
- Normal (upright and round) T waves

- The PR interval is normal (0.12 to 0.20 second), indicating that the impulse is following normal conduction pathways.
- The QRS complex is of normal duration (less than 0.12 second), representing normal ventricular impulse conduction and recovery.
- The T wave is upright in lead II, confirming that normal repolarization has taken place.
- The QT interval is within normal limits (0.36 to 0.44 second).
- No ectopic or aberrant beats occur.

That's a wrap!

Rhythm strip interpretation review

Normal P wave
- *Location*—before the QRS complex
- *Amplitude*—<0.25 mV high
- *Duration*—<0.12 second
- *Configuration*—usually rounded and upright
- *Deflection*—positive or upright in leads I, II, aV$_F$, and V$_2$ to V$_6$; usually positive but may vary in leads III and aV$_L$; negative or inverted in lead aV$_R$; biphasic or variable in lead V$_1$

Normal PR interval
- *Location*—from the beginning of the P wave to the beginning of the QRS complex
- *Duration*—0.12 to 0.20 second

Normal QRS complex
- *Location*—follows the PR interval
- *Amplitude*—5 to 30 mV (1 mm or 6 small squares high) but differs for each lead used
- *Duration*—0.06 to 0.12 second, or half the PR interval
- *Configuration*—consists of the Q wave, the R wave, and the S wave
- *Deflection*—positive in leads I, II, III, aV$_L$, aV$_F$, and V$_4$ to V$_6$ and negative in leads aV$_R$ and V$_1$ to V$_3$

Normal ST segment
- *Location*—from the S wave to the beginning of the T wave
- *Deflection*—usually isoelectric; may vary from −0.5 to +1 mm in some precordial leads

Normal T wave
- *Location*—after the S wave
- *Amplitude*—0.5 mm in leads I, II, and III and up to 10 mm in the precordial leads
- *Configuration*—typically round and smooth
- *Deflection*—usually upright in leads I, II, and V$_3$ to V$_6$; inverted in lead aV$_R$; variable in all other leads

Normal QT interval
- *Location*—from the beginning of the QRS complex to the end of the T wave
- *Duration*—varies; usually lasts from 0.36 to 0.44 second

Normal U wave
- *Location*—after T wave
- *Configuration*—typically upright and rounded
- *Deflection*—upright

Rhythm strip interpretation review *(Continued)*

Interpreting a rhythm strip: 8-step method

- Step 1: Determine the rhythm
- Step 2: Determine the rate
- Step 3: Evaluate the P wave
- Step 4: Measure the PR interval
- Step 5: Determine the QRS complex duration
- Step 6: Examine the T waves
- Step 7: Measure the QT interval duration
- Step 8: Check for ectopic beats and other abnormalities

Normal sinus rhythm

Normal sinus rhythm is the standard against which all other rhythms are compared.

Characteristics

- Regular rhythm
- Normal rate
- P wave for every QRS complex; all P waves similar in size and shape
- All QRS complexes similar in size and shape
- Normal PR and QT intervals
- Normal T waves

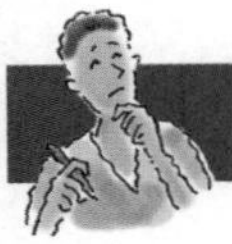

Quick quiz

1. The P wave represents:
   A. atrial repolarization.
   B. atrial depolarization.
   C. ventricular depolarization.
   D. ventricular repolarization.

Answer: B. The impulse spreading across the atria, or atrial depolarization, generates a P wave.

2. The normal duration of a QRS complex is:
   A. 0.06 to 0.10 second.
   B. 0.12 to 0.20 second.
   C. 0.24 to 0.28 second.
   D. 0.36 to 0.44 second.

Answer: A. Normal duration of a QRS complex, which represents ventricular depolarization, is 0.06 to 0.12 second.

3.   To gather information about impulse conduction from the atria to the ventricles, study the:
    A.   P wave.
    B.   PR interval.
    C.   ST segment.
    D.   T wave.

Answer: B. The PR interval measures the interval between atrial depolarization and ventricular depolarization. A normal PR interval is 0.12 to 0.20 second.

4.   The period when myocardial cells are vulnerable to extra stimuli begins with the:
    A.   end of the P wave.
    B.   start of the R wave.
    C.   start of the Q wave.
    D.   peak of the T wave.

Answer: D. The peak of the T wave represents the beginning of the relative, although not the absolute, refractory period, when the cells are vulnerable to stimuli.

5.   Atrial and ventricular rates can be determined by counting the number of small boxes between:
    A.   the end of one P wave and the beginning of another.
    B.   two consecutive P and R waves, respectively.
    C.   the middle of two consecutive T waves.
    D.   the beginning of the P wave and the end of the T wave.

Answer: B. Atrial and ventricular rates can be determined by counting the number of small boxes between two consecutive P or R waves and then dividing that number into 1,500.

Test strips

Now try these test strips. Fill in the blanks below with the particular characteristics of the strip.

Strip 1

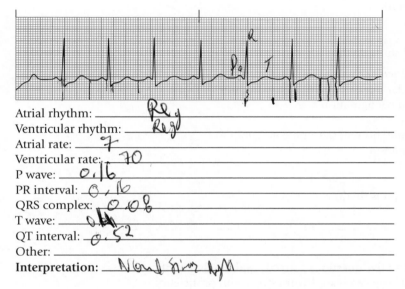

Atrial rhythm: _____ Reg _____
Ventricular rhythm: _____ Reg _____
Atrial rate: _____ 7 _____
Ventricular rate: _____ 70 _____
P wave: _____ 0.16 _____
PR interval: _____ 0.16 _____
QRS complex: _____ 0.08 _____
T wave: _____ 0.44 _____
QT interval: _____ 0.52 _____
Other: _____
Interpretation: _____ Normal sinus rhythm _____

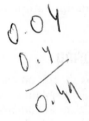

0.08
0.4
0.46

0.04
0.4
0.44

Strip 2

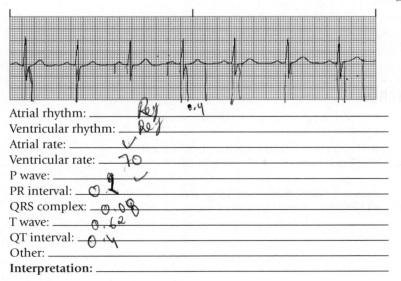

Atrial rhythm: _____ Reg _____ 0.4
Ventricular rhythm: _____ Reg _____
Atrial rate: _____ ✓ _____
Ventricular rate: _____ 70 _____
P wave: _____ 9 ✓ _____
PR interval: _____ 0.9 _____
QRS complex: _____ 0.08 _____
T wave: _____ 0.62 _____
QT interval: _____ 0.4 _____
Other: _____
Interpretation: _____

0.44

Answers to test strips

1. Rhythm: Atrial and ventricular rhythms are regular
   Rate: Atrial and ventricular rates are each 79 beats/minute
   P wave: Normal size and configuration
   PR interval: 0.12 second
   QRS complex: 0.08 second; normal size and configuration
   T wave: Normal configuration
   QT interval: 0.44 second
   Other: None
   Interpretation: Normal sinus rhythm

2. Rhythm: Atrial and ventricular rhythms are regular
   Rate: Atrial and ventricular rates are each 72 beats/minute
   P wave: Normal size and configuration
   PR interval: 0.20 second
   QRS complex: 0.10 second; normal size and configuration
   T wave: Normal configuration
   QT interval: 0.42 second
   Other: None
   Interpretation: Normal sinus rhythm

Scoring

☆☆☆   If you answered all five questions correctly and filled in all the blanks, excellent! You can read rhythm strips with proficiency.

☆☆   If you answered four questions correctly and filled in most of the blanks, very good!

☆   If you answered fewer than four questions correctly and missed most of the blanks, chin up! Review rhythm strips and the chapters and you'll be proficient shortly. The trick to learning rhythm strips is repetition.

Recommended references

Brown, D. F. M., & Martindale, J. L. (2012). *Rapid interpretation of ECG's in emergency medicine.* Philadelphia, PA: Wolters Kluwer.

García-Niebla, J. (2009). Comparison of p-wave patterns derived from correct and incorrect placement of V1-V2 electrodes. *Journal of Cardiovascular Nursing, 24*(2), 156–161.

Katritsis, D. G., Gersch, B. J., & Camm, A. J. (2013). *Clinical cardiology: Current practice guidelines.* Oxford, United Kingdom: Oxford University Press.

Mann, D. L., Zipes, D. P., Libby, P., & Bonow, R. D. (2014). *Braunwald's heart disease: A textbook of cardiovascular medicine* (10th ed.). St. Louis, MO: Saunders | Elsevier.

McLaughlin, M. A. (clinical ed.) (2014). *Cardiovascular care made incredibly easy* (3rd ed.). Philadelphia, PA: Wolters Kluwer.

Rosen, A. V., Koppikan, S., Shaw, C., & Baranchuk, A. (2014). Common ECG lead placement errors. Part 1: Limb lead reversals. *International Journal of Medical Students, 2*(3), 92–98.

Urden, L., & Stacy, K. (2013). *Critical Care Nursing.* (7th ed.). St. Louis, MO: Mosby | Elsevier.

Wagner, G. S., & Strauss, D. G. (2013). *Marriott's practical electrocardiology* (12th ed.). Philadelphia, PA: Wolters Kluwer.

Part II

Recognizing arrhythmias

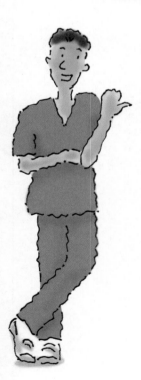

Chapter 4

Sinus node arrhythmias

Just the facts

In this chapter, you'll learn:

◆ the proper way to identify the various sinus node arrhythmias

◆ the role of the sinoatrial node in arrhythmia formation

◆ the causes, significance, treatment, and nursing implications of each arrhythmia

◆ assessment findings associated with each arrhythmia

◆ interpretation of sinus node arrhythmias on an electrocardiogram.

A look at sinus node arrhythmias

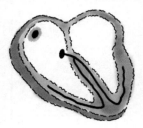

When the heart functions normally, the sinoatrial (SA) node, also called the *sinus node,* acts as the primary pacemaker. The sinus node assumes this role because its automatic firing rate exceeds that of the heart's other pacemakers. In an adult at rest, the sinus node has an inherent firing rate of 60 to 100 times per minute.

The SA node's blood supply comes from the right coronary artery or the left circumflex artery. The autonomic nervous system richly innervates the sinus node through the vagus nerve, a parasympathetic nerve, and several sympathetic nerves. Stimulation of the vagus nerve decreases the node's firing rate, and stimulation of the sympathetic system increases it.

Sinus arrhythmia

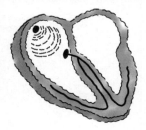

In sinus arrhythmia, the pacemaker cells of the SA node fire irregularly. Sinus arrhythmia is present when there is a sinus rhythm with variability in the cycle lengths between successive P waves. The cardiac rate stays within normal limits, but the rhythm is irregular and corresponds with the respiratory cycle. Sinus arrhythmia can occur naturally in athletes and children, but it rarely occurs in infants. Conditions unrelated to respiration may also produce sinus arrhythmia, including inferior wall myocardial infarction (MI), advanced age, use of digoxin (Lanoxin) or morphine, and conditions involving increased intracranial pressure.

How it happens

Sinus arrhythmia, the heart's normal response to respirations, results from an inhibition of reflex vagal activity, or tone. During inspiration, an increase in the flow of blood back to the heart reduces vagal tone, which increases the heart rate. ECG complexes fall closer together, which shortens the P-P interval, the time elapsed between two consecutive P waves.

During expiration, venous return decreases, which in turn increases vagal tone, slows the heart rate, and lengthens the P-P interval. (See *Breathing and sinus arrhythmia*.)

Breathing and sinus arrhythmia

When sinus arrhythmia is related to respirations, you'll see an increase in heart rate with inspiration and a decrease with expiration, as shown here.

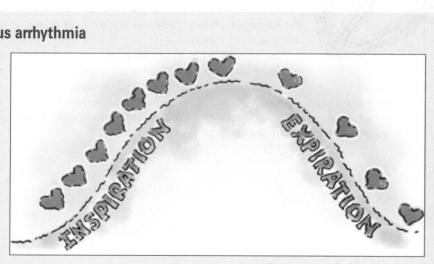

Sick sinus

Sinus arrhythmia usually isn't significant and produces no symptoms. A marked variation in P-P intervals in an older adult, however, may indicate sick sinus syndrome, a related, potentially more serious phenomenon. Sick sinus syndrome results from underlying disease of the conduction system.

What to look for

When you look for sinus arrhythmia, you'll see that the rhythm is irregular and corresponds to the respiratory cycle. (See *Identifying sinus arrhythmia.*) The difference between the shortest and longest P-P intervals—and the shortest and longest R-R intervals—exceeds 0.12 second.

The atrial and ventricular rates are within normal limits (60 to 100 beats/min) and vary with respiration—faster with inspiration, slower with expiration. All other parameters are normal, except for the QT interval, which may vary slightly but remains normal.

It's all in the breath

Look for a peripheral pulse rate that increases during inspiration and decreases during expiration. If the arrhythmia is caused by an underlying condition, you may note signs and symptoms of that condition.

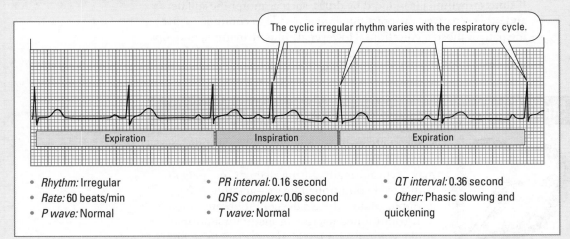

Identifying sinus arrhythmia

This rhythm strip illustrates sinus arrhythmia. Look for these distinguishing characteristics:

The cyclic irregular rhythm varies with the respiratory cycle.

Expiration   Inspiration   Expiration

- *Rhythm:* Irregular
- *Rate:* 60 beats/min
- *P wave:* Normal
- *PR interval:* 0.16 second
- *QRS complex:* 0.06 second
- *T wave:* Normal
- *QT interval:* 0.36 second
- *Other:* Phasic slowing and quickening

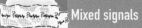

Mixed signals

A longer look at sinus arrhythmia

Don't mistake sinus arrhythmia for other rhythms. At first glance it may look like atrial fibrillation, normal sinus rhythm with premature atrial contractions, sinoatrial block, or sinus pauses. Observe the monitor and the patient's respiratory pattern for several minutes to determine the rate and rhythm. As always, check the patient's pulse.

Sinus arrhythmia is easier to detect when the heart rate is slow; it may disappear when the heart rate increases, as with exercise or after atropine administration.

How you intervene

Unless the patient is symptomatic, treatment usually isn't necessary. If sinus arrhythmia is unrelated to respirations, the underlying cause may require treatment.

When caring for a patient with sinus arrhythmia, observe the heart rhythm during respiration to determine whether the arrhythmia coincides with the respiratory cycle. Be sure to check the monitor carefully to avoid an inaccurate interpretation of the waveform. (See *A longer look at sinus arrhythmia.*)

Keep at it

If sinus arrhythmia is induced by drugs, such as morphine sulfate and other sedatives, the practitioner may decide to continue to give the patient those medications. However, if sinus arrhythmia develops suddenly in a patient taking digoxin, notify the practitioner immediately. The patient may be experiencing digoxin toxicity.

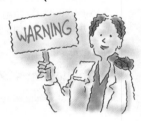

Notify the practitioner if sinus arrhythmia develops suddenly in a patient taking digoxin.

Sinus bradycardia

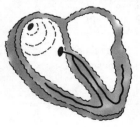

Sinus bradycardia is characterized by a sinus rate below 60 beats/min and a regular rhythm. It may occur normally during sleep or in a person with a well-conditioned heart—an athlete, for example. Many athletes develop it because their well-conditioned hearts can maintain a normal stroke volume with less-than-normal effort. Sinus bradycardia also occurs normally during sleep due to decreased metabolic demands.

How it happens

Sinus bradycardia usually occurs as the normal response to a reduced demand for blood flow. In this case, vagal stimulation increases and sympathetic stimulation decreases. (See *Causes of sinus bradycardia.*) As a result, automaticity (the tendency of cells to initiate their own impulses) in the SA node diminishes.

A tolerable condition?

Sinus bradycardia commonly occurs after an inferior wall MI that involves the right coronary artery, which supplies blood to the SA node. It can also result from numerous other conditions and the use of certain drugs.

The clinical significance of sinus bradycardia depends on how low the rate is and whether the patient is symptomatic. For example, most adults can tolerate a sinus bradycardia of 45 to 59 beats/min but are less tolerant of a rate below 45 beats/min.

No symptoms? No problem.

Usually, sinus bradycardia produces no symptoms and is insignificant. Unless the patient shows symptoms of decreased cardiac output, no treatment is necessary. (See the appendix *ACLS algorithms.*)

Symptoms? Problem!

When sinus bradycardia produces symptoms, however, prompt attention is critical. The heart of a patient with underlying cardiac disease may not be able to compensate for a drop in rate by increasing its stroke volume. The resulting drop in cardiac output produces such signs and symptoms as hypotension and dizziness. Bradycardia may also predispose some patients to more serious arrhythmias, such as ventricular tachycardia and ventricular fibrillation.

Causes of sinus bradycardia

Sinus bradycardia may be caused by
- noncardiac disorders, such as hyperkalemia, increased intracranial pressure, hypothyroidism, hypothermia, sleep, and glaucoma.
- conditions producing excess vagal stimulation or decreased sympathetic stimulation, such as sleep, deep relaxation, Valsalva's maneuver, carotid sinus massage, and vomiting.
- cardiac diseases, such as sinoatrial node disease, cardiomyopathy, myocarditis, and myocardial ischemia, immediately following an inferior wall myocardial infarction.
- certain drugs, especially beta-adrenergic blockers, digoxin (Lanoxin), calcium channel blockers, lithium (Lithobid), and antiarrhythmics, such as sotalol (Betapace), amiodarone (Cordarone), propafenone (Rythmol), and quinidine.

In a patient with acute inferior wall MI, sinus bradycardia is considered a favorable prognostic sign, unless it's accompanied by hypotension. Because sinus bradycardia rarely affects children, it's considered a poor prognostic sign in children. (See *Bradycardia and tachycardia in children*.)

What to look for

In sinus bradycardia, the atrial and ventricular rhythms are regular, as are their rates, except that they're both less than 60 beats/min. (See *Identifying sinus bradycardia*.) All other characteristics appear normal. You'll see a P wave preceding each QRS complex and a normal PR interval, QRS complex, T wave, and QT interval.

When cardiac output gets low

As long as a patient can compensate for the decreased cardiac output, they are likely to remain asymptomatic. If compensatory mechanisms fail, however, signs and symptoms of declining cardiac output, such as hypotension and dizziness, usually appear.

Palpitations and pulse irregularities may occur if the patient experiences more ectopic beats, such as premature atrial, junctional, or ventricular contractions. Diminished blood flow to the cerebrum may produce signs of decreased level of consciousness (LOC) such as confusion. Bradycardia-induced syncope (Stokes–Adams attack) may also occur.

How you intervene

If the patient is asymptomatic and vital signs are stable, treatment isn't necessary. Continue to observe the heart rhythm, monitoring the progression and duration of the bradycardia. Evaluate the patient's tolerance of the rhythm at rest and with activity. Review the drugs being taken. Check with the practitioner about stopping any medications that may be depressing the SA node, such as digoxin, beta-adrenergic blockers, or calcium channel blockers. Before giving those drugs, make sure the heart rate is within a safe range.

Identify and correct

If the patient is symptomatic, treatment aims to identify and correct the underlying cause. Meanwhile, the heart rate must be maintained with transcutaneous pacing. Use drugs such as atropine, epinephrine, or dopamine, while awaiting a pacemaker or if pacing is ineffective.

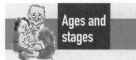

Ages and stages

Bradycardia and tachycardia in children

Evaluate bradycardia and tachycardia in children in context. Bradycardia (less than 90 beats/min) may occur in the healthy infant during sleep; tachycardia may be a normal response when the child is crying or otherwise upset. Keep in mind that because heart rate varies considerably from the neonate to the adolescent, one definition of bradycardia or tachycardia can't fit all children.

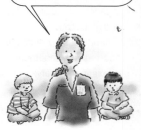

Sinus bradycardia in a child is an ominous sign.

Identifying sinus bradycardia

This rhythm strip illustrates sinus bradycardia. Look for these distinguishing characteristics:

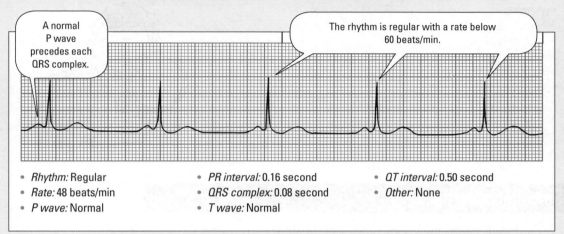

A normal P wave precedes each QRS complex.

The rhythm is regular with a rate below 60 beats/min.

- *Rhythm:* Regular
- *Rate:* 48 beats/min
- *P wave:* Normal

- *PR interval:* 0.16 second
- *QRS complex:* 0.08 second
- *T wave:* Normal

- *QT interval:* 0.50 second
- *Other:* None

Atropine is given as a 0.5 mg dose by rapid injection. The dose may be repeated every 3 to 5 minutes up to a maximum of 3 mg total. If atropine proves ineffective, administer an epinephrine infusion at a rate of 2 to 10 mcg/min. If low blood pressure accompanies bradycardia, administer a dopamine infusion at 2 to 10 mcg/kg/min. Treatment of chronic, symptom-producing sinus bradycardia requires insertion of a permanent pacemaker.

Check the ABCs

If the patient abruptly develops a significant sinus bradycardia, assess the airway, breathing, and circulation (ABCs). If these are adequate, determine whether the patient has an effective cardiac output. If not, they will become symptomatic. (See *Clues to symptomatic bradycardia,* page 78.)

When administering atropine, be sure to give the correct dose: Doses lower than 0.5 mg can have a paradoxical effect, slowing the heart rate even further. Keep in mind that a patient with a transplanted heart won't respond to atropine and may require pacing for emergency treatment.

Clues to symptomatic bradycardia

If a patient can't tolerate bradycardia, they may develop these signs and symptoms:
* hypotension
* cool, clammy skin
* altered mental status
* dizziness
* blurred vision
* crackles, dyspnea, and an S_3 heart sound, which indicate heart failure
* chest pain
* syncope

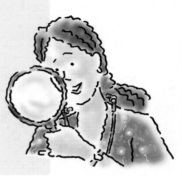

Sinus tachycardia

If sinus bradycardia is the tortoise of the sinus arrhythmias, sinus tachycardia is the hare. Sinus tachycardia in an adult is characterized by a sinus rate of more than 100 beats/min. The rate rarely exceeds 160 beats/min except during strenuous exercise; the maximum rate achievable with exercise decreases with age.

How it happens

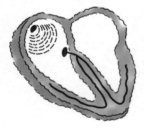

The clinical significance of sinus tachycardia depends on the underlying cause. (See *Causes of sinus tachycardia.*) The arrhythmia may be the body's response to exercise or high emotional states and may be of no clinical significance. It may also occur with hypovolemia, hemorrhage, or pain. When the stimulus for the tachycardia is removed, the arrhythmia spontaneously resolves.

Hard on the heart

Sinus tachycardia can also be a significant arrhythmia with dire consequences. Because myocardial demands for oxygen are increased at higher heart rates, tachycardia can bring on an episode of chest pain in patients with coronary artery disease. It can also be detrimental for patients with obstructive types of heart conditions, such as aortic stenosis and hypertrophic cardiomyopathy.

Sinus tachycardia occurs in about 30% of patients after acute MI and is considered a poor prognostic sign because it may be associated with massive heart damage. Persistent tachycardia may also signal impending heart failure or cardiogenic shock.

Causes of sinus tachycardia

Sinus tachycardia may be a normal response to exercise, pain, stress, fever, or strong emotions, such as fear and anxiety. It can also occur
* in certain cardiac conditions, such as heart failure, cardiogenic shock, and pericarditis.
* as a compensatory mechanism in shock, anemia, respiratory distress, pulmonary embolism, sepsis, and hyperthyroidism.
* when taking such drugs as atropine, isoproterenol (Isuprel), aminophylline, dopamine, dobutamine, epinephrine, alcohol, caffeine, nicotine, and amphetamines.

What to look for

In sinus tachycardia, atrial and ventricular rhythms are regular. (See *Identifying sinus tachycardia.*) Both rates are equal, generally 100 to 160 beats/min. As in sinus bradycardia, the P wave is of normal size and shape and precedes each QRS, but it may increase in amplitude. As the heart rate increases, the P wave may be superimposed on the preceding T wave and difficult to identify the PR interval, QRS complex and T wave are normal. The QT interval normally shortens with tachycardia.

Pulse check!

When assessing a patient with sinus tachycardia, look for a pulse rate of more than 100 beats/min but with a regular rhythm. Usually, the patient is asymptomatic. However, if the cardiac output falls and compensatory mechanisms fail, they may experience hypotension, syncope, and blurred vision. (See *What happens in tachycardia,* page 80.)

They may report chest pain and palpitations, commonly described as a pounding chest or a sensation of skipped heartbeats. They may also report a sense of nervousness or anxiety. If heart failure develops, the patient may exhibit crackles, an extra heart sound (S₃), and jugular vein distention.

> With sinus tachycardia, look for a pulse rate of more than 100 beats/min but with a regular rhythm.

Identifying sinus tachycardia

This rhythm strip illustrates sinus tachycardia. Look for these distinguishing characteristics:

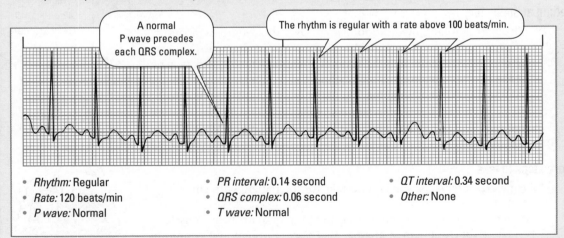

> A normal P wave precedes each QRS complex.

> The rhythm is regular with a rate above 100 beats/min.

- *Rhythm:* Regular
- *Rate:* 120 beats/min
- *P wave:* Normal
- *PR interval:* 0.14 second
- *QRS complex:* 0.06 second
- *T wave:* Normal
- *QT interval:* 0.34 second
- *Other:* None

What happens in tachycardia

Tachycardia can lower cardiac output by reducing ventricular filling time and the amount of blood pumped by the ventricles during each contraction. Normally, ventricular volume reaches 120 to 130 mL during diastole. In tachycardia, decreased ventricular volume leads to hypotension and decreased peripheral perfusion.

As cardiac output plummets, arterial pressure and peripheral perfusion decrease. Tachycardia worsens myocardial ischemia by increasing the heart's demand for oxygen and reducing the duration of diastole—the period of greatest coronary flow.

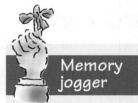

Memory jogger

To help you remember how to identify sinus bradycardia from sinus tachycardia, think of the **b** in bradycardia as **b**elow. Sinus bradycardia is **below** 60 beats/min, while sinus tachycardia is **above** 100 beats/min. Both have a normal QRS complex, preceded by a normal P wave.

How you intervene

When treating the asymptomatic patient, focus on determining the cause of the sinus tachycardia. Treatment for a symptomatic patient involves maintaining adequate cardiac output and tissue perfusion and identifying and correcting the underlying cause. For example, if the tachycardia is caused by hemorrhage, treatment includes stopping the bleeding and replacing blood and fluid.

Slow it down

If tachycardia leads to cardiac ischemia, treatment may include medications to slow the heart rate. The most commonly used drugs include beta-adrenergic blockers, such as metoprolol (Lopressor) and atenolol (Tenormin), and calcium channel blockers such as verapamil (Calan).

Getting at the history

Check the patient's medication history. Over-the-counter sympathomimetic agents, which mimic the effects of the sympathetic nervous system, may contribute to the sinus tachycardia. These agents may be contained in nose drops and cold formulas.

You should also ask about the patient's use of caffeine, nicotine, alcohol, and such recreational drugs as cocaine and amphetamines, any of which can trigger tachycardia. Advise them to avoid these substances.

More steps to take

Here are other steps you should take for the patient with sinus tachycardia:
- Because sinus tachycardia can lead to injury of the heart muscle, check for chest pain or angina. Also assess for signs and symptoms of heart failure, including crackles, an S_3 heart sound, and jugular vein distention.

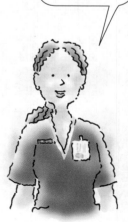

Advise the patient to avoid caffeine, nicotine, alcohol, and recreational drugs.

- Monitor intake and output as well as daily weight.
- Check the patient's LOC to assess cerebral perfusion.
- Provide the patient with a calm environment. Help to reduce fear and anxiety, which can fuel the arrhythmia.
- Teach about procedures and treatments. Include relaxation techniques in the information you provide.
- Be aware that a sudden onset of sinus tachycardia after an MI may signal extension of the infarction. Prompt recognition is vital so treatment can be started.
- Remember that tachycardia is commonly the first sign of a pulmonary embolism. Maintain suspicion, especially if your patient has risk factors for thrombotic emboli.

Sinus arrest

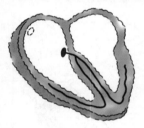

A disorder of impulse formation, sinus arrest is caused by a lack of electrical activity in the atrium, a condition called atrial standstill. (See *Causes of sinus arrest.*) During atrial standstill, the atria aren't stimulated and an entire PQRST complex will be missing from the ECG strip.

Except for this missing complex, or pause, the ECG usually remains normal. Atrial standstill is called *sinus pause* when one or two beats aren't formed and *sinus arrest* when three or more beats aren't formed.

Sinus arrest closely resembles third-degree SA block, also called *exit block,* on the ECG strip. (See *Understanding sinoatrial blocks,* pages 82 and 83.)

How it happens

Sinus arrest occurs when the SA node fails to generate an impulse. Such failure may result from a number of conditions, including acute infection, heart disease, and vagal stimulation. Sinus arrest may be associated with sick sinus syndrome.

The clinical significance of sinus arrest depends on the patient's symptoms. If the pauses are short and infrequent, the patient will most likely be asymptomatic and won't require treatment. They may have a normal sinus rhythm for days or weeks between episodes of sinus arrest. They may not be able to feel the arrhythmias at all.

Pauses of 2 to 3 seconds normally occur in healthy adults during sleep and occasionally in patients with increased vagal tone or hypersensitive carotid sinus disease.

Causes of sinus arrest

The following conditions can cause sinus arrest:
- sinus node disease, such as fibrosis and idiopathic degeneration
- increased vagal tone, as occurs with Valsalva's maneuver, carotid sinus massage, and vomiting
- digoxin (Lanoxin), quinidine, procainamide and salicylates, especially if given at toxic levels
- excessive doses of beta-adrenergic blockers, such as metoprolol (Lopressor) and propranolol (Inderal)
- cardiac disorders, such as chronic coronary artery disease, acute myocarditis, cardiomyopathy, and hypertensive heart disease
- acute inferior wall myocardial infarction
- sick sinus syndrome
- acute infection

Understanding sinoatrial blocks

In sinoatrial (SA) block, the SA node discharges impulses at regular intervals. Some of those impulses, though, are delayed on their way to the atria. Based on the length of the delay, SA blocks are divided into three categories: first-, second-, and third-degree. Second-degree block is further divided into type I and type II.

First-degree SA block consists of a delay between the firing of the sinus node and depolarization of the atria. Because the ECG doesn't show sinus node activity, you can't detect first-degree SA block. However, you can detect the other three types of SA block.

> SA blocks are divided into three categories based on the length of the delay.

Second-degree type I block

In second-degree type I block, conduction time between the sinus node and the surrounding atrial tissue becomes progressively longer until an entire cycle is dropped. The pause is less than twice the shortest P-P interval.

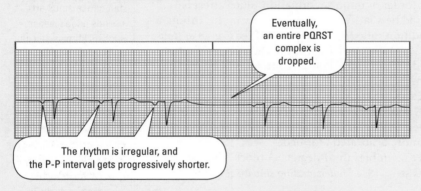

> Eventually, an entire PQRST complex is dropped.

> The rhythm is irregular, and the P-P interval gets progressively shorter.

Second-degree type II block

In second-degree type II block, conduction time between the sinus node and atrial tissue is normal until an impulse is blocked. The duration of the pause is a multiple of the P-P interval.

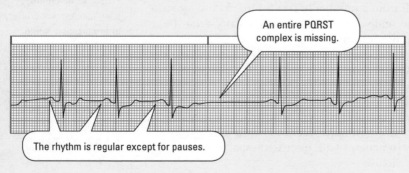

> An entire PQRST complex is missing.

> The rhythm is regular except for pauses.

Understanding sinoatrial blocks *(Continued)*

Third-degree block

In third-degree block, some impulses are blocked, causing long sinus pauses. The pause isn't a multiple of the sinus rhythm. On an ECG, third-degree SA block looks similar to sinus arrest but results from a different cause.

Third-degree SA block is caused by a failure to conduct impulses; sinus arrest results from failure to form impulses. Failure in each case causes atrial activity to stop.

In sinus arrest, the pause commonly ends with a junctional escape beat. In third-degree block, the pause lasts for an indefinite period and ends with a sinus beat.

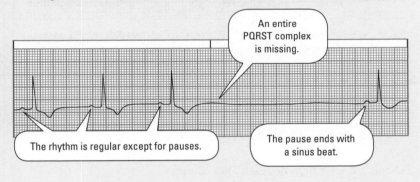

An entire PQRST complex is missing.

The rhythm is regular except for pauses.

The pause ends with a sinus beat.

Sinus arrest can cause accidents. Motor vehicle accidents are of particular concern

Too many for too long

If sinus arrest is frequent and prolonged, however, the patient will most likely have symptoms. The arrhythmias can produce syncope or near-syncopal episodes usually within 7 seconds of asystole.

During a prolonged pause, the patient may fall and injure themselves. Other situations may be just as serious. For example, a symptom-producing arrhythmia that occurs while the patient is driving a car could result in a fatal accident.

What to look for

When assessing for sinus pause, you'll find that atrial and ventricular rhythms are regular except for a missing complex at the onset of atrial standstill. (See *Identifying sinus arrest,* page 84.) The atrial and ventricular rates are equal and usually within normal limits. The rate may vary, however, as a result of the pauses.

Identifying sinus arrest

This rhythm strip illustrates sinus arrest. Look for these distinguishing characteristics:

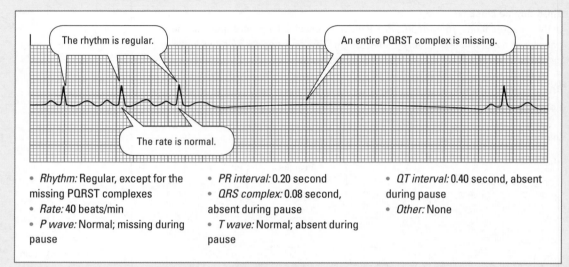

- *Rhythm:* Regular, except for the missing PQRST complexes
- *Rate:* 40 beats/min
- *P wave:* Normal; missing during pause

- *PR interval:* 0.20 second
- *QRS complex:* 0.08 second, absent during pause
- *T wave:* Normal; absent during pause

- *QT interval:* 0.40 second, absent during pause
- *Other:* None

Of normal size and shape, a P wave precedes each QRS complex but is absent during a pause. The PR interval is normal and constant when the P wave is present and not measurable when absent. The QRS complex, the T wave, and the QT interval are normal when present and are absent during a pause.

You might see junctional escape beats and premature atrial, junctional, or ventricular contractions. With sinus arrest, the length of the pause isn't a multiple of the previous R-R intervals.

Signs of recurrent pauses

You can't detect a pulse or heart sounds when sinus arrest occurs. Usually, the patient is asymptomatic. Recurrent pauses may cause signs of decreased cardiac output, such as low blood pressure, altered mental status, and cool, clammy skin. The patient may also complain of dizziness or blurred vision.

How you intervene

An asymptomatic patient needs no treatment. For a patient displaying mild symptoms, treatment focuses on maintaining cardiac output and identifying the cause of the sinus arrest. That may involve stopping

Syncope and sinus arrest

A patient with sinus arrest is at risk for syncope. Ask your patient whether they have ever passed out or felt as if they were going to pass out.

Also ask about a history of falls. If they have passed out or if they have a history of falls, obtain a detailed description of each episode, including where and how the syncope occurred.

Asking questions

If possible, check with friends and family members who witnessed the episodes to find out what happened and how long the patient remained unconscious each time.

The information you gather may help determine whether a vagal mechanism was involved. The presence of syncope or sinus pauses on an electrocardiogram may indicate the need for further electrophysiologic evaluation.

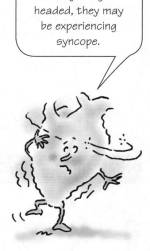

If the patient is dizzy or light-headed, they may be experiencing syncope.

medications that contribute to SA node suppression, such as digoxin, beta-adrenergic blockers, and calcium channel blockers.

Emergent treatment

A patient who develops signs of circulatory collapse needs immediate treatment. As with sinus bradycardia, emergency treatment includes using a temporary pacemaker and administration of atropine or epinephrine. A permanent pacemaker may be implanted for long-term management.

The goal for the patient with sinus arrest is to maintain adequate cardiac output and perfusion. Be sure to record and document the frequency and duration of pauses. Determine whether a pause is the result of sinus arrest or SA block.

Don't let sleeping pauses lie

Examine the circumstances under which sinus pauses occur. A sinus pause may be insignificant if detected while the patient is sleeping. If the pauses are recurrent, assess the patient for evidence of decreased cardiac output, such as altered mental status, low blood pressure, and cool, clammy skin.

Ask them whether they are dizzy or light-headed or have blurred vision. Do they feel as if they have passed out? If so, they may be experiencing syncope from a prolonged sinus arrest. (See *Syncope and sinus arrest.*)

Document the patient's vital signs and how they feel during pauses as well as what activities they were involved in when the episode(s) occurred. Activities that increase vagal stimulation, such as Valsalva's maneuver or vomiting, increase the likelihood of sinus pauses.

When matters get even worse

Assess for a progression of the arrhythmia. Notify the practitioner immediately if the patient becomes unstable. Lower the head of the bed and administer atropine or epinephrine, as ordered or as your facility's policy directs. Withhold medications that may contribute to sinus pauses and check with the practitioner about whether those drugs should be continued.

If appropriate, be alert for signs of digoxin, quinidine, or procainamide toxicity. Obtain a serum digoxin level and a serum electrolyte level. If a pacemaker is implanted, give the patient discharge instructions about pacemaker care.

Sick sinus syndrome

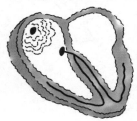

Also called *sinus node disease or sinus nodal dysfunction*, sick sinus syndrome refers to a wide spectrum of SA node abnormalities. The syndrome is caused by disturbances in the way impulses are generated or the inability to conduct impulses to the atrium.

Sick sinus syndrome usually shows up as bradycardia, with episodes of sinus arrest and SA block interspersed with sudden, brief periods of rapid atrial fibrillation. Patients are also prone to paroxysms of other atrial tachyarrhythmias, such as atrial flutter and ectopic atrial tachycardia, a condition sometimes referred to as *bradycardia–tachycardia* (or *brady–tachy*) syndrome.

Most patients with sick sinus syndrome are older than age 60, but anyone can develop the arrhythmia. It's rare in children except after open-heart surgery that results in SA node damage. The arrhythmia affects men and women equally. The onset is progressive, insidious, and chronic.

How it happens

Sick sinus syndrome results from a dysfunction of the sinus node's automaticity or abnormal conduction or blockages of impulses coming out of the nodal region. (See *Causes of sick sinus syndrome.*) These conditions, in turn, stem from a degeneration of the area's autonomic nervous system and partial destruction of the sinus node, as may occur with an interrupted blood supply after an inferior wall MI.

Blocked exits

In addition, certain conditions can affect the atrial wall surrounding the SA node and cause exit blocks. Conditions that cause inflammation

Causes of sick sinus syndrome

Sick sinus syndrome may result from

- conditions leading to fibrosis of the sinoatrial (SA) node, such as increased age, atherosclerotic heart disease, hypertension, and cardiomyopathy.
- trauma to the SA node caused by open heart surgery (especially valvular surgery), pericarditis, or rheumatic heart disease.
- autonomic disturbances affecting autonomic innervation, such as hypervagatonia and degeneration of the autonomic nervous system.
- cardioactive medications, such as digoxin (Lanoxin), beta-adrenergic blockers, and calcium channel blockers.

or degeneration of atrial tissue can also lead to sick sinus syndrome. In many patients, though, the exact cause of this syndrome is never identified.

Prognosis of the diagnosis

The significance of sick sinus syndrome depends on the patient's age, the presence of other diseases, and the type and duration of the specific arrhythmias that occur. If atrial fibrillation is involved, the prognosis is worse, most likely because of the risk of thromboembolic complications.

If prolonged pauses are involved with sick sinus syndrome, syncope may occur. The length of a pause significant enough to cause syncope varies with the patient's age, posture at the time, and cerebrovascular status. Consider significant any pause that lasts at least 2 to 3 seconds.

Long-term problems

A significant part of the diagnosis is whether the patient experiences symptoms while the disturbance occurs. Because the syndrome is progressive and chronic, a symptomatic patient needs lifelong treatment. In addition, thromboembolism may develop as a complication of sick sinus syndrome, possibly resulting in stroke or peripheral embolization.

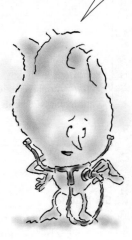

Prolonged pauses with sick sinus syndrome cause syncope. Consider significant any pause lasting 2 to 3 seconds.

What to look for

Sick sinus syndrome encompasses several potential rhythm disturbances that may be intermittent or chronic. (See *Identifying sick sinus syndrome,* page 88.) Those rhythm disturbances include one or a combination of:

- sinus bradycardia
- SA block
- sinus arrest
- sinus bradycardia alternating with sinus tachycardia
- episodes of atrial tachyarrhythmias, such as atrial fibrillation and atrial flutter
- failure of the sinus node to increase heart rate with exercise.

Check for speed bumps

Also look for an irregular rhythm with sinus pauses and abrupt rate changes. Atrial and ventricular rates may be fast, slow, or alternating periods of fast rates and slow rates interrupted by pauses.

The P wave varies with the rhythm and usually precedes each QRS complex. The PR interval is usually within normal limits but varies with changes in the rhythm. The QRS complex and T wave are usually normal, as is the QT interval, which may vary with rhythm changes.

Identifying sick sinus syndrome

This rhythm strip illustrates sick sinus syndrome. Look for these distinguishing characteristics:

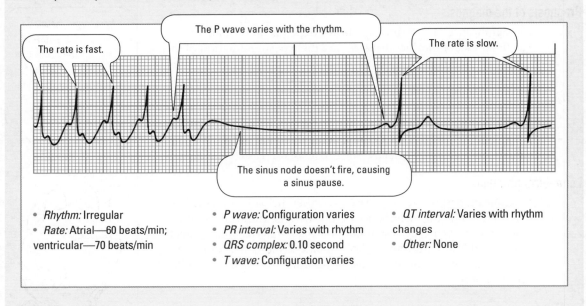

- *Rhythm:* Irregular
- *Rate:* Atrial—60 beats/min; ventricular—70 beats/min
- *P wave:* Configuration varies
- *PR interval:* Varies with rhythm
- *QRS complex:* 0.10 second
- *T wave:* Configuration varies
- *QT interval:* Varies with rhythm changes
- *Other:* None

No set pattern

The patient's pulse rate may be fast, slow, or normal, and the rhythm may be regular or irregular. You can usually detect an irregularity on the monitor or when palpating the pulse, which may feel inappropriately slow, then rapid.

If you monitor the patient's heart rate during exercise or exertion, you may observe an inappropriate response to exercise such as a failure of the heart rate to increase. You may also detect episodes of brady–tachy syndrome, atrial flutter, atrial fibrillation, SA block, or sinus arrest on the monitor.

Extra sounds

Other assessment findings depend on the patient's condition. For example, they may have crackles in the lungs, an S_3 heart sound, or a dilated and displaced left ventricular apical impulse if he has underlying cardiomyopathy.

The patient may show signs and symptoms of decreased cardiac output, such as hypotension, blurred vision, and syncope, a common experience with this arrhythmia. (See *Check mental status.*)

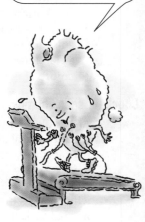

Monitoring heart rate during exercise may show an inappropriate response. Can I stop now?!

How you intervene

As with other sinus node arrhythmias, no treatment is necessary if the patient is asymptomatic. If the patient is symptomatic, however, treatment aims to alleviate signs and symptoms and correct the underlying cause of the arrhythmia.

Atropine or epinephrine may be given initially for symptomatic bradycardia. A temporary or permanent pacemaker may be used. Tachyarrhythmias may be treated with antiarrhythmic medications, such as metoprolol and digoxin.

Drugs don't always help

Unfortunately, medications used to suppress tachyarrhythmias may worsen underlying SA node disease and bradyarrhythmias. The patient may need anticoagulants if they develop sudden bursts, or paroxysms, of atrial fibrillation. The anticoagulants help prevent thromboembolism and stroke, a complication of the condition. (See *Recognizing an embolism.*)

Watch and document

When caring for a patient with sick sinus syndrome, monitor and document all arrhythmias they experience and signs or symptoms that develop. Assess how the rhythm responds to activity and pain looking for changes.

Watch the patient carefully after starting calcium channel blockers, beta-adrenergic blockers, or other antiarrhythmic medications. If treatment includes anticoagulant therapy and the insertion of a pacemaker, make sure the patient and family receive appropriate instruction.

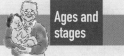

Ages and stages

Check mental status

Because the older adult with sick sinus syndrome may have mental status changes, be sure to perform a thorough assessment to rule out such disorders as stroke, delirium, or dementia.

Recognizing an embolism

When caring for a patient with sick sinus syndrome, be alert for signs and symptoms of an embolism, especially if the patient has atrial fibrillation. Any clots that form in the heart can break off and travel through the bloodstream, blocking the blood supply to the lungs, heart, brain, kidneys, intestines, or other organs.

Assess early

Assess the patient for neurologic changes, such as confusion, vision disturbances, weakness, chest pain, dyspnea, tachypnea, tachycardia, and acute onset of pain. Early recognition allows for prompt treatment.

That's a wrap!

Sinus node arrhythmias review

SA node
- Acts as primary pacemaker
- Inherent firing rate of 60 to 100 times per minute in a resting adult
- Supplied by blood from the right coronary artery and left circumflex artery

Sinus arrhythmia
Characteristics
- *Rhythms:* Irregular, corresponding to the respiratory cycle
- *Rates:* Within normal limits; vary with respiration
- *Other parameters:* QT interval variations

Treatment
- No treatment if asymptomatic
- Correction of the underlying cause

Sinus bradycardia
Characteristics
- *Rhythms:* Regular
- *Rates:* Less than 60 beats/min
- *Other parameters:* Normal

Treatment
- No treatment if asymptomatic
- Correction of the underlying cause
- Temporary pacing to increase heart rate
- Atropine or epinephrine to maintain heart rate
- Dopamine for hypotension
- Permanent pacing if necessary

Sinus tachycardia
Characteristics
- *Rhythms:* Regular
- *Rates:* Both equal, generally 100 to 160 beats/min
- *PR interval:* Normal
- *QRS complex:* Normal
- *T wave:* Normal
- *QT interval:* Shortened

Treatment
- No treatment if asymptomatic
- Correction of the underlying cause
- Beta-adrenergic blockers or calcium channel blockers if symptomatic

Sinus arrest
Characteristics
- *Rhythms:* Regular, except for missing PQRST complex
- *Rates:* Equal and usually within normal limits; may vary as a result of pauses
- *P wave:* Normal and constant when P wave is present; not measurable when P wave is absent
- *QRS complex:* Normal when present; absent during pause
- *T wave:* Normal when present; absent during pause
- *QT interval:* Normal when present; absent during pause

Treatment
- No treatment if asymptomatic
- Correction of the underlying cause

Sinus node arrhythmias review *(Continued)*

• Atropine or epinephrine to maintain heart rate
• Temporary pacemaker to maintain adequate cardiac output and perfusion
• Permanent pacemaker if necessary

Sick sinus syndrome
Characteristics
• *Rhythms:* Irregular with sinus pauses and abrupt rate changes
• *Rates:* Fast, slow, or combination of both
• *P wave:* Variations with rhythm and usually before QRS complex
• *QRS complex:* Normal

• *T wave:* Normal
• *QT interval:* Normal; variations with rhythm changes

Treatment
• No treatment if asymptomatic
• Correction of the underlying cause
• Atropine or epinephrine for symptomatic bradycardia
• Temporary or permanent pacemaker if necessary
• Antiarrhythmics, such as metoprolol and digoxin, for tachyarrhythmias
• Anticoagulants if atrial fibrillation develops

Quick quiz

1. A patient with symptomatic sinus bradycardia at a rate of 40 beats/min typically experiences:
    A.   high blood pressure.
    B.   hypotension and dyspnea.
    C.   facial flushing and ataxia.
    D.   calf pain and a dry cough.

Answer: B. A patient with symptomatic bradycardia suffers from low cardiac output, which may produce hypotension and dyspnea. The patient may also have chest pain, crackles, an S$_3$ heart sound, and a sudden onset of confusion.

2. For a patient with symptomatic sinus bradycardia, appropriate nursing interventions include establishing I.V. access to administer:
    A.   atropine.
    B.   anticoagulants.
    C.   calcium channel blocker.
    D.   beta-adrenergic blocker.

Answer: A. Atropine or epinephrine are standard treatments for sinus bradycardia.

3. A monitor shows an irregular rhythm and a rate that increases and decreases in consistent cycles. This rhythm most likely represents:
    A. sinus arrest.
    B. sinus bradycardia.
    C. normal sinus rhythm.
    D. sinus arrhythmia.

Answer: D. In sinus arrhythmia, occurring naturally in athletes and young children, the heart rate varies with the respiratory cycle and is rarely treated.

4. Treatment for symptomatic sick sinus syndrome includes:
    A. beta-adrenergic blockers.
    B. ventilatory support.
    C. pacemaker insertion.
    D. cardioversion.

Answer: C. A temporary or permanent pacemaker is commonly used to maintain a steady heart rate in patients with sick sinus syndrome.

5. Persistent tachycardia in a patient who has had an MI may signal:
    A. chronic sick sinus syndrome.
    B. pulmonary embolism or stroke.
    C. the healing process.
    D. impending heart failure or cardiogenic shock.

Answer: D. Sinus tachycardia occurs in about 30% of patients after acute MI and is considered a poor prognostic sign because it may be associated with massive heart damage.

6. Beta-adrenergic blockers, such as metoprolol and atenolol, and calcium channel blockers, such as diltiazem may be used to treat the sinus arrhythmia:
    A. sinus bradycardia.
    B. sinus tachycardia.
    C. sinus arrest.
    D. sinus arrhythmia.

Answer: B. Beta-adrenergic blockers and calcium channel blockers may be used to treat sinus tachycardia.

Test strips

Try these test strips. Interpret each strip using the 8-step method and fill in the blanks below with the particular characteristics of the strip. Then compare your answers with the answers given.

Strip 1

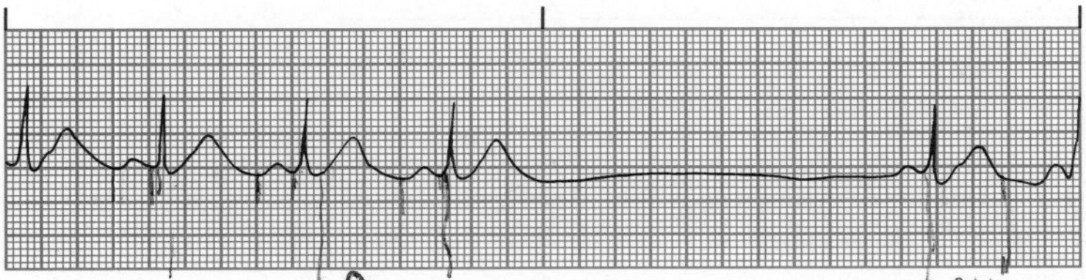

Atrial rhythm: _____ R R _____

Ventricular rhythm: _____ R _____

Atrial rate: _____ R _____

Ventricular rate: _____ 50 _____

P wave: _____ ✓ _____

PR interval: _____ 0.16 _____

QRS complex: _____ 0.12 _____

T wave: _____ 0.32 _____

QT interval: _____ 0.08 _____

Other: _____ _____

Interpretation: _____ Mobi _____

Strip 2

Atrial rhythm: _____ ll O _____
Ventricular rhythm: _____ HO _____
Atrial rate: _____ RR _____
Ventricular rate: _____ RR _____
P wave: _____ V _____
PR interval: _____ 0.14 _____
QRS complex: _____ 0.08 _____
T wave: _____ Norm _____
QT interval: _____ 0.36 _____
Other: _____ NO _____
Interpretation: _____ Sinus tach _____

Strip 3

Atrial rhythm: _____ 90 _____
Ventricular rhythm: _____ WV l _____
Atrial rate: _____ ll'g _____
Ventricular rate: _____ 90 _____
P wave: _____ V _____
PR interval: _____ 0.16 _____
QRS complex: _____ 0.08 _____
T wave: _____
QT interval: _____
Other: _____
Interpretation: _____

Answers to test strips

1. Rhythm: Regular except during pause
   Rate: Atrial and ventricular—50 beats/min
   P wave: Normal size and configuration, except when missing during pause
   PR interval: 0.16 second
   QRS complex: 0.10 second; normal size and configuration except when missing during pause
   T wave: Normal except when missing during pause
   QT interval: 0.42 second
   Other: Pause isn't a multiple of a previous sinus rhythm
   Interpretation: Sinus arrest

2. Rhythm: Regular
   Rate: Atrial and ventricular—110 beats/min
   P wave: Normal configuration
   PR interval: 0.14 second
   QRS complex: 0.08 second; normal size and configuration
   T wave: Normal configuration
   QT interval: 0.36 second
   Other: None
   Interpretation: Sinus tachycardia

3. Rhythm: Atrial and ventricular—irregular
   Rate: Atrial and ventricular—90 beats/min
   P wave: Normal
   PR interval: 0.12 second
   QRS complex: 0.10 second and normal
   T wave: Normal
   QT interval: 0.30 second
   Other: None
   Interpretation: Sinus arrhythmia

Scoring

☆☆☆ If you answered all six questions correctly and filled in all the blanks close to what we did, wow! You deserve to head down to the nearest club and tachy-brady all night long!

☆☆ If you answered five questions correctly and filled in most of the blanks pretty much as we did, super! When you get to the club, you can lead the dance parade.

☆ If you answered fewer than five questions correctly and missed most of the blanks, don't worry! A few lessons and you'll be tachy-brading with the best of 'em.

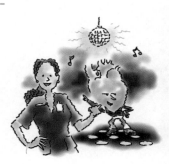

Recommended references

Brown, D. F. M., & Martindale, J. L. (2012). *Rapid interpretation of ECG's in emergency medicine.* Philadelphia, PA: Wolters Kluwer.

Crisel, R. K., Farzaneh-Far, R., Na, B., & Whooley, M. A. (2011). First-degree atrioventricular block is associated with heart failure and death in persons with stable coronary artery disease: Data from the Heart and Soul Study. *European Heart Journal, 32*(15), 1875–1880.

García-Niebla, J. (2009). Comparison of P-wave patterns derived from correct and incorrect placement of V1-V2 electrodes. *Journal of Cardiovascular Nursing, 24*(2), 156–161.

Katritsis, D. G., Gersch, B. J., & Camm, A. J. (2013). *Clinical cardiology: Current practice guidelines.* Oxford, United Kingdom: Oxford University Press.

Kulig, J., & Koplan, B. (2013). Wolff-Parkinson-white syndrome and accessory pathways. *Circulation, 122,* 480–483.

McLaughlin, M. A. (clinical ed.) (2014). *Cardiovascular care made incredibly easy* (3rd ed.). Philadelphia, PA: Wolters Kluwer.

Neumar, R. W., Otto, C. W., Link, M. S., Kronick, S. L., Shuster, M., Callaway, C.W., … Morrison, L. J. (2010). American heart association guidelines for ardiovascular resuscitation and emergency cardiovascular care science, Part 8.4: Management of symptomatic bradycardia and tachycardia. *Circulation, 122,* S746–S757.

Strauss, D. G., & Wagner, G. S. (2013). *Marriott's practical electrocardiology* (12th ed.). Philadelphia, PA: Wolters Kluwer.

Chapter 5

Atrial arrhythmias

Just the facts

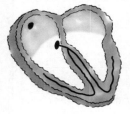

In this chapter, you'll learn:

◆ the proper way to identify the various atrial arrhythmias

◆ the causes, significance, treatment, and nursing implications of each arrhythmia

◆ assessment findings associated with each arrhythmia

◆ interpretation of atrial arrhythmias on an ECG.

A look at atrial arrhythmias

Atrial arrhythmias, the most common cardiac rhythm disturbances, result from impulses originating in areas outside the sinoatrial (SA) node. These arrhythmias can affect ventricular filling time and diminish the strength of the atrial kick, a contraction that normally provides the ventricles with about 15% to 25% of their blood.

Triple play

Atrial arrhythmias are thought to result from three mechanisms—enhanced automaticity, re-entry, and afterdepolarization. Let's take a look at each cause and review specific atrial arrhythmias:

• *Enhanced automaticity*—An increase in the automaticity (the ability of cardiac cells to initiate impulses on their own) of the atrial fibers can trigger abnormal impulses. Causes of increased automaticity include extracellular factors, such as hypoxia, acidosis, hypocalcemia, and digoxin toxicity, and conditions in which the function of the heart's normal pacemaker, the SA node, is diminished. For example, increased vagal tone or hypokalemia can increase the refractory period of the SA node and allow atrial fibers to fire impulses.

- *Re-entry*—In re-entry, an electrical stimulus is conducted in a circular loop that is large enough to allow the tissue to repolarize and be able to accept a new electrical stimulus. This process continues until something interrupts the continuous cycle. Re-entry may occur with coronary artery disease, cardiomyopathy, myocardial infarction (MI), or with structural abnormalities of the heart.
- *Triggered activity*—An injured cell sometimes only partly repolarizes. Partial repolarization can lead to a repetitive ectopic firing called *triggered activity.* The depolarization produced by triggered activity is known as *afterdepolarization* and can lead to atrial or ventricular tachycardia. Afterdepolarization can occur with cell injury, digoxin toxicity, and other conditions. Now let's examine each atrial arrhythmia in detail.

Premature atrial contractions

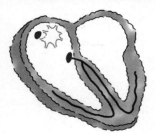

Premature atrial contractions (PACs) originate outside the SA node and usually result from an irritable spot, or focus, in the atria that take over as pacemaker for one or more beats. Before the SA node can fire an impulse an irritable atrial focus jumps in, firing its own impulse causing an early beat.

PACs may be conducted through the atrioventricular (AV) node and the rest of the heart, depending on their prematurity and the status of the AV and intraventricular conduction system. Nonconductor or blocked PACs don't conduct through the AV node or trigger a QRS complex.

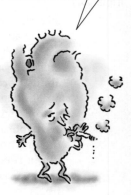

The nicotine in cigarettes can cause PACs. Yuk!

How it happens

PACs occur commonly in a normal heart and are very common in people who are 50 years old or older. PACs can be triggered by alcohol, nicotine, anxiety, fatigue, fever, and infectious diseases. A patient who eliminates or controls those factors can correct the arrhythmias.

PACs may also be associated with coronary or valvular heart disease, acute respiratory failure, hypoxia, pulmonary disease, digoxin toxicity, and certain electrolyte imbalances.

PACs are rarely dangerous in a patient who doesn't have heart disease. In fact, they commonly cause no symptoms and can go unrecognized for years. The patient may perceive PACs as normal palpitations or skipped beats.

Early warning sign

However, in patients with heart disease, PACs may lead to more serious arrhythmias, such as atrial fibrillation and atrial flutter. In a patient with an acute MI, PACs can serve as an early sign of heart failure or an electrolyte imbalance. PACs can also result from the release of the neurohormone catecholamine during episodes of pain or anxiety.

What to look for

The hallmark ECG characteristic of a PAC is a premature (early) P wave with an abnormal shape when compared with a sinus P wave. (See *Nonconducted PACs and second-degree AV block.*)

When the PAC is conducted, the QRS complex appears similar to the underlying QRS complex. PACs are commonly followed by a pause.

The PAC depolarizes the SA node early, causing it to reset itself and disrupt the normal cycle. The next sinus beat occurs sooner than it normally would, causing the P-P interval between two normal beats that have been interrupted by a PAC to be shorter than three consecutive sinus beats, an occurrence referred to as non-compensatory. (See *Identifying premature atrial contractions,* page 100.)

Lost in the T

When examining a PAC on an ECG, look for irregular atrial and ventricular rhythms. The underlying rhythm is usually regular. An irregular rhythm results from the PAC and its corresponding pause. The P wave is premature and abnormally shaped and may be lost in the previous T wave, distorting that wave's configuration. (The T wave might be bigger or have an extra bump.) Varying configurations of the P wave indicate more than one ectopic site.

The PR interval can be normal, shortened, or slightly prolonged, depending on the origin of the ectopic focus. If no QRS complex follows the premature P wave, a nonconducted PAC has occurred.

PACs may occur in bigeminy (every other beat is a PAC), trigeminy (every third beat is a PAC), or couplets (two PACs in a row).

The patient will have an irregular peripheral or apical pulse rhythm when the PACs occur. He may have no symptoms or he may complain of palpitations, skipped beats, or a fluttering sensation.

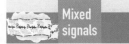

Mixed signals

Nonconducted PACs and second-degree AV block

Don't confuse nonconducted PACs with type II second-degree atrioventricular (AV) block. In type II second-degree AV block, the P-P interval is regular and all Ps look exactly the same. A nonconducted PAC, however, is an atrial impulse that arrives early to the AV node, when the node isn't yet repolarized.

As a result, the premature P wave fails to be conducted to the ventricle. The rhythm strip below shows an abnormally shaped P wave embedded in the preceding T wave.

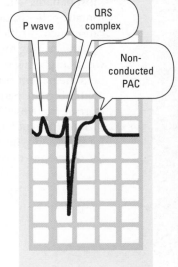

Identifying premature atrial contractions

This rhythm strip illustrates PAC. Look for these distinguishing characteristics:

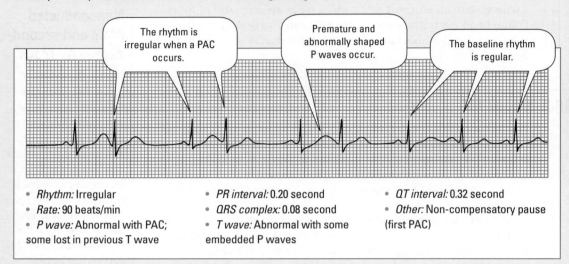

The rhythm is irregular when a PAC occurs.

Premature and abnormally shaped P waves occur.

The baseline rhythm is regular.

- *Rhythm:* Irregular
- *Rate:* 90 beats/min
- *P wave:* Abnormal with PAC; some lost in previous T wave

- *PR interval:* 0.20 second
- *QRS complex:* 0.08 second
- *T wave:* Abnormal with some embedded P waves

- *QT interval:* 0.32 second
- *Other:* Non-compensatory pause (first PAC)

In a patient with heart disease, signs and symptoms of decreased cardiac output—such as hypotension and syncope—may rarely occur.

How you intervene

Most patients who are asymptomatic don't need treatment. In symptomatic patients, however, treatment may focus on eliminating the cause, such as caffeine, alcohol, and nicotine.

When caring for a patient with PACs, assess him to help determine what's triggering the ectopic beats. Tailor your patient teaching to help the patient correct or avoid the underlying cause. For example, if applicable, the patient should eliminate caffeine, nicotine, alcohol or learn stress reduction techniques to lessen his anxiety.

If the patient has ischemic or valvular heart disease, monitor him for signs and symptoms of heart failure, electrolyte imbalances, and the development of more severe atrial arrhythmias.

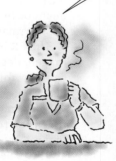

PACs may be caused by too much caffeine or alcohol.

Atrial tachycardia

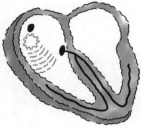

Atrial tachycardia is a supraventricular tachycardia, which means the impulses driving the rapid rhythm originate above the ventricles. Atrial tachycardia has an atrial rate from 150 to 250 beats/min. The rapid rate shortens diastole, resulting in a loss of atrial kick, reduced cardiac output, reduced coronary perfusion, and potentially causing ischemic myocardial changes.

Three types of atrial tachycardia exist: atrial tachycardia with block, multifocal atrial tachycardia (MAT), and paroxysmal atrial tachycardia (PAT).

How it happens

Atrial tachycardia can occur in patients with normal hearts. In those cases, the condition is commonly related to excessive use of caffeine or other stimulants, marijuana use, electrolyte imbalances, hypoxia, and physical or psychological stress. However, this arrhythmia is usually associated with primary or secondary cardiac problems.

Cardiac conditions that can cause atrial tachycardia include MI, cardiomyopathy, congenital anomalies, Wolff–Parkinson–White syndrome, and valvular heart disease. This rhythm may also be a component of sick sinus syndrome. Other problems resulting in atrial tachycardia include cor pulmonale, hyperthyroidism, systemic hypertension, and digoxin toxicity, which is the most common cause of atrial tachycardia. (See *Signs of digoxin toxicity.*)

An ominous sign?

In a healthy person, atrial tachycardia is usually benign. However, this rhythm may be a forerunner of a more serious ventricular arrhythmia, especially if it occurs in a patient with an underlying heart condition.

The increased ventricular rate of atrial tachycardia results in a decrease in the time allowed for the ventricles to fill, an increase in myocardial oxygen consumption, and a decrease in oxygen supply. Angina, heart failure, ischemic myocardial changes, and even MI can occur as a result.

What to look for

Atrial tachycardia is characterized by three or more successive ectopic atrial beats at a rate of 150 to 250 beats/min. If the P wave is visible, it will be a different shape than the sinus P, is usually upright, and is followed by a narrow QRS complex.

Signs of digoxin toxicity

With digoxin toxicity, atrial tachycardia isn't the only change you might see in your patient. Be alert for the following signs and symptoms, especially if the patient is taking digoxin and his potassium level is low or he's also taking amiodarone (Cordarone) (because both combinations can increase the risk of digoxin toxicity):
* *CNS:* fatigue, general muscle weakness, agitation, hallucinations
* *EENT:* yellow-green halos around visual images, blurred vision
* *GI:* anorexia, nausea, vomiting
* *CV:* arrhythmias (most commonly, conduction disturbances with or without atrioventricular block, premature ventricular contractions, and supraventricular arrhythmias), increased severity of heart failure, hypotension (Digoxin's toxic effects on the heart may be life-threatening and always require immediate attention.)

Keep in mind that atrial beats may be conducted on a 1:1 basis to the ventricles (meaning that each P wave has a QRS complex), so atrial and ventricular rates will be equal. In other cases, atrial beats may be conducted only periodically, meaning the AV node blocks conduction of some of the atrial impulses. The AV node stops the ventricles from receiving every impulse and beating at a very high rate.

Think of the AV node as a gatekeeper or doorman. Sometimes it lets atrial impulses through to the ventricles regularly (every impulse or every other impulse, for instance), and sometimes it lets them through irregularly (two impulses might get through, for instance, and then three, and then one).

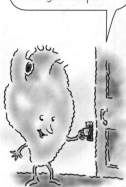

Think of the AV node as a doorman or gatekeeper!

Fast but regular

When assessing a rhythm strip for atrial tachycardia, you'll see that atrial rhythm is regular, and ventricular rhythm is regular when the block is constant and irregular when it isn't. (See *Identifying atrial tachycardia*.) The rate consists of three or more successive ectopic atrial beats at a rate of 150 to 250 beats/min. The ventricular rate varies according to the AV conduction ratio.

The P wave has a 1:1 ratio with the QRS complex unless a block is present. The P wave may not be discernible because of the rapid rate and may be hidden in the previous ST segment or T wave. You may not be able to measure the PR interval if the P wave can't be distinguished from the preceding T wave.

Identifying atrial tachycardia

This rhythm strip illustrates atrial tachycardia. Look for these distinguishing characteristics:

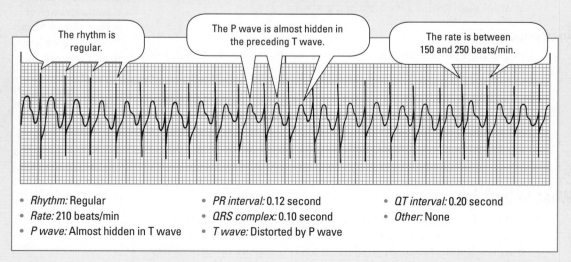

The rhythm is regular.

The P wave is almost hidden in the preceding T wave.

The rate is between 150 and 250 beats/min.

- *Rhythm:* Regular
- *Rate:* 210 beats/min
- *P wave:* Almost hidden in T wave
- *PR interval:* 0.12 second
- *QRS complex:* 0.10 second
- *T wave:* Distorted by P wave
- *QT interval:* 0.20 second
- *Other:* None

The QRS complex is usually normal, unless the impulses are being conducted abnormally through the ventricles. (See *Identifying types of atrial tachycardia.*) The T wave may be normal or inverted if ischemia is present. The QT interval is usually within normal limits but may be shorter because of the rapid rate. ST-segment and T-wave changes may appear if ischemia occurs with a prolonged arrhythmia.

Check out the outward signs

The patient with atrial tachycardia has a rapid apical or peripheral pulse rate. The rhythm may be regular or irregular, depending on the type of atrial tachycardia. A patient with PAT may complain that his heart suddenly starts to beat faster or that he suddenly feels palpitations.

Identifying types of atrial tachycardia

Atrial tachycardia comes in three varieties. Here's a quick rundown of each.

Atrial tachycardia with block

Atrial tachycardia with block is caused by increased automaticity of the atrial tissue. As the atrial rate speeds up and atrioventricular (AV) conduction becomes impaired, a 2:1 block typically occurs. Occasionally a type I (Wenckebach) second-degree AV block may be seen. Look for these distinguishing characteristics:

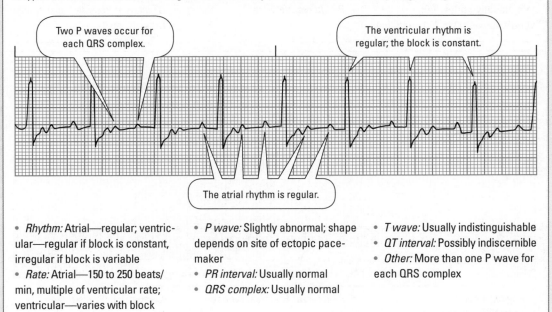

Two P waves occur for each QRS complex.

The ventricular rhythm is regular; the block is constant.

The atrial rhythm is regular.

- *Rhythm:* Atrial—regular; ventricular—regular if block is constant, irregular if block is variable
- *Rate:* Atrial—150 to 250 beats/min, multiple of ventricular rate; ventricular—varies with block
- *P wave:* Slightly abnormal; shape depends on site of ectopic pacemaker
- *PR interval:* Usually normal
- *QRS complex:* Usually normal
- *T wave:* Usually indistinguishable
- *QT interval:* Possibly indiscernible
- *Other:* More than one P wave for each QRS complex

(continued)

Identifying types of atrial tachycardia *(Continued)*

Multifocal atrial tachycardia

In MAT, atrial tachycardia occurs with numerous atrial foci firing intermittently. MAT produces varying P waves on the strip and occurs most commonly in patients with chronic pulmonary disease. The irregular baseline in this strip is caused by movement of the chest wall. Look for these distinguishing characteristics:

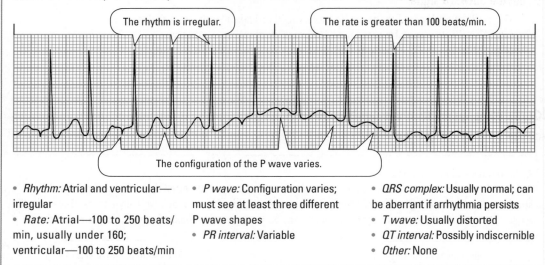

> The rhythm is irregular.

> The rate is greater than 100 beats/min.

> The configuration of the P wave varies.

- *Rhythm:* Atrial and ventricular—irregular
- *Rate:* Atrial—100 to 250 beats/min, usually under 160; ventricular—100 to 250 beats/min
- *P wave:* Configuration varies; must see at least three different P wave shapes
- *PR interval:* Variable
- *QRS complex:* Usually normal; can be aberrant if arrhythmia persists
- *T wave:* Usually distorted
- *QT interval:* Possibly indiscernible
- *Other:* None

Paroxysmal atrial tachycardia

A type of paroxysmal supraventricular tachycardia, PAT features brief periods of tachycardia that alternate with periods of normal sinus rhythm. PAT starts and stops suddenly as a result of rapid firing of an ectopic focus. It commonly follows frequent PACs, one of which initiates the tachycardia. Look for these distinguishing characteristics:

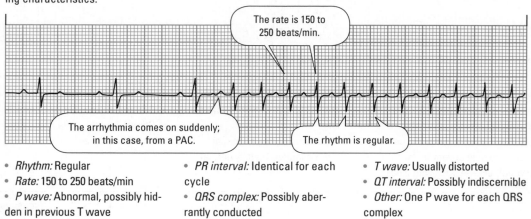

> The rate is 150 to 250 beats/min.

> The arrhythmia comes on suddenly; in this case, from a PAC.

> The rhythm is regular.

- *Rhythm:* Regular
- *Rate:* 150 to 250 beats/min
- *P wave:* Abnormal, possibly hidden in previous T wave
- *PR interval:* Identical for each cycle
- *QRS complex:* Possibly aberrantly conducted
- *T wave:* Usually distorted
- *QT interval:* Possibly indiscernible
- *Other:* One P wave for each QRS complex

Persistent tachycardia and rapid ventricular rate cause decreased cardiac output, which can lead to blurred vision, syncope, and hypotension.

How you intervene

Treatment depends on the type of tachycardia, the width of the QRS complex, and the clinical stability of the patient. Digoxin toxicity is one of the most common causes of atrial tachycardia so assessing the patient for signs and symptoms of toxicity and monitoring serum digoxin levels are important.

Valsalva's maneuver or carotid sinus massage may be used to treat atrial tachycardia. (See *No massage for elderly patients* and *Understanding carotid sinus massage.*) Keep in mind that vagal stimulation can result in bradycardia, ventricular arrhythmias, and asystole. If vagal maneuvers are used, make sure that resuscitative equipment is readily available.

Understanding carotid sinus massage

Carotid sinus massage may be used to diagnose or treat atrial tachycardias. Massaging the carotid sinus stimulates the vagus nerve, which then inhibits firing of the sinoatrial (SA) node and slows atrioventricular node conduction. As the rate slows down the atrial arrhythmia can more easily be identified. Sometimes carotid massage will convert the rhythm back to sinus as the SA node resumes its job as primary pacemaker. Risks of carotid sinus massage include decreased heart rate, vasodilation, ventricular arrhythmias, stroke, and cardiac standstill.

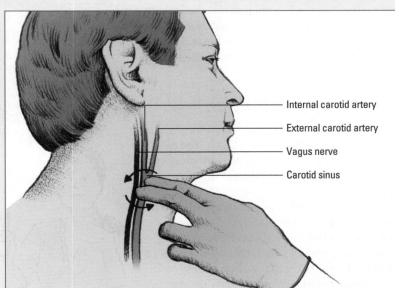

- Internal carotid artery
- External carotid artery
- Vagus nerve
- Carotid sinus

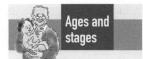

Ages and stages

No massage for elderly patients

Older adults may have undiagnosed carotid atherosclerosis and carotid bruits may be absent, even with significant disease. As a result, you shouldn't perform cardiac sinus massage in late middle-aged and older patients.

Remember, don't perform carotid sinus massage on older patients.

Optimal treatment options

Drug therapy may be used, including adenosine (Adeocard), amiodarone (Cordarone), beta-adrenergic blockers, and calcium channel blockers. When other treatments fail, or if the patient is clinically unstable, synchronized cardioversion may be used.

Atrial overdrive pacing may also be used to stop the arrhythmia. This treatment helps suppress the depolarization of the ectopic pacemaker and permits the SA node to resume its normal role. Radiofrequency ablation or surgical ablation may be needed for patients who continue to have atrial tachycardia in spite of routine treatment.

Monitor the strip

When caring for a patient with atrial tachycardia, carefully monitor his rhythm. Doing so may provide information about the cause of atrial tachycardia, which can facilitate treatment. In addition, monitor the patient for chest pain, indications of decreased cardiac output, and signs and symptoms of heart failure or myocardial ischemia.

Atrial flutter

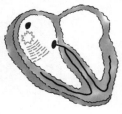

Atrial flutter, a supraventricular tachycardia, is characterized by an atrial rate of 250 to 350 beats/min, although it's generally around 300 beats/min. Originating in a single atrial focus, this rhythm results from re-entry and possibly increased automaticity.

On an ECG, the P waves lose their distinction due to the rapid atrial rate. The waves blend together in a sawtoothed appearance and are called *flutter waves*. These waves are the hallmark of atrial flutter. The distance from one R wave to the next is regular in atrial flutter.

> Atrial flutter is commonly associated with AV nodal block.

How it happens

Atrial flutter is commonly associated with AV nodal block. The AV node prevents the conduction of every impulse to the ventricles. As a result, the ventricular rate is slower than the atrial rate. This protects the ventricles from excessive rates.

Atrial flutter may be caused by conditions that enlarge atrial tissue and elevate atrial pressures. It's commonly found in patients with heart failure, severe mitral valve disease, hyperthyroidism, alcoholism, pericardial disease, and primary myocardial disease. The rhythm is also sometimes encountered in patients after cardiac surgery or in patients with acute MI, chronic obstructive pulmonary disease (COPD), pulmonary embolus, and systemic arterial hypoxia. Atrial flutter rarely occurs in healthy people. When it does, it may indicate intrinsic cardiac disease.

Rating the ratio

The clinical significance of atrial flutter is determined by the number of impulses conducted through the node—expressed as a conduction ratio, for example, 2:1 or 4:1—and the resulting ventricular rate. If the ventricular rate is too slow (fewer than 40 beats/min) or too fast (more than 150 beats/min), cardiac output can be seriously compromised.

Usually the faster the ventricular rate, the more dangerous the arrhythmia. The rapid rate reduces ventricular filling time and coronary perfusion, which can cause angina, heart failure, pulmonary edema, hypotension, and syncope.

What to look for

Atrial flutter is characterized by abnormal P waves that produce a saw-toothed appearance, the hallmark flutter-wave appearance. (See *Identifying atrial flutter.*) Varying degrees of AV block produce ventricular rates one half to one fourth of the atrial rate.

The AV node usually won't accept more than 180 impulses/min and allows every second, third, or fourth impulse to be conducted, the ratio of which determines the ventricular rate.

> Saw-toothed flutter waves are the hallmark of atrial flutter.

Identifying atrial flutter

This rhythm strip illustrates atrial flutter. Look for these distinguishing characteristics:

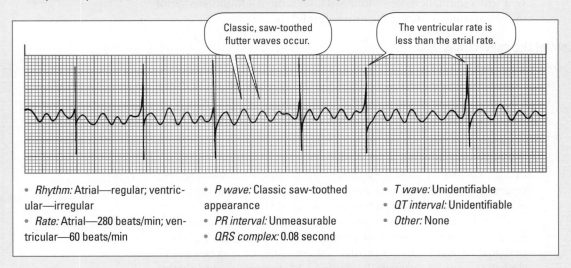

Classic, saw-toothed flutter waves occur.

The ventricular rate is less than the atrial rate.

- *Rhythm:* Atrial—regular; ventricular—irregular
- *Rate:* Atrial—280 beats/min; ventricular—60 beats/min
- *P wave:* Classic saw-toothed appearance
- *PR interval:* Unmeasurable
- *QRS complex:* 0.08 second
- *T wave:* Unidentifiable
- *QT interval:* Unidentifiable
- *Other:* None

The most common ventricular rate is 150 beats/min. With an atrial rate of 300, that rhythm is referred to as a 2:1 block. (See *Atrial flutter and sinus tachycardia.*)

The QRS complex is usually normal but may be widened if flutter waves are buried in the complex. You won't be able to identify a T wave, nor will you be able to measure the QT interval.

The atrial rhythm may vary between fibrillatory waves and flutter waves, an arrhythmia commonly referred to as *atrial fibrillation and flutter.*

Misleading pulses

When caring for a patient with atrial flutter, you may note that their peripheral or apical pulse is normal in rate and rhythm. That's because the pulse reflects the number of ventricular contractions, not the number of atrial impulses.

If the ventricular rate is normal, the patient may be asymptomatic. However, if the ventricular rate is rapid, the patient may exhibit signs and symptoms of reduced cardiac output and cardiac decompensation.

How you intervene

If the patient is hemodynamically unstable, synchronized electrical cardioversion should be administered immediately. Cardioversion delivers electrical current to the heart to correct an arrhythmia. It's synchronized to discharge at the peak of the R wave. Synchronizing the energy current delivery with the R wave ensures that the current won't be delivered on the vulnerable T wave, which could initiate ventricular tachycardia or ventricular fibrillation. Procedural sedation is often administered prior to cardioversion to reduce the discomfort for the patient.

Control and convert operation

The focus of treatment for hemodynamically stable patients includes controlling the rate and converting the rhythm. Specific interventions depend on the patient's cardiac function, whether pre-excitation syndromes are involved, and the duration (less than or greater than 48 hours) of the arrhythmia.

For example, in atrial flutter with normal cardiac function and duration, synchronized cardioversion may be considered; for duration greater than 48 hours, synchronized cardioversion wouldn't be considered because it increases the risk of thromboembolism unless the patient has been adequately anticoagulated.

If synchronized cardioversion is not indicated, to treat atrial flutter medications may be used. Diltiazem (Cardizem), verapamil (Calan), or digoxin can slow the ventricular rate. Amiodarone may be used to slow the rate and to convert the rhythm back to normal sinus rhythm.

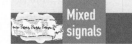

Mixed signals

Atrial flutter and sinus tachycardia

Whenever you see sinus tachycardia with a rate of 150 beats/min, take another look. That rate is a common one for atrial flutter with 2:1 conduction. Look closely for flutter waves, which may be difficult to see if they're hidden in the QRS complex. You may need to check another lead to clearly see them. Another hint is that sometimes if you turn the rhythm strip upside down you may be able to see the flutter waves more easily.

Stay alert

Because atrial flutter may indicate intrinsic cardiac disease, monitor the patient closely for signs and symptoms of low cardiac output. If cardioversion is necessary, prepare the patient for I.V. administration of a sedative or anesthetic as ordered. Keep resuscitative equipment at the bedside. Also be alert for bradycardia because cardioversion can decrease the heart rate.

Atrial fibrillation

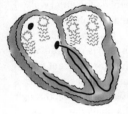

Atrial fibrillation, sometimes called *A-fib*, is defined as chaotic, asynchronous, electrical activity in atrial tissue. It's the most common arrhythmia, affecting an estimated 2.3 million people in the United States. Atrial fibrillation stems from the firing of a number of impulses in multiple re-entry pathways. As with atrial flutter, atrial fibrillation results in a loss of atrial kick. The ectopic impulses may fire at a rate of 400 to 600 times/min, causing the atria to quiver instead of contract.

The ventricles respond only to those impulses that make it through the AV node. On an ECG, atrial activity is no longer represented by P waves but by erratic baseline waves called *fibrillatory waves*, or *f waves*. This rhythm may be either sustained or paroxysmal (occurring in bursts). It can be either preceded by or be the result of PACs.

The irregular conduction of impulses through the AV node produces a characteristic irregularly irregular ventricular response. If you see no P waves and ventricular rhythm that is irregularly irregular, suspect atrial fibrillation.

> Whenever I lose my kick, I jump start it with a little exercise. Loss of atrial kick may require something else!

How it happens

Atrial fibrillation occurs more commonly than atrial flutter or atrial tachycardia. Atrial fibrillation can occur following cardiac surgery, or it can be caused by long-standing hypertension, diabetes, obesity, obstructive sleep apnea, smoking, pulmonary embolism, COPD, electrolyte imbalances, mitral insufficiency, mitral stenosis, hyperthyroidism, infection, coronary artery disease, acute MI, pericarditis, hypoxia, and atrial septal defects.

The rhythm may also occur in a healthy person who uses coffee, alcohol, or nicotine to excess or who's fatigued and under stress. Catecholamine release during exercise may also trigger the arrhythmia.

Where have all the atrial kicks gone?

As with other atrial arrhythmias, atrial fibrillation eliminates atrial kick. That loss, combined with the decreased filling times associated with rapid rates, can lead to clinically significant problems. If the ventricular response is greater than 100 beats/min—a condition called *uncontrolled atrial fibrillation*—the patient may develop heart failure, angina, or syncope.

Patients with pre-existing cardiac disease, such as hypertrophic obstructive cardiomyopathy, mitral stenosis, rheumatic heart disease, and mitral prosthetic valves, tend to tolerate atrial fibrillation poorly and may develop shock and severe heart failure.

Left untreated, atrial fibrillation can lead to cardiovascular collapse, thrombus formation, and systemic arterial or pulmonary embolism. (See *Risk of restoring sinus rhythm.*)

What to look for

Atrial fibrillation is distinguished by the absence of P waves and an irregular ventricular response. When several ectopic sites in the atria fire impulses, depolarization can't spread in an organized manner. (See *Identifying atrial fibrillation.*)

Small sections of the atria are activated individually, which results in the atrial muscle quivering instead of contracting. On an ECG, you'll see uneven baseline and f waves rather than clearly distinguishable P waves.

That fabulous filter

The AV node protects the ventricles from the 400 to 600 erratic atrial impulses that occur each minute by acting as a filter and blocking some of the impulses. The AV node itself doesn't receive all the impulses, however. If muscle tissue around the AV node is in a refractory state, impulses from other areas of the atria can't reach the AV node, which further reduces the number of atrial impulses conducted through to the ventricles.

Those two factors help explain the characteristic wide variation in R-R intervals in atrial fibrillation.

Barely measurable

The atrial rate is indiscernible but is usually greater than 400 impulses/min. It is important to note that with atrial fibrillation atrial response is chaotic without any organized atrial contraction. The ventricular rate usually varies from 100 to 150 beats/min but can be lower or higher. When the ventricular response rate is below 100, atrial fibrillation is considered controlled. When it exceeds 100, the rhythm is considered uncontrolled.

Risk of restoring sinus rhythm

A patient with atrial fibrillation is at increased risk for developing atrial thrombus and systemic arterial embolism. Because the atria don't contract, blood may pool on the atrial wall, and thrombi can form.

If normal sinus rhythm is restored and the atria contract normally, clots can break away and travel through the pulmonary or systemic circulation with potentially disastrous results.

Identifying atrial fibrillation

This rhythm strip illustrates atrial fibrillation. Look for these distinguishing characteristics:

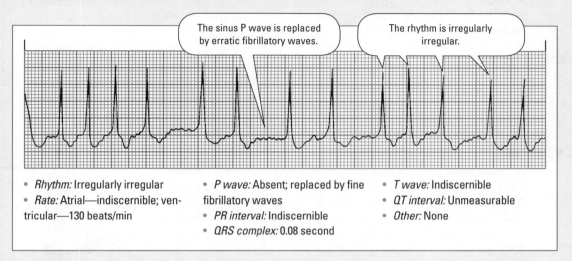

The sinus P wave is replaced by erratic fibrillatory waves.

The rhythm is irregularly irregular.

- *Rhythm:* Irregularly irregular
- *Rate:* Atrial—indiscernible; ventricular—130 beats/min
- *P wave:* Absent; replaced by fine fibrillatory waves
- *PR interval:* Indiscernible
- *QRS complex:* 0.08 second
- *T wave:* Indiscernible
- *QT interval:* Unmeasurable
- *Other:* None

Atrial fibrillation is called *coarse* if the f waves are pronounced and *fine* if they aren't. Atrial fibrillation and flutter may also occur. Look for a configuration that varies between fibrillatory waves and flutter waves.

Pulse differences

When caring for a patient with atrial fibrillation, you may find that the radial pulse rate is slower than the apical rate. That's because, unlike the stronger contractions, the weaker contractions of the heart don't produce a palpable peripheral pulse.

The pulse rhythm will be irregular. If the ventricular rate is rapid, the patient may show signs and symptoms of decreased cardiac output, including hypotension and light-headedness. Their heart may be able to compensate for the decrease if the fibrillation lasts long enough to become chronic. In those cases, however, the patient is at greater-than-normal risk for developing pulmonary, cerebral, or other emboli and may exhibit signs of those conditions.

How you intervene

The major therapeutic goal in treating atrial fibrillation is to reduce the ventricular rate to below 80 beats/min, some patients may tolerate a heart rate as fast as 110 beats/min. The faster rate is OK if the patient doesn't have symptoms of decreased cardiac output. This may be accomplished either by drugs that control the ventricular response or by cardioversion and drugs in combination to convert the rhythm to sinus.

Atrial fibrillation is treated following the same guidelines as atrial flutter.

Timing is everything

Electrical cardioversion is most successful if used within the first 48 hours of treatment and less successful if the rhythm has existed for a long time. If the patient shows signs of more severe angina or of decreased cardiac output, emergency measures are necessary.

Cardioversion

A symptomatic patient needs immediate synchronized cardioversion. The patient should receive appropriate anticoagulation therapy first because cardioversion can cause emboli to be released from the atrial wall, especially in a patient with chronic or paroxysmal atrial fibrillation.

A conversion to normal sinus rhythm will cause forceful atrial contractions to resume abruptly. If a thrombus forms in the atria, the resumption of contractions can result in systemic emboli. (See *How synchronized cardioversion works.*)

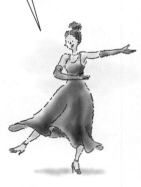

Immediate synchronized cardioversion reestablishes normal sinus rhythm in a symptomatic patient. Rhythm is very important!

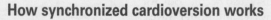

How synchronized cardioversion works

A patient whose arrhythmia causes low cardiac output and hypotension may be a candidate for synchronized cardioversion. This may be an elective or emergency procedure. For instance, it may be used to make a person with atrial fibrillation more comfortable or to save the life of a patient with ventricular tachycardia.

Synchronize the energy
Synchronized cardioversion is similar to defibrillation except that cardioversion generally requires lower energy levels. In synchronized cardioversion, the R wave on the patient's electrocardiogram is synchronized with the cardioverter (defibrillator). After the firing buttons have been pressed, the defibrillator discharges energy when it senses the next R wave.

When the stimulus hits
To stop atrial depolarization and re-establish normal sinus rhythm, electrical stimulation must occur during the R wave. Stimulation that hits a T wave increases the risk of fatal arrhythmias. Keep in mind that there's a slight delay between the time the firing button is pressed and the moment the energy is actually discharged. Call, "All clear," and observe that no one is touching the patient until the energy is actually discharged.

Digoxin toxicity warning
Be aware that synchronized cardioversion carries the risk of lethal arrhythmias when used in patients with digoxin toxicity.

Re-establishing its role

Drugs such as metoprolol (Lopressor), atenolol (Tenormin), esmolol (Brevibloc), propranolol (Inderal), diltiazem (Cardizem), verapamil (Calan), and amiodarone (Cordarone), can be given after successful cardioversion to maintain normal sinus rhythm and to control the ventricular rate in chronic atrial fibrillation. Some of these drugs prolong the atrial refractory period, giving the SA node an opportunity to re-establish its role as the heart's pacemaker, whereas others primarily slow AV node conduction, controlling the ventricular rate. Symptomatic atrial fibrillation that doesn't respond to routine treatment may be treated with radiofrequency ablation therapy or surgical removal of the area in the left atrium causing atrial fibrillation.

When assessing a patient with atrial fibrillation, assess both the peripheral and apical pulses. If the patient isn't on a cardiac monitor, be alert for an irregular pulse and differences in the apical and radial pulse rates.

Assess for symptoms of decreased cardiac output and heart failure. If drug therapy is used, monitor serum drug levels and observe the patient for evidence of toxicity. Tell the patient to report pulse rate changes, syncope or dizziness, chest pain, or signs of heart failure, such as increasing dyspnea and peripheral edema.

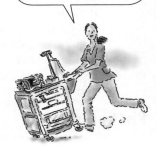

Meds to the rescue! Drugs can help maintain normal sinus rhythm after cardioversion.

Wandering pacemaker

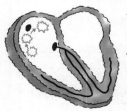

A wandering pacemaker is an irregular rhythm that results when the heart's pacemaker changes its focus from the SA node to another area above the ventricles. The origin of the impulse may wander beat to beat from the SA node to other atrial sites or to the AV junction. The P wave and PR interval vary from beat to beat as the pacemaker site changes.

How it happens

Wandering pacemaker may be caused by:
- increased vagal tone
- digoxin toxicity
- organic heart disease such as rheumatic carditis.

The arrhythmia may be normal in young patients and is common in athletes who have slow heart rates. It may be difficult to identify because the arrhythmia is commonly transient. Although wandering pacemaker is rarely serious, chronic arrhythmias are a sign of heart disease and should be monitored.

What to look for

The rhythm on an ECG strip will look slightly irregular because sites of impulse initiation vary. The rate is usually normal—60 to 100 beats/min—but it may be slower. The P waves are different shapes as the pacemaker site changes. There will be at least three differently shaped P waves.

Impulses may originate in the SA node, atria, or AV junction. If an impulse originates in the AV junction, the P wave may come before, during, or after the QRS complex. The PR interval will also vary from beat to beat as the pacemaker site changes, but it will always be less than 0.20 second.

Mind the PRs and QRSs

The variation in PR interval will cause a slightly irregular R-R interval. If the impulse originates in the AV junction, the PR interval will be less than 0.12 second. Ventricular depolarization is normal, so the QRS complex will be less than 0.12 second. The T wave and QT interval will usually be normal, although the QT interval can vary. (See *Identifying wandering pacemaker.*)

Patients are generally asymptomatic and unaware of the arrhythmia. The pulse rate and rhythm may be normal or irregular.

Identifying wandering pacemaker

This rhythm strip illustrates wandering pacemaker. Look for these distinguishing characteristics:

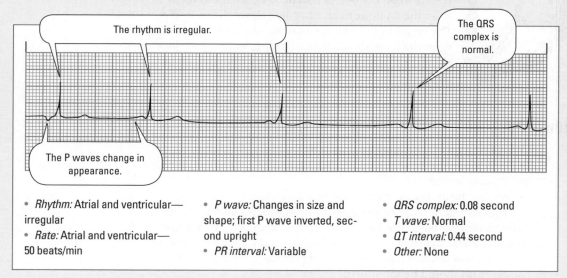

- *Rhythm:* Atrial and ventricular— irregular
- *Rate:* Atrial and ventricular— 50 beats/min
- *P wave:* Changes in size and shape; first P wave inverted, second upright
- *PR interval:* Variable
- *QRS complex:* 0.08 second
- *T wave:* Normal
- *QT interval:* 0.44 second
- *Other:* None

How you intervene

Usually, no treatment is needed. If the patient is symptomatic, however, the underlying cause should be treated.

You'll need to monitor the patient's heart rhythm and assess for signs of decreased cardiac output. Also assess blood pressure, mental status, and skin color.

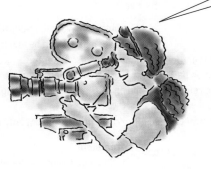

Usually, no treatment is needed for a wandering pacemaker, but monitor my rhythm and keep a close eye on the patient.

That's a wrap!

Atrial arrhythmias review

PACs

Characteristics
- *Rhythms:* Irregular as a result of PACs
- *P wave:* Premature with an abnormal configuration; may be buried in the previous T wave
- *PR interval:* Usually normal; may be slightly shortened or prolonged
- *QRS complex:* Similar to the underlying QRS complex when PAC is conducted; may not follow the premature P wave when a nonconducted PAC occurs

Treatment
- No treatment if asymptomatic
- Correction of the underlying cause

Atrial tachycardia

Characteristics
- *Rhythms:* Atrial—regular, irregular in MAT; ventricular—regular when the block is constant and irregular when it isn't
- *Rates:* Atrial—three or more successive ectopic atrial beats at a rate of 150 to 250 beats/min; ventricular—varies

- *P wave:* A 1:1 ratio with QRS complex (unless a block is present); may not be discernible; may be hidden in previous ST segment or T wave; in MAT, at least three different P waves seen
- *PR interval:* Sometimes not measurable; varies in MAT
- *QRS complex:* Usually normal
- *T wave:* Normal or inverted
- *QT interval:* Usually within normal limits; may be shorter
- *ST-segment and T-wave changes:* Sometimes with ischemia

Treatment
- Correction of underlying cause
- Monitoring of blood digoxin levels for toxicity
- Valsalva's maneuver or carotid sinus massage
- Calcium channel blocker, beta-adrenergic blocker, or digoxin; synchronized cardioversion
- Atrial overdrive pacing to stop arrhythmia

(continued)

Atrial arrhythmias review *(Continued)*

Atrial flutter
Characteristics
- *Rhythms:* Atrial—regular; ventricular—depends on the AV conduction pattern
- *Rates:* Atrial—250 to 350; ventricular—less than atrial
- *P waves:* Abnormal with saw-toothed appearance
- *QRS complex:* Usually normal; may be widened if flutter waves are buried in complex
- *T wave:* Unidentifiable
- *QT interval:* Unmeasurable

Treatment
- Anticoagulation therapy before converting rhythm if flutter is present for more than 48 hours
- Diltiazem, verapamil or digoxin, or amiodarone to control rate if heart function is impaired; synchronized cardioversion or amiodarone to convert rhythm if less than 48 hours

Atrial fibrillation
Characteristics
- *Rhythms:* Irregularly irregular
- *Rates:* Atrial—greater than 400 impulses/min, unable to measure; ventricular—varies from 100 to 150 beats/min but can be lower or higher
- *P waves:* Absent
- *f waves:* Seen as uneven baseline on ECG rather than distinguishable P waves
- *R-R intervals:* Irregularly irregular

Treatment
- Same guidelines as for atrial flutter

Wandering pacemaker
Characteristics
- *Rhythms:* Irregular
- *Rates:* Usually normal or below 60 beats/min
- *P wave:* At least three P waves of different size and shape
- *PR interval:* Varies; always less than 0.20 second
- *QRS complex:* Usually normal; less than 0.12 second
- *QT interval:* Sometimes varies

Treatment
- No treatment if asymptomatic
- Correction of the underlying cause

Quick quiz

1. The hallmark of a PAC is:
   A. regular atrial rhythm.
   B. premature, abnormally shaped P wave.
   C. P wave followed by an aberrantly conducted QRS complex.
   D. regular ventricular rhythm.

   Answer: B. Because PACs originate outside the SA node, the P wave comes earlier in the cycle and has a different configuration than the sinus P wave.

2. In atrial flutter, the key consideration in determining treatment is the:
   A. atrial rate.
   B. ventricular rate.
   C. configuration of the flutter waves.
   D. QT interval.

Answer: B. If the ventricular rate is too fast or too slow, cardiac output will be compromised. A rapid ventricular rate may require immediate cardioversion.

3. In controlled atrial fibrillation, the ventricular response rate is:
   A. less than 60 beats/min.
   B. less than or equal to 80 beats/min.
   C. greater than 100 beats/min.
   D. greater than 120 beats/min.

Answer: B. Atrial fibrillation with a ventricular response rate less than or equal to 80 is considered controlled and usually requires no treatment. A rate greater than 110 is considered uncontrolled and may cause symptoms and require cardioversion or other treatment.

4. Carotid sinus massage is used to:
   A. prevent the continued development of PACs.
   B. increase the ventricular rate in AV block.
   C. convert atrial tachycardia to sinus rhythm.
   D. suppress the development of flutter waves.

Answer: C. Carotid sinus massage slows the atrial rate by inhibiting firing of the SA node and slowing AV conduction. This allows the SA node to re-establish itself as the primary pacemaker. In atrial flutter, the technique may increase the block and slow the ventricular rate but won't convert the rhythm.

5. For atrial fibrillation, electrical cardioversion is most successful if used:
   A. during the first 48 hours after the onset of the arrhythmia.
   B. during the first 2 weeks of treatment for the arrhythmia.
   C. during the first 4 months after the onset of the arrhythmia.
   D. anytime during the first year after the onset of the arrhythmia.

Answer: A. Electrical cardioversion is most successful if used within the first 48 hours of treatment and less successful if the rhythm has existed for a long time.

6. In a patient with wandering pacemaker, the ECG strip will show:
   A. an early beat causing irregularity.
   B. a regular rhythm of 40 beats/min.
   C. slight irregularity because sites of impulse initiation vary.
   D. a regular rhythm and a rate of 60 to 100 beats/min.

Answer: C. Wandering pacemaker is an irregular rhythm that results when the heart's pacemaker changes its focus from the SA node to another area above the ventricles. So, the rhythm on the ECG strip will look slightly irregular due to the variation of the impulse sites.

Test strips

Try these test strips. Interpret each strip using the 8-step method and fill in the blanks below with the particular characteristics of the strip. Then compare your answers with the answers given.

Strip 1

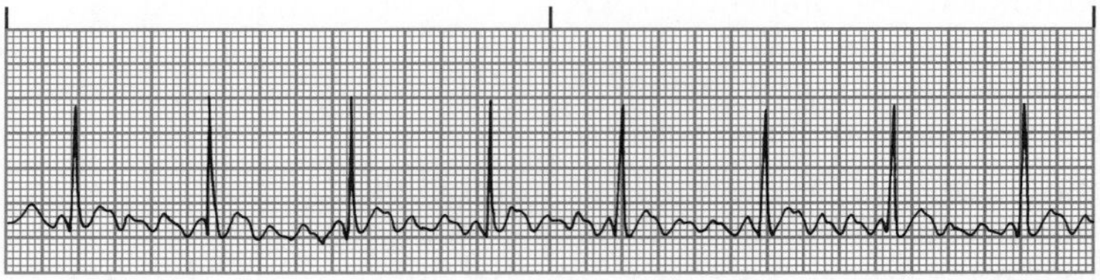

Atrial rhythm: _____

Ventricular rhythm: _____

Atrial rate: _____

Ventricular rate: _____

P wave: _____

PR interval: _____

QRS complex: _____

T wave: _____

QT interval: _____

Other: _____

Interpretation: _____

Strip 2

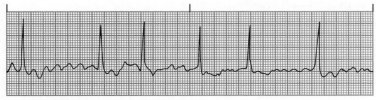

Atrial rhythm: _____

Ventricular rhythm: _____

Atrial rate: _____

Ventricular rate: _____

P wave: _____

PR interval: _____

QRS complex: _____

T wave: _____

QT interval: _____

Other: _____

Interpretation: _____

Strip 3

Atrial rhythm: _____

Ventricular rhythm: _____

Atrial rate: _____

Ventricular rate: _____

P wave: _____

PR interval: _____

QRS complex: _____

T wave: _____

QT interval: _____

Other: _____

Interpretation: _____

Answers to test strips

1. Rhythm: Regular
   Rate: Atrial—310 beats/min; ventricular—80 beats/min
   P wave: Saw-toothed
   PR interval: Unmeasurable
   QRS complex: 0.08 second
   T wave: Normal configuration
   QT interval: 0.36 second
   Other: None
   Interpretation: Atrial flutter

2. Rhythm: Irregular
   Rate: Atrial and ventricular—80 beats/min
   P wave: Normal configuration, early P's look different than the sinus P's
   PR interval: 0.14 second
   QRS complex: 0.08 second
   T wave: Normal configuration
   QT interval: 0.36 second
   Other: every other beat is a PAC
   Interpretation: Normal sinus rhythm with bigeminal PACs

3. Rhythm: Irregular
   Rate: Atrial—undetermined; ventricular—60 beats/min
   P wave: Absent; coarse fibrillatory waves present
   PR interval: Indiscernible
   QRS complex: 0.12 second
   T wave: Indiscernible
   QT interval: Unmeasurable
   Other: None
   Interpretation: Atrial fibrillation

Scoring

☆☆☆ If you answered all six questions correctly and filled in all the blanks close to what we did, outstanding! You're the MVP of the Atrial World Series.

☆☆ If you answered five questions correctly and filled in most of the blanks, terrific! You're an up-and-coming power hitter, destined for the Atrial Hall of Fame.

☆ If you answered fewer than five questions correctly and missed most of the blanks, hang in there. With a bit of batting practice, you'll be smacking home runs outta Atrial Park in no time.

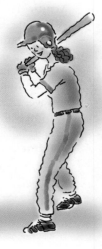

Recommended references

Beinart, S. C. (2014). Junctional rhythm treatment and management. Retrieved from http://emedicine.medscape.com/article/155146

Brown, D. F. M., & Borczuk, P. (2014). Emergent management of atrial flutter. Retrieved from http://emedicine.medscape.com/article/151066-overview

Brown, D. F. M., & Martindale, J. L. (2012). *Rapid interpretation of ECG's in emergency medicine.* Philadelphia, PA: Wolters Kluwer.

Budzikowski, A. S., & Rottman, J. (2014). Atrial tachycardia Ppractice Eessentials. Retrieved from http://emedicine.medscape.com/article/151456-overview

García-Niebla, J. (2009). Comparison of P-wave patterns derived from correct and incorrect placement of V1-V2 electrodes. *Journal of Cardiovascular Nursing, 24*(2), 156–161.

January, C. T., Wann, L. S., Alpert, J. S., Calkins, H., Cleveland, J. C., Jr., Cigarroa J. E., … Yancy, C. W. (2014). 2014 AHA/ACC/HRS Guideline for the management of patients with atrial fibrillation: Executive summary: A report of the American College of Cardiology/American Heart Association Task Force on practice guidelines and the heart rhythm society. *Journal of the American College of Cardiology, 64*(21), 2246–2280.

Katritsis, D. G., Gersch, B. J., & Camm, A. J. (2013). *Clinical cardiology: Current practice guidelines.* Oxford, United Kingdom: Oxford University Press.

Nainggolan, L. (2012). Multispecialty: Risk factors identified for premature atrial contractions. Retrieved from http://emedicine.medscape.com/viewarticle/755891_2

Neumar, R. W., Otto, C. W., Link, M. S., Kronick, S. L., Shuster, M., Callaway, C. W., … Morrison, L. J. (2010). American heart association guidelines for cardiovascular resuscitation and emergency cardiovascular care science, Part 8.4: Management of symptomatic bradycardia and tachycardia. *Circulation, 122,* S746–S757.

Chapter 6

Junctional arrhythmias

Just the facts

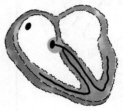

In this chapter, you'll learn:

◆ the proper way to identify various junctional arrhythmias

◆ the causes, significance, treatment, and nursing implications of each arrhythmia

◆ assessment findings associated with each arrhythmia

◆ interpretation of junctional arrhythmias on an ECG.

A look at junctional arrhythmias

Junctional arrhythmias originate in the atrioventricular (AV) junction—the area around the AV node and the bundle of His. The arrhythmias occur when the sinoatrial (SA) node, a higher pacemaker, is suppressed and fails to conduct impulses or when a block occurs in conduction. Electrical impulses may then be initiated by pacemaker cells in the AV junction.

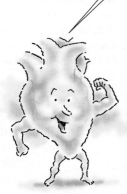

Normal impulses keep the blood pumping.

Just your normal impulse

In normal impulse conduction, the AV node slows transmission of the impulse from the atria to the ventricles, which gives the atria time to contract and pump as much blood as they can into the ventricles before the ventricles contract. However, impulses aren't always conducted normally. (See *Conduction in Wolff–Parkinson–White syndrome*, page 124.)

Which way did the impulse go?

Because the AV junction is located in the lower part of the right atrium near the tricuspid valve, impulses generated in this area cause the heart to be depolarized in an abnormal way. The impulse moves upward and causes backward, or *retrograde*, depolarization of the atria. P waves

Now I get it!

Conduction in Wolff–Parkinson–White syndrome

Conduction doesn't always take place in a normal way. In Wolff–Parkinson–White syndrome, for example, an extra conduction pathway develops outside the atrioventricular (AV) junction and connects the atria with the ventricles, as shown. Wolff–Parkinson–White syndrome is typically a congenital rhythm disorder that occurs mainly in young children and adults of ages 20 to 35.

Rapidly conducted

The bypass formed in Wolff–Parkinson–White syndrome, known as the *bundle of Kent,* conducts impulses to the atria or the ventricles. Impulses aren't delayed at the AV node, so conduction is abnormally fast. Retrograde conduction, circus re-entry, and re-entrant tachycardia can result.

Checking the ECG

This syndrome causes a shortened PR interval (less than 0.10 second) and a widened QRS complex (greater than 0.10 second). The beginning of the QRS complex may look slurred because of altered ventricular depolarization. This hallmark sign of Wolff–Parkinson–White syndrome is called a *delta wave,* shown in the inset.

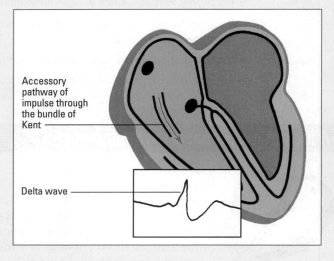

Accessory pathway of impulse through the bundle of Kent

Delta wave

When to treat

This syndrome must be treated if tachyarrhythmias, such as atrial fibrillation and atrial flutter, occur. First, electrophysiology studies are done to determine the location of the conduction pathway and evaluate specific treatments. Radiofrequency ablation may be used with tachyarrhythmias that are resistant to medications such as adenosine or amiodarone.

might not be seen, but if they are, look for them to be inverted in leads II, III, and aV$_F$, leads in which you would normally see upright P waves. (See *Finding the P wave.*)

The impulse also moves down toward the ventricles, causing forward, or antegrade, depolarization of the ventricles and an upright QRS complex. Since this is the normal conduction pathway to, and through, the ventricles, the QRS complex has a normal configuration and duration and the T wave and QT interval are usually normal.

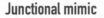 Mixed signals

Finding the P wave

When the pacemaker fires in the atrioventricular junction, the impulse may reach either the atria or the ventricles first. Therefore, the inverted P wave and the following QRS complex won't have a consistent relationship. These rhythm strips show the various positions the P wave can take in junctional rhythms.

Atria first
If the atria are depolarized first, the P wave will occur before the QRS complex.

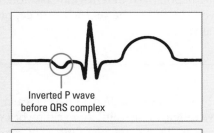

Inverted P wave
before QRS complex

Ventricles first
If the ventricles are depolarized first, the QRS complex will come before the P wave.

Inverted P wave
before QRS complex

Simultaneous
If the ventricles and atria are depolarized simultaneously, the P wave will be hidden in the QRS complex.

Inverted P wave hidden
in QRS complex

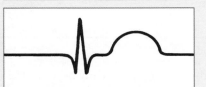

Don't mistake an atrial arrhythmia for a junctional arrhythmia. Check the PR interval.

Junctional mimic

Atrial arrhythmias are sometimes mistaken for junctional arrhythmias because impulses are generated so low in the atria that they cause retrograde depolarization and inverted P waves. Looking at the PR interval will help you determine whether an arrhythmia is atrial or junctional.

An arrhythmia with an inverted P wave before the QRS complex and a normal PR interval (0.12 to 0.20 second) originated in the atria. An arrhythmia with a PR interval less than 0.12 second originated in the AV junction.

Premature junctional contraction

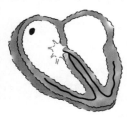

A premature junctional contraction (PJC) is a beat that occurs before a normal beat and causes an irregular rhythm. This ectopic beat occurs when an irritable location within the AV junction acts as a pacemaker and fires either prematurely or out of sequence.

As with all beats produced by the AV junction, the atria are depolarized in retrograde fashion, causing an inverted P wave. The ventricles are depolarized normally.

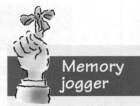

Memory jogger

To help you remember what a PJC is, think of "beat before" for premature, "normal beat" for junctional, and "causing irregular rhythm" for contraction.

How it happens

PJCs may be caused by toxic levels of digoxin (level greater than 2.5 mg/mL), excessive caffeine intake, inferior wall myocardial infarction (MI), rheumatic heart disease, valvular disease, hypoxia, heart failure, swelling of the AV junction after heart surgery, or other causes of inflammation or ischemia.

The beat goes on

Although PJCs themselves usually aren't dangerous, you'll need to monitor the patient carefully and assess him for other signs of intrinsic pacemaker failure.

What to look for

A PJC appears on a rhythm strip as an early beat causing an irregularity. The rest of the strip may show regular atrial and ventricular rhythms, depending on the patient's underlying rhythm.

P wave inversion

Look for an inverted P wave in leads II, III, and aV$_F$. Depending on when the impulse occurs, the P wave may fall before, during, or after the QRS complex. (See *Identifying a PJC.*) If it falls during the QRS complex, it's hidden. If it comes before the QRS complex, the PR interval is less than 0.12 second.

Because the ventricles are usually depolarized normally, the QRS complex has a normal configuration and a normal duration of less than 0.12 second. The T wave and the QT interval are usually normal.

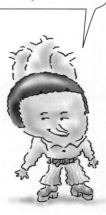

There's an early beat on the wave form with a PJC. I prefer it when the beat goes on... the beat goes on...

Identifying a PJC

This rhythm strip illustrates PJC. Look for these distinguishing characteristics:

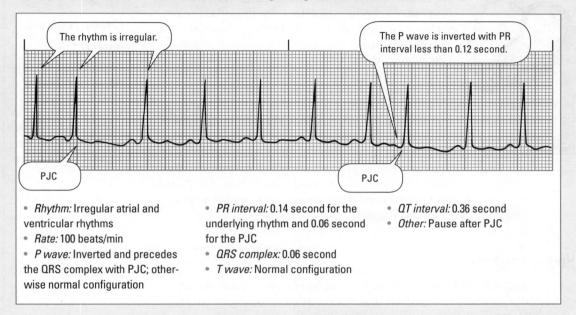

The rhythm is irregular.

The P wave is inverted with PR interval less than 0.12 second.

PJC

PJC

- *Rhythm:* Irregular atrial and ventricular rhythms
- *Rate:* 100 beats/min
- *P wave:* Inverted and precedes the QRS complex with PJC; otherwise normal configuration

- *PR interval:* 0.14 second for the underlying rhythm and 0.06 second for the PJC
- *QRS complex:* 0.06 second
- *T wave:* Normal configuration

- *QT interval:* 0.36 second
- *Other:* Pause after PJC

That quickening feeling

The patient may be asymptomatic or he may complain of palpitations or a feeling of quickening in the chest. You may be able to palpate an irregular pulse. If the PJCs are frequent enough, the patient may have hypotension from a transient decrease in cardiac output.

How you intervene

PJCs usually don't require treatment unless symptoms occur. In those cases, the underlying cause should be treated. If digoxin toxicity is the culprit, the medication should be discontinued and serum digoxin (Lanoxin) levels monitored.

You should also monitor the patient for hemodynamic instability. If ectopic beats are frequent, the patient should decrease or eliminate his caffeine intake.

Junctional escape rhythm

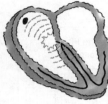

A junctional escape rhythm is a string of beats that occurs after a conduction delay from the atria. The normal intrinsic firing rate for cells in the AV junction is 40 to 60 beats/min.

Remember that the AV junction can take over as the heart's pacemaker if higher pacemaker sites slow down or fail to fire or conduct. The junctional escape beat is an example of this compensatory mechanism. Because junctional escape beats prevent ventricular standstill, they should never be suppressed.

Backward and upside down

In a junctional escape rhythm, as in all junctional arrhythmias, the atria are depolarized by means of retrograde conduction. The P waves are inverted, and impulse conduction through the ventricles is normal. (See *Check age and lifestyle.*)

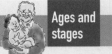

Ages and stages

Check age and lifestyle

Junctional escape beats may occur in healthy children during sleep. They may also occur in healthy athletic adults. In these situations, no treatment is necessary.

How it happens

A junctional escape rhythm can be caused by any condition that disturbs SA node function or enhances AV junction automaticity. Common causes of the arrhythmia include:
- sick sinus syndrome
- vagal stimulation
- electrolyte imbalances
- digoxin toxicity
- inferior wall MI
- rheumatic heart disease.

The great escape

Whether junctional escape rhythm harms the patient depends on how well the patient's heart tolerates a decreased heart rate and decreased cardiac output. The less tolerant the heart is, the more significant the effects of the arrhythmia.

What to look for

A junctional escape rhythm shows a regular rhythm of 40 to 60 beats/min on an ECG strip. Look for inverted P waves in leads II, III, and aV$_F$.

The P waves occur before, after, or hidden within the QRS complex. The PR interval is less than 0.12 second and is measurable only if the P wave comes before the QRS complex. (See *Identifying junctional escape rhythm.*)

Just as junctional escape beats should never be suppressed, neither should escapes to the beach!

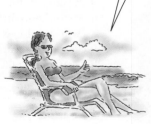

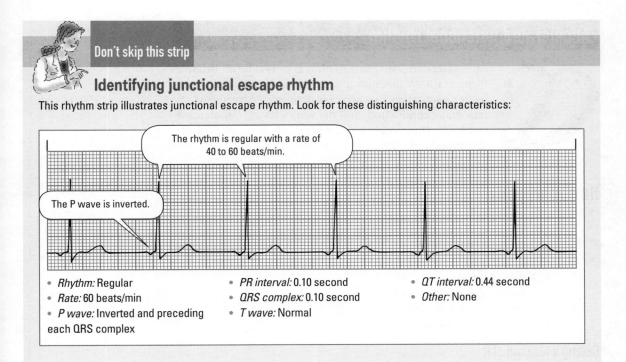

Don't skip this strip

Identifying junctional escape rhythm

This rhythm strip illustrates junctional escape rhythm. Look for these distinguishing characteristics:

The rhythm is regular with a rate of 40 to 60 beats/min.

The P wave is inverted.

- *Rhythm:* Regular
- *Rate:* 60 beats/min
- *P wave:* Inverted and preceding each QRS complex

- *PR interval:* 0.10 second
- *QRS complex:* 0.10 second
- *T wave:* Normal

- *QT interval:* 0.44 second
- *Other:* None

The rest of the ECG waveform—including the QRS complex, T wave, and QT interval—should appear normal because impulses through the ventricles are usually conducted normally.

It may be slow, but at least it's regular

A patient with a junctional escape rhythm has a slow, regular pulse rate of 40 to 60 beats/min. The patient may be asymptomatic. However, pulse rates less than 60 beats/min may lead to inadequate cardiac output, causing hypotension, syncope, or decreased urine output.

How you intervene

Treatment for a junctional escape rhythm involves correcting the underlying cause; for example, digoxin may be withheld. Atropine may be given to stimulate the sympathetic nervous system and increase the heart rate, or a temporary or permanent pacemaker may be inserted if the patient remains symptomatic.

Nursing care includes monitoring the patient's serum digoxin and electrolyte levels and watching for signs of decreased cardiac output, such as hypotension, syncope, or decreased urine output. If the patient is hypotensive, lower the head of his bed as far as he can tolerate it and keep atropine at the bedside. Discontinue digoxin if indicated.

Accelerated junctional rhythm

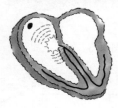

An accelerated junctional rhythm is caused by an irritable focus in the AV junction that speeds up to take over as the heart's pacemaker. The atria are depolarized by means of retrograde conduction, and the ventricles are depolarized normally. The accelerated rate is usually between 60 and 100 beats/min.

How it happens

Conditions that affect SA node or AV node automaticity can cause accelerated junctional rhythm. These conditions include:

- digoxin toxicity
- hypokalemia
- hypercalcemia
- inferior or posterior wall MI
- rheumatic heart disease
- valvular heart disease.

Getting a kick out of it

This arrhythmia is significant if the patient has symptoms of decreased cardiac output—hypotension, syncope, and decreased

Identifying accelerated junctional rhythm

This rhythm strip illustrates accelerated junctional rhythm. Look for these distinguishing characteristics:

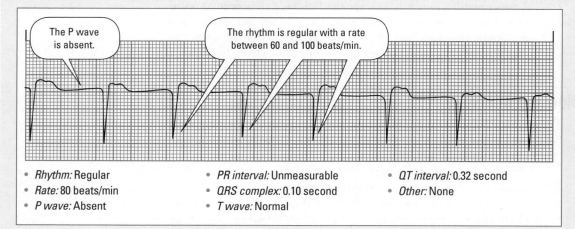

The P wave is absent.

The rhythm is regular with a rate between 60 and 100 beats/min.

- *Rhythm:* Regular
- *Rate:* 80 beats/min
- *P wave:* Absent
- *PR interval:* Unmeasurable
- *QRS complex:* 0.10 second
- *T wave:* Normal
- *QT interval:* 0.32 second
- *Other:* None

urine output. These can occur if the atria are depolarized after the QRS complex, which prevents blood ejection from the atria into the ventricles, or atrial kick.

What to look for

With an accelerated junctional rhythm, look for a regular rhythm and a rate of 60 to 100 beats/min. (See *Identifying accelerated junctional rhythm.*) If the P wave is present, it will be inverted in leads II, III, and aV_F and will occur before or after the QRS complex or be hidden in it. If the P wave comes before the QRS complex, the PR interval will be less than 0.12 second. The QRS complex, T wave, and QT interval all appear normal. (See *Escape rate higher in young children.*)

Low-down, dizzy, and confused

The patient may be asymptomatic because accelerated junctional rhythm has the same rate as sinus rhythm. However, the atria may not be able to fill completely before contracting or not be able to empty sufficiently into the ventricles, lowering the cardiac output. The patient may become dizzy, hypotensive, and confused and have weak peripheral pulses.

How you intervene

Treatment for accelerated junctional arrhythmia involves correcting the underlying cause. Nursing interventions include observing the patient to see how well he tolerates this arrhythmia, monitoring his serum digoxin level, and withholding his digoxin dose as ordered.

You should also assess potassium and other electrolyte levels and administer supplements as ordered; monitor vital signs for hemodynamic instability; and observe for signs of decreased cardiac output. Temporary pacing may be necessary if the patient is symptomatic.

Junctional tachycardia

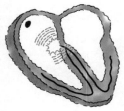

In junctional tachycardia, three or more PJCs occur in a row. This supraventricular tachycardia occurs when an irritable focus from the AV junction has enhanced automaticity, overriding the SA node to function as the heart's pacemaker.

In this arrhythmia, the atria are depolarized by means of retrograde conduction, and conduction through the ventricles is normal. The rate is usually 100 to 200 beats/min. (See *Identifying junctional tachycardia,* page 132.)

Escape rate higher in young children

Up to age 3, the atrioventricular nodal escape rhythm is 50 to 80 beats/min. Consequently, a junctional rhythm is considered accelerated in infants and toddlers only when greater than 80 beats/min.

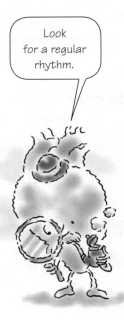

Look for a regular rhythm.

Identifying junctional tachycardia

This rhythm strip illustrates junctional tachycardia. Look for these distinguishing characteristics:

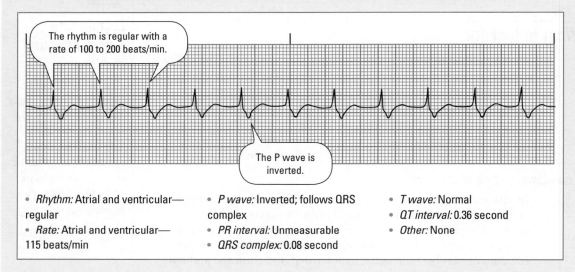

- *Rhythm:* Atrial and ventricular—regular
- *Rate:* Atrial and ventricular—115 beats/min
- *P wave:* Inverted; follows QRS complex
- *PR interval:* Unmeasurable
- *QRS complex:* 0.08 second
- *T wave:* Normal
- *QT interval:* 0.36 second
- *Other:* None

How it happens

Possible causes of junctional tachycardia include:
- digoxin toxicity (most common cause), which can be enhanced by hypokalemia
- inferior or posterior wall MI or ischemia
- congenital heart disease in children
- swelling of the AV junction after heart surgery.

Compromisin' rhythm

The significance of junctional tachycardia depends on the rate, underlying cause, and severity of the accompanying cardiac disease. At higher ventricular rates, junctional tachycardia may compromise cardiac output by decreasing the amount of blood filling the ventricles with each beat. Higher rates also result in the loss of atrial kick.

What to look for

When assessing a rhythm strip for junctional tachycardia, look for a rate of 100 to 200 beats/min. The P wave is inverted in leads II, III, and aV$_F$ and can occur before, during (hidden P wave), or after the QRS complex.

Measurement of the PR interval depends on whether the P wave falls before, in, or after the QRS complex. If it comes before the QRS complex, the only time the PR interval can be measured, it will always be less than 0.12 second.

The QRS complexes look normal, as does the T wave, unless a P wave occurs in it or the rate is so fast that the T wave can't be detected. (See *Junctional and supraventricular tachycardia.*)

Rapid rate = instability

Patients with rapid heart rates may have decreased cardiac output and hemodynamic instability. The pulse will be rapid, and dizziness, low blood pressure, and other signs of decreased cardiac output may be present.

How you intervene

The underlying cause should be treated. If the cause is digoxin toxicity, the digoxin should be discontinued. Vagal maneuvers and medications such as I.V. adenosine may slow the heart rate for the symptomatic patient. Oral diltiazem may also be used along with a beta-blocker. (See *Comparing junctional rates.*)

If the patient recently had an MI or heart surgery, he may need a temporary pacemaker to reset the heart's rhythm. A child with a permanent arrhythmia may be resistant to drug therapy and require surgery. The patient with recurrent junctional tachycardia may be

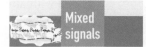

Junctional and supraventricular tachycardia

If a tachycardia has a narrow QRS complex, you may have trouble deciding whether its source is junctional or atrial. When the rate approaches 150 beats/min, a formerly visible P wave is hidden in the previous T wave, so you won't be able to use the P wave to determine where the rhythm originated.

In these cases, call the rhythm *supraventricular* tachycardia, a general term that refers to the origin as being above the ventricles. Examples of supraventricular tachycardia include atrial flutter, multifocal atrial tachycardia, and junctional tachycardia.

Comparing junctional rates

The names given to junctional rhythms vary according to rate. The illustration below shows how each rhythm's name and rate are correlated.

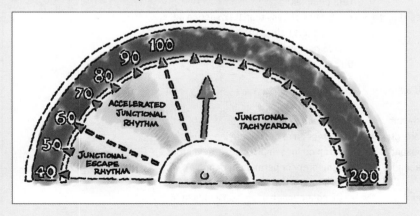

treated with ablation therapy, followed by permanent pacemaker insertion.

Monitor patients with junctional tachycardia for signs of decreased cardiac output. You should also check serum digoxin and potassium levels and administer potassium supplements, as ordered. If symptoms are severe and digoxin is the culprit, the practitioner may order digoxin immune fab, a digoxin-binding drug.

That's a wrap!

Junctional arrhythmias review

Overview of junctional arrhythmias
- Originate in the AV junction
- Occur when the SA node is suppressed or conduction is blocked
- Impulses cause retrograde atrial depolarization and inverted P waves in leads II, III, and aV$_F$

Wolff–Parkinson–White syndrome
Characteristics
- *PR interval:* Less than 0.10 second
- *QRS complex:* Greater than 0.10 second; beginning of complex may have slurred appearance (delta wave)

Treatment
- No treatment if asymptomatic
- Treatment of tachyarrhythmias as indicated
- Radiofrequency ablation if resistant to other treatments

PJC
Characteristics
- *Rhythms:* Irregular with PJC appearance
- *Rates:* Vary with underlying rhythm
- *P wave:* Inverted; occurs before, during, or after QRS complex; may be absent
- *PR interval:* Less than 0.12 second or unmeasurable
- *QRS complex:* Usually normal

- *T wave:* Usually normal
- *QT interval:* Usually normal
- *Other:* Sometimes a compensatory pause after PJC

Treatment
- No treatment if asymptomatic
- Correction of the underlying cause
- Discontinuation of digoxin if indicated
- Reduction or elimination of caffeine intake

Junctional escape rhythm
Characteristics
- *Rhythms:* Regular
- *Rates:* 40 to 60 beats/min
- *P wave:* Inverted in leads II, III, and aV$_F$; can occur before, during, or after QRS complex
- *PR interval:* Less than 0.12 second if P wave comes before QRS complex
- *QRS complex:* Normal; less than 0.12 second
- *T wave:* Normal
- *QT interval:* Normal

Treatment
- Correction of the underlying cause
- Atropine for symptomatic bradycardia
- Temporary or permanent pacemaker insertion if arrhythmia refractory to drugs
- Discontinuation of digoxin if indicated

Junctional arrhythmias review *(Continued)*

Accelerated junctional rhythm
Characteristics
- *Rhythms:* Regular
- *Rates:* 60 to 100 beats/min
- *P wave:* Inverted in leads II, III, and aV$_F$ (if present); occurs before, during, or after QRS complex
- *PR interval:* Measurable only with P wave that comes before QRS complex; 0.12 second or less
- *QRS complex:* Normal
- *T wave:* Normal
- *QT interval:* Normal

Treatment
- Correction of the underlying cause
- Discontinuation of digoxin if indicated
- Temporary pacemaker insertion if symptomatic
- Antiarrhythmic medications generally not indicated

Junctional tachycardia
Characteristics
- *Rhythms:* Regular
- *Rates:* 100 to 200 beats/min
- *P wave:* Inverted in leads II, III, and aV$_F$; location varies around QRS complex
- *PR interval:* Shortened at less than 0.12 second or unmeasurable
- *QRS complex:* Normal
- *T wave:* Usually normal; may contain P wave
- *QT interval:* Usually normal

Treatment
- Correction of the underlying cause
- Discontinuation of digoxin if indicated
- Temporary or permanent pacemaker insertion if symptomatic
- Vagal maneuvers or drugs such as adenosine to slow heart rate if symptomatic

Quick quiz

1. In a junctional escape rhythm, the P wave can occur:
    - A. within the T wave.
    - B. on top of the preceding Q wave.
    - C. before, during, or after the QRS complex.
    - D. earlier than expected.

    Answer: C. In all junctional arrhythmias, the P wave is inverted in leads II, III, and aV$_F$ and may appear before, during, or after the QRS complex.

2.   In an accelerated junctional rhythm, the QRS complex appears:
   A.   narrowed.
   B.   widened.
   C.   damped.
   D.   normal.

Answer: D. Because the ventricles are usually depolarized normally in this rhythm, the QRS complex has a normal configuration and a normal duration of less than 0.12 second.

3.   The normal slowing of impulses as they pass through the AV node allows the atria to:
   A.   fill completely with blood from the venae cava.
   B.   pump the maximum amount of blood possible into the ventricles.
   C.   remain insensitive to ectopic impulse formation outside the sinus node.
   D.   contract simultaneously.

Answer: B. In normal impulse conduction, the AV node slows impulse transmission from the atria to the ventricles and allows the atria to pump as much blood as possible into the ventricles before the ventricles contract.

4.   If the ventricles are depolarized first in a junctional rhythm, the P wave will:
   A.   appear before the QRS complex.
   B.   appear within the QRS complex.
   C.   appear after the QRS complex.
   D.   not be apparent.

Answer: C. If the ventricles are depolarized first, the P wave will come after the QRS complex.

Test strips

Try these test strips. Interpret each strip using the 8-step method and
fill in the blanks below with the particular characteristics of the strip.
Then compare your answers with the answers given.

Strip 1

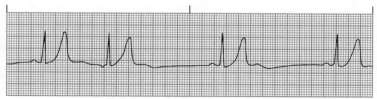

Atrial rhythm: _____

Ventricular rhythm: _____

Atrial rate: _____

Ventricular rate: _____

P wave: _____

PR interval: _____

QRS complex: _____

T wave: _____

QT interval: _____

Other: _____

Interpretation: _____

Strip 2

Atrial rhythm: _____

Ventricular rhythm: _____

Atrial rate: _____

Ventricular rate: _____

P wave: _____

PR interval: _____

QRS complex: _____

T wave: _____

QT interval: _____

Other: _____

Interpretation: _____

Strip 3

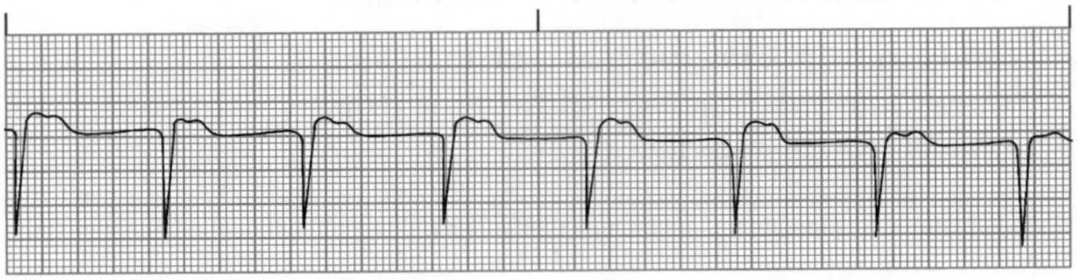

Atrial rhythm: _____

Ventricular rhythm: _____

Atrial rate: _____

Ventricular rate: _____

P wave: _____

PR interval: _____

QRS complex: _____

T wave: _____

QT interval: _____

Other: _____

Interpretation: _____

Answers to test strips

1. Rhythm: Regular
   Rate: 47 beats/min
   P wave: Inverted
   PR interval: 0.08 second
   QRS complex: 0.06 second
   T wave: Normal configuration
   QT interval: 0.42 second
   Other: None
   Interpretation: Junctional escape rhythm

2. Rhythm: Atrial and ventricular—irregular
   Rate: 40 beats/min
   P wave: Normal configuration except inverted on second complex
   PR interval: 0.16 second on beat 1, 3, and 4; 0.08 second beat 2
   QRS complex: 0.08 second
   T wave: Tall and peaked
   QT interval: 0.48 second
   Other: Second beat conducted early
   Interpretation: Sinus bradycardia with PJCs

3. Rhythm: Regular
Rate: 75 beats/min
P wave: Abnormal within T wave
PR interval: Unmeasurable
QRS complex: 0.08 second
T wave: Distorted by P wave
QT interval: Unmeasurable
Other: None
Interpretation: Accelerated junctional rhythm

Scoring

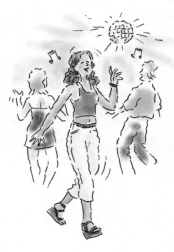

☆☆☆ If you answered all four questions correctly and correctly filled in all the blanks, we're impressed! Dance away to that hot new band, the Junctional Escape Rhythms.

☆☆ If you answered three questions correctly and correctly filled in most of the blanks, wow! You've clearly got that accelerated junctional rhythm.

☆ If you answered fewer than three questions correctly and missed most of the blanks, we still think your heart is in the right place.

Recommended references

Beinart, S. C. (2014). Junctional rhythm treatment and management. Retrieved from http://emedicine.medscape.com/article/155146

Katritsis, D. G., Gersh, B. J., & Camm, A. J. (2013). *Clinical cardiology: Current practice guidelines.* Oxford, United Kingdom: Oxford University Press. Retrieved from http://www.books.google.com/books?isbn=0191508519

Kulig, J., & Koplan, B. A. (2010). Cardiology patient page. Wolff-Parkinson-White syndrome and accessory pathways. *Circulation, 122*, e480–e483.

Chapter 7

Ventricular arrhythmias

Just the facts

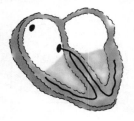

In this chapter, you'll learn:

◆ the proper way to identify various ventricular arrhythmias

◆ the role of the ventricles in arrhythmia formation

◆ the causes, significance, treatment, and nursing implications of each arrhythmia

◆ assessment findings associated with each arrhythmia

◆ interpretation of ventricular arrhythmias on an ECG.

A look at ventricular arrhythmias

Ventricular arrhythmias originate in the ventricles below the bundle of His. They occur when electrical impulses depolarize the myocardium using a different pathway from normal impulses.

Ventricular arrhythmias appear on an ECG in characteristic ways. The QRS complex is wider than normal (>0.10) because of the prolonged conduction time through the ventricles. The T wave and the QRS complex deflect in opposite directions because of the difference in the action potential during ventricular depolarization and repolarization. Also, the P wave is absent because atrial depolarization doesn't occur.

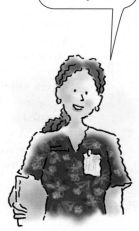

Ventricular arrhythmias appear on an ECG in characteristic ways.

No kick from the atria

When electrical impulses are generated from the ventricles instead of the atria, atrial kick is lost and cardiac output decreases by as much as 30%. Patients with ventricular arrhythmias may show signs and symptoms of cardiac decompensation, including hypotension, angina, syncope, and respiratory distress.

Potential to kill

Although ventricular arrhythmias may be benign, they're potentially deadly because the ventricles are ultimately responsible for cardiac output. Rapid recognition and treatment of ventricular arrhythmias increases the chance for successful resuscitation.

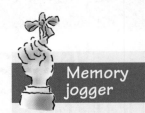

Premature ventricular contraction

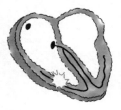

A premature ventricular contraction (PVC) is an ectopic beat that may occur in healthy people without causing problems. PVCs may occur singly, in clusters of two or more, or in repeating patterns, such as bigeminy or trigeminy. (See *Identifying PVCs.*) When PVCs occur in patients with underlying heart disease, they may indicate impending lethal ventricular arrhythmias.

How it happens

PVCs are usually caused by electrical irritability in the ventricular conduction system or muscle tissue. This irritability may be provoked by anything that disrupts normal electrolyte shifts during cell depolarization and repolarization. Conditions that can disrupt electrolyte shifts include:
- electrolyte imbalances, such as hypokalemia, hyperkalemia, hypomagnesemia, and hypocalcemia
- metabolic acidosis
- hypoxia
- myocardial ischemia and infarction
- drug intoxication, particularly cocaine, amphetamines, and tricyclic antidepressants
- enlargement of the ventricular chambers
- increased sympathetic stimulation
- myocarditis
- caffeine or alcohol ingestion
- proarrhythmic effects of some antiarrhythmic
- tobacco use.

People with damaged hearts are more likely to develop serious arrhythmias.

This could get serious

PVCs are significant for two reasons. First, they can lead to more serious arrhythmias, such as ventricular tachycardia or ventricular fibrillation. The risk of developing a more serious arrhythmia increases in patients with ischemic or damaged hearts.

PVCs also decrease cardiac output, especially if the ectopic beats are frequent or sustained. Decreased cardiac output is caused by

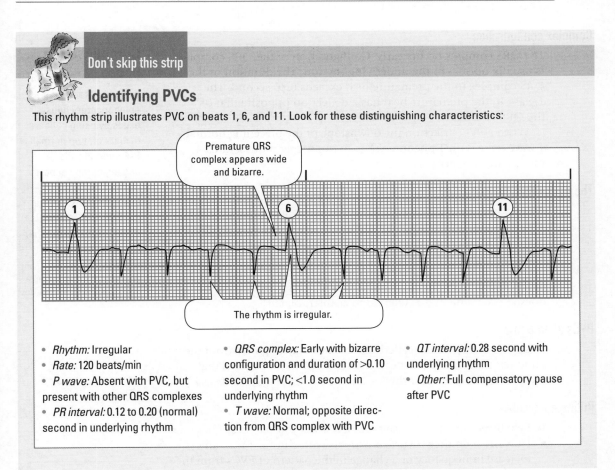

Don't skip this strip

Identifying PVCs

This rhythm strip illustrates PVC on beats 1, 6, and 11. Look for these distinguishing characteristics:

Premature QRS complex appears wide and bizarre.

The rhythm is irregular.

- *Rhythm:* Irregular
- *Rate:* 120 beats/min
- *P wave:* Absent with PVC, but present with other QRS complexes
- *PR interval:* 0.12 to 0.20 (normal) second in underlying rhythm

- *QRS complex:* Early with bizarre configuration and duration of >0.10 second in PVC; <1.0 second in underlying rhythm
- *T wave:* Normal; opposite direction from QRS complex with PVC

- *QT interval:* 0.28 second with underlying rhythm
- *Other:* Full compensatory pause after PVC

reduced ventricular diastolic filling time and a loss of atrial kick. The clinical impact of PVCs hinges on how well perfusion is maintained and how long the abnormal rhythm lasts.

What to look for

On the ECG strip, PVCs look wide and bizarre and appear as early beats causing atrial and ventricular irregularity. The rate follows the underlying rhythm, which is usually regular.

The P wave is usually absent. Retrograde P waves may be stimulated by the PVC and cause distortion of the ST segment. The PR interval and QT interval aren't measurable on a premature beat, only on the normal beats.

Complex configuration

The QRS complex occurs early. Configuration of the QRS complex is usually normal in the underlying rhythm. The duration of the QRS complex in the premature beat exceeds 0.10 second. The T wave in the premature beat has a deflection opposite that of the QRS complex.

When a PVC strikes on the downslope of the preceding normal T wave—the R-on-T phenomenon—it can trigger more serious rhythm disturbances.

The pause that compensates

A horizontal baseline called a full *compensatory pause* may follow the T wave of the PVC. When a compensatory pause appears, the interval between two normal sinus beats containing a PVC equals two normal sinus intervals. (See *Compensatory pause.*) This pause occurs because the ventricle is refractory and can't respond to the next regularly timed P wave from the sinus node. When a compensatory pause doesn't occur, the PVC is referred to as interpolated.

PVCs all in a row

PVCs that look alike are called *uniform* and may originate from the same ectopic focus. These beats may also appear in patterns that can progress to more lethal arrhythmias. (See *When PVCs spell danger.*)

Ruling out trouble

To help determine the seriousness of PVCs, ask yourself these questions:
- How often do they occur? In patients with chronic PVCs, an increase in frequency or a change in the pattern of PVCs from the baseline rhythm may signal a more serious condition.
- What pattern do they occur in? If the ECG shows a dangerous pattern—such as paired PVCs, PVCs with more than one shape, bigeminy, or R-on-T phenomenon—the patient may require immediate treatment.
- Are they really PVCs? Make sure the complex you see is a PVC, not another, less dangerous arrhythmia. (See *Deciphering PVCs.*) Don't delay treatment, however, if the patient is unstable.

Outward signs tell a story

The patient with PVCs will have a much weaker pulse wave after the premature beat and a longer-than-normal pause between pulse waves. At times, you won't be able to palpate any pulse after the PVC. If the carotid pulse is visible, however, you may see a weaker pulse wave after the premature beat. When auscultating for heart sounds, you'll hear an abnormally early heart sound and a diminished amplitude with each premature beat.

Compensatory pause

You can determine if a compensatory pause exists by using calipers to mark off two normal P-P intervals. Place one leg of the calipers on the sinus P wave that comes just before the PVC. If the pause is compensatory, the other leg of the calipers will fall precisely on the P wave that comes after the pause.

Ask yourself specific questions to determine the seriousness of PVCs.

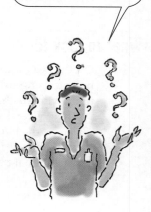

When PVCs spell danger

Here are some examples of patterns of dangerous PVCs.

Paired PVCs

Two PVCs in a row are called a pair, or *couplet* (see highlighted areas). A pair can produce ventricular tachycardia because the second depolarization usually meets refractory tissue. Three or more PVCs in a row is considered ventricular tachycardia. If the patient spontaneously converts to underlying rhythm, it is called a run of V-tach. Measure the rate of the V-tach. Not all V-tach are the same.

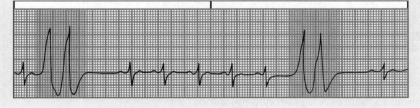

Multiform PVCs

PVCs that look different from one another arise from different sites or from the same site with abnormal conduction (see highlighted areas). Multiform PVCs may indicate increased ventricular irritability. Review patients baseline to confirm this is new for the patient. With increasing age, some patients have PVCs as part of their baseline rhythm, it has been assessed in the past and deemed benign.

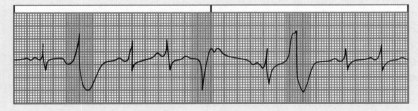

Bigeminy and trigeminy

PVCs that occur every other beat (bigeminy) or every third beat (trigeminy) may indicate increased ventricular irritability (see highlighted areas).

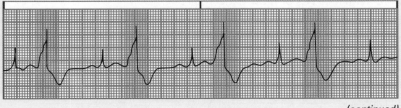

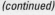
(continued)

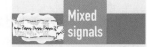
Mixed signals

Deciphering PVCs

To determine whether the rhythm you're assessing is a PVC or some other beat, ask yourself these questions:

- Are you seeing ventricular escape beats rather than PVCs? Escape beats act as a safety mechanism to protect the heart from ventricular standstill. The ventricular escape beat will be late, rather than premature.
- Are you seeing normal beats with aberrant ventricular conduction? Some supraventricular impulses may take an abnormal pathway through the ventricular conduction system, causing the QRS complex to appear abnormal. This aberrantly conducted beat will have a P wave, whereas a PVC doesn't.

When PVCs spell danger *(Continued)*

R-on-T phenomenon
In R-on-T phenomenon, the PVC occurs so early that it falls on the T wave of the preceding beat (see highlighted area). Because the cells haven't fully repolarized, ventricular tachycardia or ventricular fibrillation can result.

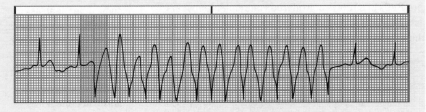

Patients with frequent PVCs may complain of palpitations and may also experience hypotension or syncope.

How you intervene

If the patient is asymptomatic, the arrhythmia probably won't require treatment. If he has symptoms or a dangerous form of PVCs, the type of treatment depends on the cause of the problem.

The practitioner may order amiodarone (Cordarone), or lidocaine if symptomatic. I.V. Potassium chloride may be given I.V. or orally to correct hypokalemia, and magnesium sulfate I.V. may be given to correct hypomagnesemia. Other treatments may be aimed at adjusting drug therapy or correcting acidosis, hypothermia, or hypoxia.

Stat assessment

Patients who have recently developed PVCs need prompt assessment, especially if they have underlying heart disease or complex medical problems. Those with chronic PVCs should be observed closely for the development of more frequent PVCs or more dangerous PVC patterns.

Until effective treatment is begun, a patient with PVCs accompanied by serious symptoms should have continuous ECG monitoring and ambulate only with assistance. If the patient is discharged from the healthcare facility on antiarrhythmic drugs, family members should know how to contact the emergency medical service (EMS) and how to perform cardiopulmonary resuscitation (CPR).

Idioventricular rhythms

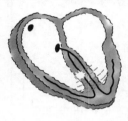

Called the *rhythms of last resort*, idioventricular rhythms act as safety mechanisms to prevent ventricular stand-still when no impulses are conducted to the ventricles from above the bundle of His. The cells of the His–Purkinje system take over and act as the heart's pacemaker to generate electrical impulses.

Idioventricular rhythms can occur as ventricular escape beats, idioventricular rhythm (a term used to designate a specific type of idioventricular rhythm), or accelerated idioventricular rhythm.

How it happens

Idioventricular rhythms occur when all of the heart's other pacemakers have failed to function or when supraventricular impulses can't reach the ventricles because of a block in the conduction system. The arrhythmias may accompany third-degree heart block or be caused by

- myocardial ischemia
- myocardial infarction (MI)
- digoxin toxicity
- beta-adrenergic blockers
- pacemaker failure
- metabolic imbalances.

Conduction foibles and pacemaker failures

Idioventricular rhythms signal a serious conduction defect with a failure of the primary pacemaker. The slow ventricular rate of these arrhythmias and the loss of atrial kick markedly reduce cardiac output. Patients require close observation because this problem can progress to more lethal arrhythmias. Idioventricular arrhythmias also commonly occur in dying patients.

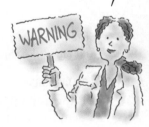

Carefully monitor patients who have idioventricular rhythms.

What to look for

If just one idioventricular beat is generated, it's called a *ventricular escape beat*. (See *Identifying idioventricular rhythm*, page 148.) The beat appears late in the conduction cycle, when the rate drops to 40 beats/min.

Consecutive ventricular beats on the ECG strip make up idioventricular rhythm. When this arrhythmia occurs, atrial rhythm and rate can't be determined. The ventricular rhythm is usually regular at 20 to 40 beats/min, the inherent rate of the ventricles. If the rate is

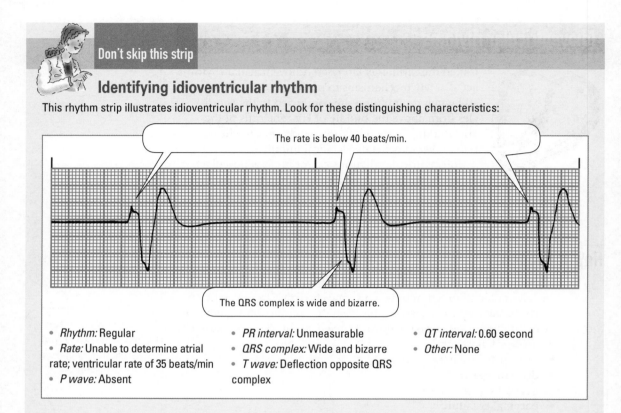

Don't skip this strip

Identifying idioventricular rhythm

This rhythm strip illustrates idioventricular rhythm. Look for these distinguishing characteristics:

The rate is below 40 beats/min.

The QRS complex is wide and bizarre.

- *Rhythm:* Regular
- *Rate:* Unable to determine atrial rate; ventricular rate of 35 beats/min
- *P wave:* Absent

- *PR interval:* Unmeasurable
- *QRS complex:* Wide and bizarre
- *T wave:* Deflection opposite QRS complex

- *QT interval:* 0.60 second
- *Other:* None

faster, it's called an *accelerated idioventricular rhythm.* (See *Accelerated idioventricular rhythm.*)

A tell–tale arrhythmia

Distinguishing characteristics of idioventricular rhythm include an absent P wave or one that can't conduct through to the ventricles. This makes the PR interval unmeasurable.

Because of abnormal ventricular depolarization, the QRS complex has a duration of longer than 0.10 second, with a wide and bizarre configuration. The T-wave deflection will be opposite the QRS complex. The QT interval is usually prolonged, indicating delayed depolarization and repolarization.

The patient may complain of palpitations, dizziness, or light-headedness, or he may have a syncopal episode. If the arrhythmia persists, hypotension, weak peripheral pulses, decreased urine output, or confusion can occur.

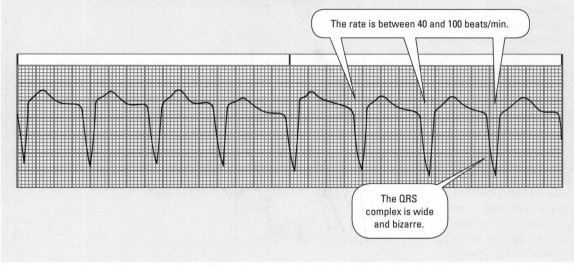

Don't skip this strip

Accelerated idioventricular rhythm

An accelerated idioventricular rhythm has the same characteristics as an idioventricular rhythm except that it's faster. The rate shown here varies between 40 and 100 beats/min.

The rate is between 40 and 100 beats/min.

The QRS complex is wide and bizarre.

How you intervene

If the patient is symptomatic, treatment should be initiated immediately to increase the heart rate, improve cardiac output, and establish a normal rhythm. Atropine may be prescribed to increase the heart rate by increasing sinus node automaticity but will not work to increase ventricular rate if the normal conduction system is not intact since vagus nerve intervention is at the level of the bundle. Atropine antagonizes the effects of acetylcholine.

If atropine isn't effective or if the patient develops hypotension or other signs of instability, a pacemaker may be needed to re-establish a heart rate that provides enough cardiac output to perfuse organs properly. A transcutaneous pacemaker may be used in an emergency until a temporary or permanent transvenous pacemaker can be inserted. Also, direct acting catecholamine drips may be used to increase heart rate. These include dopamine and epinephrine drips. (See *Transcutaneous pacemaker,* page 150.)

Remember: The goal of treatment doesn't include suppressing the idioventricular rhythm because it acts as a safety mechanism to protect the heart from standstill. *Idioventricular rhythm should never*

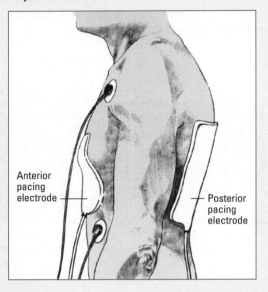

I can't waste time

Transcutaneous pacemaker

In life-threatening situations in which time is critical, a transcutaneous pacemaker may be used to regulate heart rate. This device sends an electrical impulse from the pulse generator to the heart by way of two electrodes placed on the patient's chest and back, as shown.

The electrodes are placed at heart level, on either side of the heart, so the electrical stimulus has only a short distance to travel to the heart. Transcutaneous pacing is quick and effective, but it may be painful. It's used only until transvenous pacing/epinephrine or dopamine drip can be started.

Anterior pacing electrode

Posterior pacing electrode

be treated with lidocaine or other antiarrhythmic that would suppress that safety mechanism.

Continuous monitoring needed

Patients with idioventricular rhythms need continuous ECG monitoring and constant assessment until treatment restores hemodynamic stability. Keep pacemaker equipment at the bedside and have atropine readily available. Enforce bed rest until a permanent system is in place for maintaining an effective heart rate.

Be sure to tell the patient and his family about the serious nature of this arrhythmia and all aspects of treatment. If a permanent pacemaker is inserted, teach the patient and his family how it works, how to recognize problems, when to contact the practitioner, and how pacemaker function will be monitored.

Teach the patient about how a pacemaker works and when to contact the practitioner.

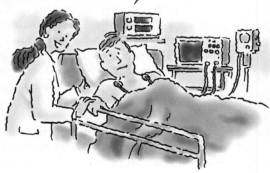

Ventricular tachycardia

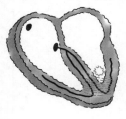

In ventricular tachycardia, commonly called *V-tach*, three or more PVCs occur in a row and the ventricular rate exceeds 100 beats/min. This arrhythmia may precede ventricular fibrillation and sudden cardiac death, especially if the patient isn't in a healthcare facility.

Ventricular tachycardia is an extremely unstable rhythm. It can occur in short, paroxysmal bursts lasting fewer than 30 seconds and causing few or no symptoms. Alternatively, it can be sustained, requiring immediate treatment to prevent death, even in patients initially able to maintain adequate cardiac output, 30% to 50% will have no pulse.

> V-tach may be unstable and can occur in short paroxysmal bursts.

How it happens

Ventricular tachycardia usually results from increased myocardial irritability, which may be triggered by enhanced automaticity or re-entry within the Purkinje system or by PVCs initiating the R-on-T phenomenon. Conditions that can cause ventricular tachycardia include

- myocardial ischemia
- MI
- coronary artery disease
- valvular heart disease
- heart failure
- cardiomyopathy
- electrolyte imbalances such as hypokalemia
- drug intoxication from digoxin (Lanoxin), procainamide, quinidine, cocaine or meta-amphetamines
- proarrhythmic effects of some antiarrhythmic.

Unpredictable V-tach

Ventricular tachycardia is significant because of its unpredictability and potential to cause death. A patient may be stable with a normal pulse and adequate hemodynamics or unstable with hypotension and no detectable pulse. Because of reduced ventricular filling time and the drop in cardiac output, the patient's condition can quickly deteriorate to ventricular fibrillation and complete cardiac collapse.

What to look for

On the ECG strip, the atrial rhythm and rate can't be determined. The ventricular rhythm is usually regular but may be slightly irregular. The ventricular rate is usually rapid—100 to 250 beats/min.

The P wave is usually absent but may be obscured by the QRS complex. Retrograde P waves may be present. Because the P wave can't be seen in most cases, you can't measure the PR interval. The QRS complex is wide and bizarre, usually with an increased amplitude and a duration of longer than 0.12 second.

All about uniformity

QRS complexes in monomorphic ventricular tachycardia have a uniform shape. In polymorphic ventricular tachycardia, the shape of the QRS complex constantly changes. If the T wave is visible, it occurs opposite the QRS complex. The QT interval isn't measurable. (See *Identifying ventricular tachycardia.*)

Torsades de pointes is a special variation of polymorphic ventricular tachycardia. (See *Torsades de pointes* and *Pediatric torsades de pointes.*)

Don't skip this strip

Identifying ventricular tachycardia

This rhythm strip illustrates ventricular tachycardia. Look for these distinguishing characteristics:

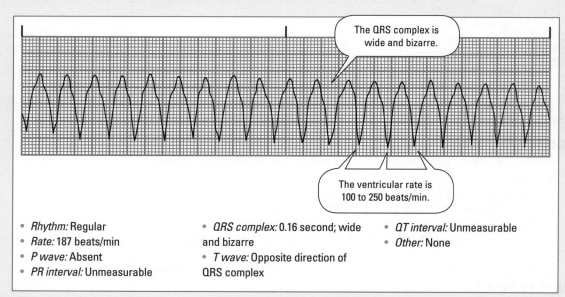

The QRS complex is wide and bizarre.

The ventricular rate is 100 to 250 beats/min.

- *Rhythm:* Regular
- *Rate:* 187 beats/min
- *P wave:* Absent
- *PR interval:* Unmeasurable

- *QRS complex:* 0.16 second; wide and bizarre
- *T wave:* Opposite direction of QRS complex

- *QT interval:* Unmeasurable
- *Other:* None

Quick work prevents collapse

Although some patients have only minor symptoms at first, they still need rapid intervention and treatment to prevent cardiac collapse.

Don't skip this strip

Torsades de pointes

Torsades de pointes, which means "twisting about the points," is a special form of polymorphic ventricular tachycardia. The hallmark characteristics of this rhythm, shown below, are QRS complexes that rotate about the baseline, deflecting downward and upward for several beats.

The rate is 150 to 250 beats/min, usually with an irregular rhythm, and the QRS complexes are wide with changing amplitude. The P wave is usually absent.

Paroxysmal rhythm
This arrhythmia may be paroxysmal, starting and stopping suddenly, and may deteriorate into ventricular fibrillation. It should be considered when ventricular tachycardia doesn't respond to antiarrhythmic therapy or other treatments.

Reversible causes
The cause of this form of ventricular tachycardia is usually reversible. The most common causes are drugs that lengthen the QT interval, such as amiodarone, ibutilide, erythromycin, haloperidol, droperidol, and sotalol. Other causes include myocardial ischemia and electrolyte abnormalities, such as hypokalemia, hypomagnesaemia, and hypocalcemia.

Going into overdrive
Torsades de pointes is treated by correcting the underlying cause, especially if the cause is related to specific drug therapy. The practitioner may order mechanical overdrive pacing, which overrides the ventricular rate and breaks the triggered mechanism for the arrhythmia. Magnesium sulfate may also be effective. Electrical cardioversion may be used when torsades de pointes doesn't respond to other treatment or defibrillation if patient has no pulse.

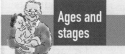

Ages and stages

Pediatric torsades de pointes

Torsades de pointes at an early age is usually due to congenital long QT syndrome. Ask the parents about a family history of sudden cardiac death or sudden infant death syndrome.

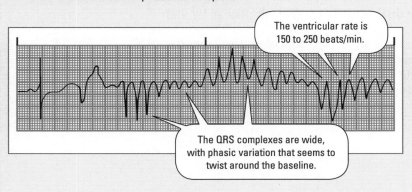

The ventricular rate is 150 to 250 beats/min.

The QRS complexes are wide, with phasic variation that seems to twist around the baseline.

Most patients with ventricular tachycardia have weak or absent pulses. Low cardiac output will cause hypotension and a decreased level of consciousness (LOC) leading to unresponsiveness. Ventricular tachycardia may precipitate angina, heart failure, or a substantial decrease in organ perfusion.

How you intervene

Treatment depends on whether the patient's pulse is detectable or undetectable. A patient with pulseless ventricular tachycardia receives the same treatment as one with ventricular fibrillation and requires immediate defibrillation and CPR. Treatment for the patient with a detectable pulse depends on whether his condition is stable or unstable and has monomorphic or polymorphic QRS complexes.

Unstable patients generally have heart rates greater than 150 beats/min. They may also have hypotension, shortness of breath, an altered LOC, heart failure, angina, or MI—conditions that indicate cardiac decompensation. These patients are treated immediately with direct-current synchronized cardioversion.

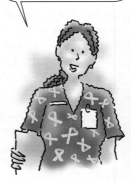

Treatment for the patient in V-tach depends on whether his pulse is detectable or undetectable.

Typical tachycardia complex

A hemodynamically stable patient with monomorphic ventricular tachycardia is treated differently. First, administer amiodarone following advanced cardiac life support (ACLS) protocols to correct the rhythm disturbance. If the drug doesn't correct the disturbance, prepare the patient for synchronized cardioversion.

If the patient has polymorphic ventricular tachycardia with a normal QT interval, correct ischemia and electrolyte imbalances. Then administer amiodarone, lidocaine, beta-adrenergic blockers, following ACLS protocol. Again, if drug therapy is unsuccessful, synchronized cardioversion is performed.

Correct electrolyte abnormalities in the patient with polymorphic ventricular tachycardia with a prolonged QT interval and administer magnesium I.V. If the rhythm persists, prepare the patient for overdrive pacing.

Patients with chronic, recurrent episodes of ventricular tachycardia who are unresponsive to drug therapy may have a cardioverter-defibrillator implanted. This device is a more permanent solution to recurrent episodes of ventricular tachycardia. (For more information about the implantable cardioverter-defibrillator [ICD], see Chapter 9.)

Always assume the worst

Any wide QRS complex tachycardia should be treated as ventricular tachycardia until definitive evidence is found to establish another diagnosis, such as supraventricular tachycardia with abnormal ventricular conduction. *Always assume that the patient has ventricular tachycardia and treat him accordingly. Rapid intervention will prevent cardiac decompensation or the onset of more lethal arrhythmias.*

Teacher, teacher

Be sure to teach the patient and his family about the serious nature of this arrhythmia and the need for prompt treatment. If your patient is undergoing cardioversion, tell him he'll be given an analgesic or a sedative to help prevent discomfort.

If a patient will be discharged with an ICD or a prescription for long-term antiarrhythmic drugs, teach his family how to contact the EMS and how to perform CPR.

Ventricular fibrillation

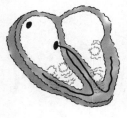

Ventricular fibrillation, commonly called *V-fib*, is a chaotic pattern of electrical activity in the ventricles in which electrical impulses arise from many different foci. It produces no effective muscular contraction and no cardiac output. Untreated ventricular fibrillation causes most cases of sudden cardiac death in people outside of a hospital.

How it happens

Causes of ventricular fibrillation include
- myocardial ischemia
- MI
- untreated ventricular tachycardia
- underlying heart disease
- acid–base imbalance
- electric shock
- severe hypothermia
- electrolyte imbalances, such as hypokalemia, hyperkalemia, and hypercalcemia
- drug toxicity, including digoxin
- severe hypoxia.

Quivering ventricles

With ventricular fibrillation, the ventricles quiver instead of contract, so cardiac output falls to zero. If ventricular fibrillation continues, it leads to ventricular standstill and death.

What to look for

On the ECG strip, ventricular activity appears as fibrillatory waves with no recognizable pattern. Atrial rate and rhythm can't be determined, nor can ventricular rhythm because no pattern or regularity occurs.

As a result, the ventricular rate, P wave, PR interval, QRS complex, T wave, and QT interval can't be determined. Larger, or coarse, fibrillatory waves are easier to convert to a normal rhythm than are smaller waves because larger waves indicate a greater degree of electrical activity in the heart. (See *Identifying ventricular fibrillation.*)

No greater urgency

The patient in ventricular fibrillation is in full cardiac arrest, unresponsive, and without a detectable blood pressure or carotid or femoral pulse. Whenever you see a pattern resembling ventricular fibrillation, check the patient immediately, check the rhythm in another lead, and start treatment.

Be aware that other factors can mimic ventricular fibrillation on an ECG strip. Interference from an electric razor is one such mimic, as is muscle movement from shivering.

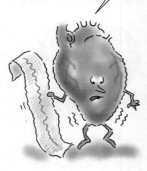

With V-fib, the ventricles quiver instead of contract, so no pattern or regularity can be detected on the ECG strip.

How you intervene

Defibrillation is the most effective treatment for ventricular fibrillation. (See "Pulseless arrest" in the appendix ACLS algorithms.) CPR must be performed until the defibrillator arrives to preserve oxygen supply to the brain, heart, and other vital organs. Assist with endotracheal intubation. Such drugs as epinephrine or vasopressin may help the heart respond better to defibrillation. Drugs such as amiodarone, lidocaine, and magnesium sulfate may also be given.

A shock for life

During defibrillation, hands-free patches or paddles direct an electric current through the patient's heart. The current causes the myocardium to depolarize, which, in turn, encourages the sinoatrial node to resume normal control of the heart's electrical activity.

Don't skip this strip

Identifying ventricular fibrillation

The following rhythm strips illustrate coarse ventricular fibrillation (first strip) and fine ventricular fibrillation (second strip). Look for these distinguishing characteristics:

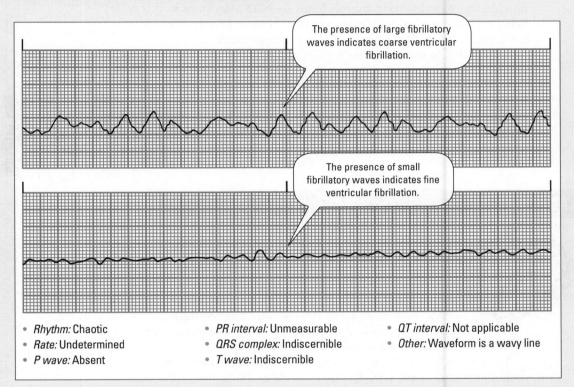

The presence of large fibrillatory waves indicates coarse ventricular fibrillation.

The presence of small fibrillatory waves indicates fine ventricular fibrillation.

- *Rhythm:* Chaotic
- *Rate:* Undetermined
- *P wave:* Absent
- *PR interval:* Unmeasurable
- *QRS complex:* Indiscernible
- *T wave:* Indiscernible
- *QT interval:* Not applicable
- *Other:* Waveform is a wavy line

One paddle is placed to the right of the upper sternum, and one is placed over the fifth or sixth intercostal space at the left anterior axillary line. A hands-free methodology, places large patches in the location where paddles were placed. These patches can be used to monitor the patient's rhythm, defibrillate, and even transcutaneously pace the patient (3-lead ECG required for pacing). During cardiac surgery, internal paddles are placed directly on the myocardium.

Automated external defibrillators are increasingly being used to provide early defibrillation. In this method, electrode pads are placed on the patient's chest and a microcomputer in the unit interprets the cardiac rhythm, providing the caregiver with step-by-step instructions on how to proceed. These defibrillators can be used by people without medical experience.

Speed is the key

For the patient with ventricular fibrillation, successful resuscitation requires rapid recognition of the problem and prompt defibrillation (<2 minutes per AHA). Many healthcare facilities and EMS providers have established protocols based on ACLS algorithms to help healthcare workers initiate prompt treatment. Make sure you know where your facility keeps its emergency equipment, be proficient in its use, and know how to recognize and deal with lethal arrhythmias.

You'll also need to teach your patient and his family how to contact the EMS. Family members need instruction in CPR. Teach them about long-term therapies that prevent recurrent episodes of ventricular fibrillation, including chronic antiarrhythmic drugs and implantation of an ICD.

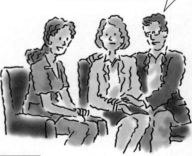

Patients and their families need to know when to contact EMS, how to perform CPR, and what long-term therapies are available, such as chronic antiarrhythmic drugs and ICDs.

Asystole

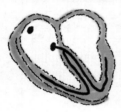

Asystole is ventricular standstill. The patient is completely unresponsive, with no electrical activity in the heart and no cardiac output. This arrhythmia results most commonly from a prolonged period of cardiac arrest without effective resuscitation. It's extremely important to distinguish asystole from fine ventricular fibrillation, which is managed differently. Therefore, asystole must be confirmed in more than one ECG lead.

Asystole has been called the *arrhythmia of death*. The patient is in cardiopulmonary arrest. Without rapid initiation of CPR and appropriate treatment, the situation quickly becomes irreversible.

How it happens

Anything that causes inadequate blood flow to the heart may lead to asystole, including
- MI
- severe electrolyte disturbances such as hyperkalemia
- massive pulmonary embolism
- prolonged hypoxemia
- severe, uncorrected acid–base disturbances
- electric shock

- drug intoxication such as cocaine overdose
- cardiac tamponade
- hypothermia.

What to look for

On the ECG strip, asystole looks like a nearly flat line (except for changes caused by chest compressions during CPR). No electrical activity is evident, except possibly P waves for a time. Atrial and ventricular activity is at a standstill, so no intervals can be measured. (See *Identifying asystole.*)

In the patient with a pacemaker, pacer spikes may be evident on the strip, but no P wave or QRS complex occurs in response to the stimulus.

The patient will be unresponsive, without any discernible pulse or blood pressure.

How you intervene

The immediate treatment for asystole is CPR. (See "Pulseless arrest" in the appendix ACLS algorithms.) Start CPR as soon as you determine that the patient has no pulse. Then verify the presence of asystole by checking two different ECG leads.

Don't skip this strip

Identifying asystole

This rhythm strip illustrates asystole, the absence of electrical activity in the ventricles. Except for a few P waves or pacer spikes, nothing appears on the waveform and the line is almost flat.

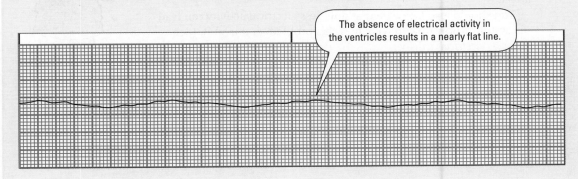

The absence of electrical activity in the ventricles results in a nearly flat line.

Pulseless electrical activity

In pulseless electrical activity, the heart muscle loses its ability to contract even though electrical activity is preserved. As a result, the patient goes into cardiac arrest.

On an electrocardiogram, you'll see evidence of organized electrical activity, but you won't be able to palpate a pulse or measure the blood pressure.

Causes

This condition requires rapid identification and treatment. Causes include hypovolemia, hypoxia, acidosis, tension pneumothorax, cardiac tamponade, massive pulmonary embolism, hypothermia, hyperkalemia, massive acute myocardial infarction, and an overdose of drugs such as tricyclic antidepressants.

Treatment

CPR is the immediate treatment, along with epinephrine. Atropine may be given to patients with bradycardia. Subsequent treatment focuses on identifying and correcting the underlying cause.

Give repeated doses of epinephrine and atropine, as ordered. Transcutaneous pacing should be initiated as soon as possible. Subsequent treatment for asystole focuses on identifying and either treating or removing the underlying cause.

Quick recognition

Your job is to recognize this life-threatening arrhythmia and start resuscitation right away. Unfortunately, most patients with asystole can't be resuscitated, especially after a prolonged period of cardiac arrest.

You should also be aware that pulseless electrical activity can lead to asystole. Know how to recognize this problem and treat it. (See *Pulseless electrical activity.*)

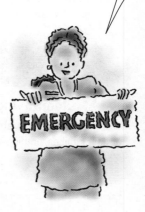

Arrhythmias can be life threatening. If asystole occurs, start CPR immediately.

That's a wrap!

Ventricular arrhythmias review

Overview of ventricular arrhythmias
- Originate in the ventricles, below the bundle of His
- Loss of atrial kick, decreasing cardiac output
- Potentially fatal without treatment or resuscitation

Characteristics
- QRS complex—wider than normal
- T wave and QRS complex deflect in opposite directions
- P wave is absent

Premature ventricular contraction
Characteristics
- *Rhythms:* Irregular during PVC; underlying rhythm may be regular
- *Rates:* Patterned after underlying rhythm
- *P wave:* Absent
- *PR interval:* Unmeasurable
- *QRS complex:* Wide and bizarre
- *T wave:* Opposite direction from QRS complex
- *QT interval:* Unmeasurable
- *Other:* Possible compensatory pause

Treatment
- Correction of the underlying cause
- Discontinuation of drug that may be causing toxicity
- Correction of electrolyte imbalances
- Amiodarone, or lidocaine if warranted

Idioventricular rhythms
- Act as safety mechanism to prevent ventricular standstill
- Occur as escape beats, idioventricular rhythm, or accelerated idioventricular rhythm

Characteristics
- *Rhythms:* Atrial—undetermined; ventricular—usually regular
- *Rates:* Atrial—unmeasurable; ventricular—20 to 40 beats/min
- *P wave:* Absent
- *PR interval:* Unmeasurable
- *QRS complex:* Wide and bizarre
- *T wave:* Deflection opposite that of QRS complex
- *QT interval:* Greater than 0.44 second

Treatment
- Atropine to increase heart rate, dopamine or epinephrine drips to increase heart rate
- Temporary or permanent pacemaker if arrhythmia is refractory to drugs
- Avoidance of drugs that suppress the idioventricular rhythm, such as lidocaine and other antiarrhythmics

Ventricular tachycardia
Characteristics
- *Rhythms:* Atrial—can't be determined; ventricular—regular or slightly irregular
- *Rates:* Atrial—can't be determined; ventricular—100 to 250 beats/min
- *P wave:* Absent or hidden by QRS complex
- *PR interval:* Unmeasurable
- *QRS complex:* Wide and bizarre, with increased amplitude; duration greater than 0.12 second
- *T wave:* Opposite direction of QRS complex
- *Other:* Possible torsades de pointes

Treatment
ACLS protocols:
- Amiodarone; if patient is stable with monomorphic QRS complexes and drugs are unsuccessful, cardioversion
- Beta-adrenergic blockers, lidocaine, amiodarone, if patient's ECG shows polymorphic QRS complexes and normal QT interval; cardioversion if unsuccessful
- Magnesium sulfate I.V. if patient shows polymorphic QRS and QT interval is prolonged, then overdrive pacing if rhythm persists (possibly also isoproterenol)

(continued)

Ventricular arrhythmias review (Continued)

- Defibrillation; CPR, endotracheal intubation, and epinephrine or vasopressin, if patient is pulseless (possibly also consider amiodarone, lidocaine, or magnesium sulfate)
- Cardioverter-defibrillator possibly implanted for recurrent ventricular tachycardia

Torsades de pointes
- A form of polymorphic ventricular tachycardia
- Sometimes deteriorates into ventricular fibrillation

Characteristics
- *Rhythms:* Ventricular—irregular
- *Rates:* 150 to 250 beats/min
- *P wave:* Usually absent
- *PR interval:* Unmeasurable
- *QRS complex:* Wide; rotates around the baseline; deflection downward and upward for several beats

Treatment
- Correction of the underlying cause
- Discontinuation of offending drug (usually one that lengthens the QT interval)
- Overdrive pacing
- Magnesium sulfate (per ACLS)
- Cardioversion if unresponsive to other treatment

Ventricular fibrillation
- Electrical impulses arise from many different foci in the ventricles
- Produces no effective muscular contraction and no cardiac output
- If untreated, it causes most cases of sudden cardiac death out of hospital

Characteristics
- *Rhythms:* Can't be determined
- *Rates:* Can't be determined
- *P wave:* Can't be determined
- *PR interval:* Can't be determined
- *QRS complex:* Can't be determined
- *T wave:* Can't be determined

- *QT interval:* Isn't applicable
- *Other:* Variations in size of fibrillatory waves

Treatment
ACLS protocols:
- Defibrillation
- Initiation of CPR
- Endotracheal intubation and administration of epinephrine or vasopressin (consider amiodarone, lidocaine, or magnesium sulfate)
- Implantation of cardioverter-defibrillator if patient is at risk for recurrent ventricular fibrillation

Asystole
- Characterized by ventricular standstill and cardiac arrest
- Fatal without prompt CPR and treatment

Characteristics
- Lack of electrical activity seen on ECG as a nearly flat line

Treatment
ACLS protocols:
- Initiation of CPR
- Endotracheal intubation, transcutaneous pacing, and epinephrine

Pulseless electrical activity
Characteristics
- Electrical activity is present on ECG but heart muscle can't contract
- Result is no palpable pulse or blood pressure and cardiac arrest

Treatment
ACLS protocols:
- Initiation of CPR
- Epinephrine
- Atropine for bradycardia
- Correction of the underlying cause

Quick quiz

1. PVCs are most dangerous if they:
    A. are multiformed and increase in frequency.
    B. appear wide and bizarre.
    C. occur after the T wave.
    D. are uniform and wide.

Answer: A. PVCs that have different shapes (multiformed) and increase in frequency may signal increased ventricular irritability and progress to a lethal arrhythmia.

2. The treatment of choice for a patient with ventricular fibrillation is:
    A. defibrillation.
    B. transesophageal pacing.
    C. synchronized cardioversion.
    D. administration of epinephrine.

Answer: A. Patients with ventricular fibrillation are in cardiac arrest and require defibrillation.

3. Patients with a slow idioventricular rhythm that doesn't respond to atropine should receive:
    A. lidocaine.
    B. dobutamine.
    C. synchronized cardioversion.
    D. transcutaneous pacing.

Answer: D. Transcutaneous pacing is a temporary way to increase the rate and ensure adequate cardiac output.

4. A compensatory pause occurs after a PVC because the:
    A. atria conduct a retrograde impulse.
    B. ventricle is refractory at that point.
    C. bundle of His blocks sinus impulses to the ventricles.
    D. atria are refractory and can't respond.

Answer: B. A compensatory pause occurs because the ventricle is refractory and can't respond to the next regularly timed P wave from the sinus node.

5. The term *pulseless electrical activity* refers to a condition in which there's:
   A. an extremely slow heart rate but no pulse.
   B. asystole on a monitor or rhythm strip.
   C. electrical activity in the heart but no actual contraction.
   D. asystole and a palpable pulse and blood pressure.

Answer: C. Pulseless electrical activity is electrical activity without mechanical contraction. The patient is in cardiac arrest, with no blood pressure or pulse.

Test strips

Ready for a few test strips? Interpret the two strips below using the 8-step method. Fill in the blanks below with the particular characteristics of the strip and then check your answers with ours.

Strip 1

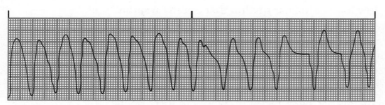

Atrial rhythm: _____

Ventricular rhythm: _____

Atrial rate: _____

Ventricular rate: _____

P wave: _____

PR interval: _____

QRS complex: _____

T wave: _____

QT interval: _____

Other: _____

Interpretation: _____

Strip 2

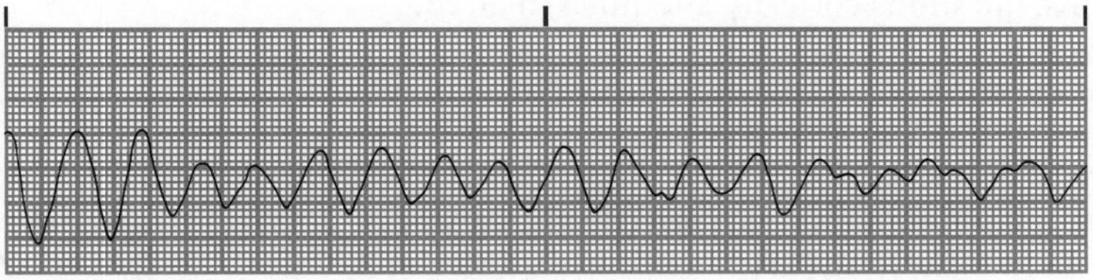

Atrial rhythm: _____

Ventricular rhythm: _____

Atrial rate: _____

Ventricular rate: _____

P wave: _____

PR interval: _____

QRS complex: _____

T wave: _____

QT interval: _____

Other: _____

Interpretation: _____

Answers to test strips

1. Rhythm: Irregular ventricular rhythm
   Rate: Ventricular rate is 130 beats/min
   P wave: Absent
   PR interval: Unmeasurable
   QRS complex: Wide and bizarre with varying duration
   T wave: Opposite QRS complex
   QT interval: Unmeasurable
   Other: None
   Interpretation: Ventricular tachycardia

2. Rhythm: Chaotic ventricular rhythm
   Rate: Can't be determined
   P wave: Indiscernible
   PR interval: Indiscernible
   QRS complex: Indiscernible
   T wave: Indiscernible
   QT interval: Indiscernible
   Other: None
   Interpretation: Ventricular fibrillation

Scoring

★★★   If you answered all five questions correctly and filled in all the blanks as we did, sensational! You're simply V-best.

★★   If you answered four questions correctly and filled in most of the blanks pretty much as we did, super! You've got a great eye for those tricky ventricular rhythms.

★   If you answered fewer than four questions correctly and missed most of the blanks, that's okay. Read this chapter again and you'll get de pointes.

Recommended references

Brown, D. F. M., & Martindale, J. L. (2012). *Rapid interpretation of ECG's in emergency medicine.* Philadelphia, PA: Wolters Kluwer.

Katritsis, D. G., Gersch, B. J., & Camm, A. J. (2013). *Clinical cardiology: Current practice guidelines.* Oxford, United Kingdom: Oxford University Press.

Mann, D. L., Zipes, D. P., Libby, P., & Bonow, R. D. (2014). *Braunwald's heart disease: A textbook of cardiovascular medicine* (10th ed.). St. Louis, MO: Saunders | Elsevier.

McLaughlin, M. A. (clinical ed.) (2014). *Cardiovascular care made incredibly easy* (3rd ed.). Philadelphia, PA: Wolters Kluwer.

Neumar, R. W., Otto, C. W., Link, M. S., Kronick, S. L., Shuster, M., Callaway, C. W., & Morrison, L. J. (2010). American Heart Association Guidelines for Cardiovascular Resuscitation and Emergency Cardiovascular Care Science, Part 8.4: Management of Symptomatic Bradycardia and Tachycardia. *Circulation, 122*: S746–S757.

Keep going...you're halfway through this book!

Chapter 8

Atrioventricular blocks

Just the facts

In this chapter, you'll learn:

◆ the proper way to identify the various forms of atrioventricular (AV) block and interpret their rhythms
◆ the reason that AV block is a significant arrhythmia
◆ patients who at risk for developing AV block
◆ signs and symptoms of AV block
◆ nursing care for patients with AV block.

A look at AV block

Atrioventricular (AV) heart block results from an interruption in the conduction of impulses between the atria and ventricles. AV block can be total or partial or it may delay conduction. The block can occur at the AV node, the bundle of His, or the bundle branches.

The heart's electrical impulses normally originate in the sinoatrial (SA) node, so when those impulses are blocked at the AV node, atrial rates are commonly normal (60 to 100 beats/min). The clinical effect of the block depends on how many impulses are completely blocked, how slow the ventricular rate is as a result, and how the block ultimately affects the heart. A slow ventricular rate can decrease cardiac output, possibly causing light-headedness, hypotension, and confusion.

The cause before the block

Various factors can lead to AV block, including underlying heart conditions, use of certain drugs, congenital anomalies, and conditions that disrupt the cardiac conduction system. (See *Causes of AV block*, page 168.)

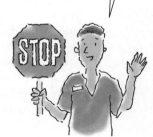

In AV block, the impulses between the atria and ventricles are totally stopped, partially stopped, or delayed.

Causes of AV block

Atrioventricular (AV) blocks can be temporary or permanent. Here's a look at causes of each kind of AV block.

Causes of temporary block
- Myocardial infarction (MI), usually inferior wall MI
- Digoxin (Lanoxin) toxicity
- Acute myocarditis
- Calcium channel blockers
- Beta-adrenergic blockers
- Cardiac surgery

Causes of permanent block
- Changes associated with aging
- Congenital abnormalities
- MI, usually anteroseptal MI
- Cardiomyopathy
- Cardiac surgery

Typical examples include
- myocardial ischemia, which impairs cellular function so cells repolarize more slowly or incompletely. The injured cells, in turn, may conduct impulses slowly or inconsistently. Relief of the ischemia can restore normal function to the AV node.
- myocardial infarction (MI), in which cell death occurs. If the necrotic cells are part of the conduction system, they no longer conduct impulses and a permanent AV block occurs.
- excessive dosage of, or an exaggerated response to, a drug which can cause AV block or increase the likelihood that a block will develop. Although many antiarrhythmic medications can have this effect, the drugs more commonly known to cause or exacerbate AV blocks include digoxin, beta-adrenergic blockers, and calcium channel blockers.
- congenital anomalies such as congenital ventricular septal defect that involve cardiac structures and affect the conduction system. Anomalies of the conduction system, such as an AV node that doesn't conduct impulses, can also occur in the absence of structural defects. (See *AV block in elderly patients.*)

Under the knife

AV block may also be caused by inadvertent damage to the heart's conduction system during cardiac surgery. Damage is most likely to occur in surgery involving the mitral or tricuspid valve or in the closure of a ventricular septal defect. If the injury involves tissues

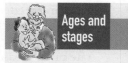
Ages and stages

AV block in elderly patients

In elderly patients, atrioventricular (AV) block may be due to fibrosis of the conduction system. Other causes include use of digoxin and the presence of aortic valve calcification.

adjacent to the surgical site and the conduction system isn't physically disrupted, the block may be only temporary. If a portion of the conduction system itself is severed, a permanent block results.

Radio blackout

Similar disruption of the conduction system can occur from a procedure called *radiofrequency ablation.* In this invasive procedure, a transvenous catheter is used to locate the area within the heart that participates in initiating or perpetuating certain tachyarrhythmias.

Radiofrequency energy is then delivered to the myocardium through this catheter to produce a small area of necrosis. The damaged tissue can no longer cause or participate in the tachyarrhythmia. If the energy is delivered close to the AV node, bundle of His, or bundle branches, block can occur.

Degrees of block

AV blocks are classified according to their severity, not their location. That severity is measured according to how well the node conducts impulses and is separated by degrees—first, second, and third. Let's take a look at them one at a time.

First-degree AV block

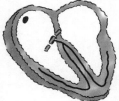

First-degree AV block occurs when impulses from the atria are consistently delayed during conduction through the AV node. All atrial impulses reach the ventricle however the conduction delay occurs within the AV node. Conduction eventually occurs; it just takes longer than normal. It's as if people are walking in a line through a doorway, but each person hesitates before crossing the threshold.

How it happens

First-degree AV block may appear normally in a healthy person or result from myocardial ischemia or infarction, myocarditis, or degenerative changes in the heart. The condition may also be caused by medications, such as digoxin, calcium channel blockers, and beta-adrenergic blockers.

First-degree AV block may be temporary, particularly if it stems from medications or ischemia early in the course of an MI. The presence of first-degree block, the least dangerous type of AV block, indicates some kind of problem in the conduction system.

Identifying first-degree AV block

This rhythm strip illustrates first-degree atrioventricular (AV) block. Look for these distinguishing characteristics:

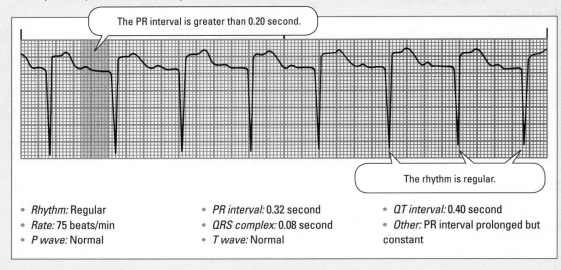

The PR interval is greater than 0.20 second.

The rhythm is regular.

- *Rhythm:* Regular
- *Rate:* 75 beats/min
- *P wave:* Normal

- *PR interval:* 0.32 second
- *QRS complex:* 0.08 second
- *T wave:* Normal

- *QT interval:* 0.40 second
- *Other:* PR interval prolonged but constant

Because first-degree AV block can progress to a more severe block, it should be monitored for changes.

What to look for

In general, a rhythm strip with this block looks like normal sinus rhythm except that the PR interval is longer than normal. (See *Identifying first-degree AV block.*) The rhythm will be regular, with one normal P wave for every QRS complex.

The PR interval will be greater than 0.20 second and will be consistent for each beat. The QRS complex is usually normal, although sometimes a bundle-branch block may occur along with first-degree AV block and cause a widening of the QRS complex.

No signs of block

Most patients with first-degree AV block show no symptoms of the block because cardiac output isn't significantly affected. If the PR interval is extremely long, a longer interval between S_1 and S_2 may be noted on cardiac auscultation.

How you intervene

Usually, just the underlying cause will be treated, not the conduction disturbance itself. For example, if a medication is causing the block, the dosage may be reduced or the medication may be discontinued. Close monitoring helps to detect progression of first-degree AV block to a more serious form of block.

When caring for a patient with first-degree AV block, evaluate him for underlying causes that can be corrected, such as medications or ischemia. Observe the ECG for progression of the block to a more severe form of block. Administer digoxin, calcium channel blockers, or beta-adrenergic blockers cautiously.

Type I second-degree AV block

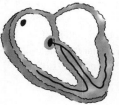

Also called *Mobitz type I block or Wenckebach,* type I second-degree AV block occurs when each successive impulse from the SA node is delayed slightly longer than the previous impulse. That pattern continues until an impulse fails to be conducted to the ventricles, and the cycle then repeats. The block generally will occur at the AV node but can also occur in the Bundle of His or the Purkinje system. It's like a line of people trying to get through a doorway, each one taking longer and longer until finally one can't get through.

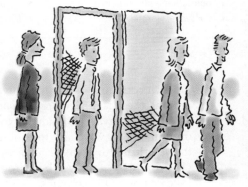

How it happens

Causes of type I second-degree AV block include coronary artery disease, inferior wall MI, and rheumatic fever. It may also be due to cardiac medications, such as beta-adrenergic blockers, digoxin, and calcium channel blockers. Increased vagal stimulation can also cause this type of block.

Type I second-degree AV block may occur normally in an otherwise healthy person. Almost always temporary, this type of block resolves when the underlying condition is corrected. Although an asymptomatic patient with this block has a good prognosis, the block may progress to a more serious form, especially if it occurs early during an MI.

What to look for

When monitoring a patient with type I second-degree AV block, you'll note that because the SA node isn't affected by this lower

Identifying type I second-degree AV block

This rhythm strip illustrates type I second-degree atrioventricular (AV) block. Look for these distinguishing characteristics:

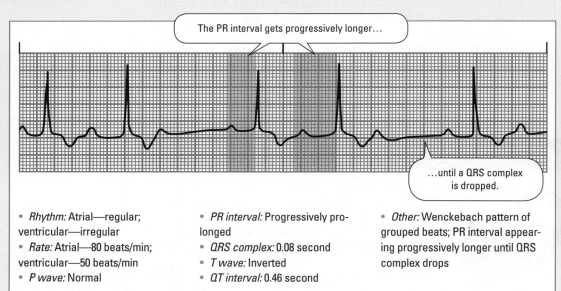

The PR interval gets progressively longer...

...until a QRS complex is dropped.

- *Rhythm:* Atrial—regular; ventricular—irregular
- *Rate:* Atrial—80 beats/min; ventricular—50 beats/min
- *P wave:* Normal

- *PR interval:* Progressively prolonged
- *QRS complex:* 0.08 second
- *T wave:* Inverted
- *QT interval:* 0.46 second

- *Other:* Wenckebach pattern of grouped beats; PR interval appearing progressively longer until QRS complex drops

block, it continues its normal activity. As a result, the atrial rhythm is normal. (See *Identifying type I second-degree AV block.*)

The PR interval gets gradually longer with each successive beat until finally a P wave fails to conduct to the ventricles. This makes the ventricular rhythm irregular, with a repeating pattern of groups of QRS complexes followed by a dropped beat in which the P wave isn't followed by a QRS complex.

Famous footprints

The pattern of grouped beating is sometimes referred to as the *footprints of Wenckebach.* (Karel Frederik Wenckebach was a Dutch internist who, at the turn of the century and long before the introduction of the ECG, described the two forms of what's now known as *second-degree AV block* by analyzing waves in the jugular venous pulse. Following the introduction of the ECG, German cardiologist Woldemar Mobitz clarified Wenckebach's findings as type I and type II.)

As you've probably noticed by now, rhythm strips have distinctive patterns. (See *Rhythm strip patterns.*)

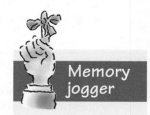

Memory jogger

To help you identify type I second-degree AV block, think of the phras e "longer, longer, drop," which describes the progressively prolonged PR intervals and the missing QRS complex. (The QRS complexes, by the way, are usually normal because the delays occur in the AV node.)

Rhythm strip patterns

The more you look at rhythm strips, the more you'll notice patterns. The symbols below represent some of the patterns you might see as you study rhythm strips.

Normal, regular (as in normal sinus rhythm)	♥ ♥ ♥ ♥ ♥ ♥
Slow, regular (as in sinus bradycardia)	♥ ♥ ♥
Fast, regular (as in sinus tachycardia)	♥ ♥ ♥ ♥ ♥ ♥ ♥ ♥ ♥ ♥ ♥ ♥
Premature (as in a premature ventricular contraction)	♥ ♥ ♥ ♥ ♥ ♥
Grouped (as in type I second-degree AV block)	♥ ♥ ♥ ♥ ♥ ♥ ♥ ♥ ♥
Irregularly irregular (as in atrial fibrillation)	♥ ♥♥ ♥ ♥ ♥♥♥ ♥ ♥
Paroxysm or burst (as in paroxysmal atrial tachycardia)	♥ ♥ ♥ ♥♥♥♥♥♥♥♥

Lonely Ps, light-headed patients

Usually asymptomatic, a patient with type I second-degree AV block may show signs and symptoms of decreased cardiac output, such as light-headedness or hypotension. Symptoms may be especially pronounced if the ventricular rate is slow.

How you intervene

No treatment is needed if the patient is asymptomatic. For a symptomatic patient, atropine may improve AV node conduction. A temporary pacemaker may be required for long-term relief of symptoms until the rhythm resolves.

When caring for a patient with this block, assess his tolerance for the rhythm and the need for treatment to improve cardiac output. Evaluate the patient for possible causes of the block, including the use of certain medications or the presence of ischemia.

Check the ECG frequently to see if a more severe type of AV block develops. Make sure the patient has a patent I.V. line. Teach him about his temporary pacemaker, if indicated.

Type II second–degree AV block

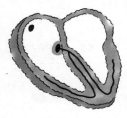

Type II second-degree AV block, also known as *Mobitz type II block,* is less common than type I but more serious. It occurs when occasional impulses from the SA node fail to conduct to the ventricles.

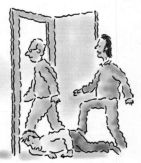

On an ECG, you won't see the PR interval lengthen before the impulse fails to conduct, as you do with type I second-degree AV block. You'll see, instead, consistent AV node conduction and an occasional dropped beat. This block is like a line of people passing through a doorway at the same speed, except that, periodically, one of them just can't get through.

How it happens

Type II second-degree AV block is usually caused by an anterior wall MI, degenerative changes in the conduction system, or severe coronary artery disease. The arrhythmia indicates a problem at the level of the bundle of His or bundle branches.

Type II block is more serious than type I because the ventricular rate tends to be slower and the cardiac output diminished. It's also more likely to cause symptoms, particularly if the sinus rhythm is slow and the ratio of conducted beats to dropped beats is low such as 2:1. (See *2:1 AV block.*) Usually chronic, type II second-degree AV block may progress to a more serious form of block. (See *High-grade AV block.*)

2:1 AV block

In 2:1 second-degree atrioventricular (AV) block, every other QRS complex is dropped, so there are always two P waves for every QRS complex. The resulting ventricular rhythm is regular.

Keep in mind that type II block is more likely to impair cardiac output, lead to symptoms such as syncope, and progress to a more severe form of block. Be sure to monitor the patient carefully.

Don't skip this strip

High-grade AV block

When two or more successive atrial impulses are blocked, the conduction disturbance is called *high-grade atrioventricular (AV) block*. Expressed as a ratio of atrial-to-ventricular beats, this block will be at least 3:1. With the prolonged refractory period of this block, latent pacemakers can discharge. As a result, you'll commonly see escape rhythms develop.

Complications

High-grade AV block causes severe complications. For instance, decreased cardiac output and reduced heart rate can combine to cause Stokes–Adams syncopal attacks. In addition, high-grade AV block usually progresses quickly to third-degree block. Look for these distinguishing characteristics:

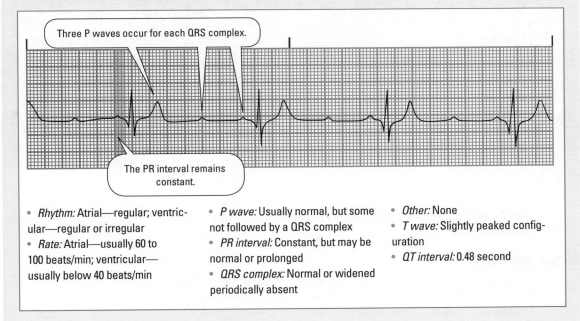

Three P waves occur for each QRS complex.

The PR interval remains constant.

- *Rhythm:* Atrial—regular; ventricular—regular or irregular
- *Rate:* Atrial—usually 60 to 100 beats/min; ventricular—usually below 40 beats/min

- *P wave:* Usually normal, but some not followed by a QRS complex
- *PR interval:* Constant, but may be normal or prolonged
- *QRS complex:* Normal or widened periodically absent

- *Other:* None
- *T wave:* Slightly peaked configuration
- *QT interval:* 0.48 second

What to look for

When monitoring a rhythm strip, look for an atrial rhythm that's regular and a ventricular rhythm that may be regular or irregular, depending on the block. (See *Identifying type II second-degree AV block,* page 176.) If the block is intermittent, the rhythm is irregular. If the block is constant, such as 2:1 or 3:1, the rhythm is regular.

Overall, the strip will look as if someone erased some QRS complexes. The PR interval will be constant for all conducted beats but

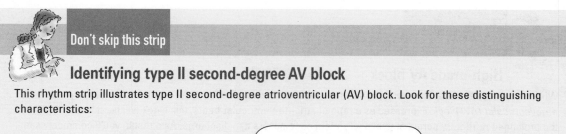

Identifying type II second-degree AV block

This rhythm strip illustrates type II second-degree atrioventricular (AV) block. Look for these distinguishing characteristics:

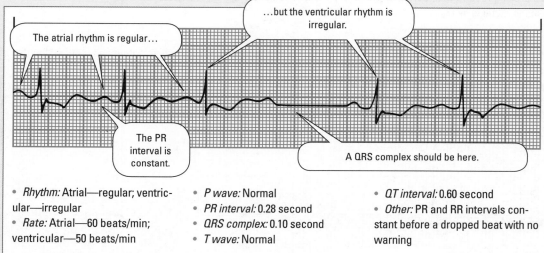

- *Rhythm:* Atrial—regular; ventricular—irregular
- *Rate:* Atrial—60 beats/min; ventricular—50 beats/min

- *P wave:* Normal
- *PR interval:* 0.28 second
- *QRS complex:* 0.10 second
- *T wave:* Normal

- *QT interval:* 0.60 second
- *Other:* PR and RR intervals constant before a dropped beat with no warning

may be prolonged. The QRS complex is usually wide, but normal complexes may occur.

Jumpin' palpitations!

Most patients who experience a few dropped beats remain asymptomatic as long as cardiac output is maintained. As the number of dropped beats increases, patients may experience palpitations, fatigue, dyspnea, chest pain, or light-headedness. On physical examination, you may note hypotension, and the pulse may be slow and regular or irregular.

How you intervene

If the dropped beats are infrequent and the patient shows no symptoms of decreased cardiac output, the practitioner may choose only to observe the rhythm, particularly if the cause is thought to be reversible. If the patient is hypotensive, treatment aims to improve cardiac output by increasing the heart rate. Atropine, dopamine, or epinephrine may be given for symptomatic bradycardia. Discontinue digoxin, if it's the cause of the arrhythmia.

Because the conduction block occurs in the His–Purkinje system, transcutaneous pacing should be initiated quickly.

Pacemaker place

Type II second-degree AV block commonly requires placement of a pacemaker. A temporary pacemaker may be used until a permanent pacemaker can be placed.

When caring for a patient with type II second-degree block, assess his tolerance for the rhythm and the need for treatment to improve cardiac output. Evaluate for possible correctable causes such as ischemia.

Keep the patient on bed rest, if indicated, to reduce myocardial oxygen demands. Administer oxygen therapy as ordered. Observe the patient for progression to a more severe form of AV block. If the patient receives a pacemaker, teach him and his family about its use.

Third-degree AV block

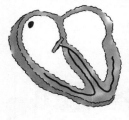

Also called *complete heart block,* third-degree AV block occurs when impulses from the atria are completely blocked at the AV node and can't be conducted to the ventricles. Maintaining our doorway analogy, this form of block is like a line of people waiting to go through a doorway, but no one can go through.

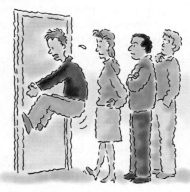

Beats of different drummers

Acting independently, the atria, generally under the control of the SA node, tend to maintain a regular rate of 60 to 100 beats/min. The ventricular rhythm can originate from the AV node and maintain a rate of 40 to 60 beats/min. Most typically, it originates from the Purkinje system in the ventricles and maintains a rate of 20 to 40 beats/min. The QRS complexes often resemble an escape rhythm.

The rhythm strip will look like a strip of P waves laid independently over a strip of QRS complexes. Note that the P wave doesn't conduct the QRS complex that follows it.

How it happens

Third-degree AV block that originates at the level of the AV node is most commonly a congenital condition. This block may also be caused by coronary artery disease, an anterior or inferior wall MI, degenerative changes in the heart, digoxin toxicity, calcium channel blockers, beta-adrenergic blockers, or surgical injury. It may be temporary or permanent. (See *Heart block after congenital heart repair.*)

Because the ventricular rate is so slow, third-degree AV block presents a potentially life-threatening situation because cardiac output can drop dramatically. In addition, the patient loses his atrial kick—extra 30% of blood flow pushed into the ventricles by atrial contraction. That happens as a result of the loss of synchrony between the atrial and ventricular contractions. The loss of atrial kick further decreases cardiac output. Any exertion on the part of the patient can worsen symptoms.

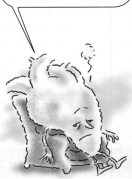

In third-degree AV block, the patient loses his atrial kick, which presents a potentially life-threatening situation.

What to look for

When analyzing an ECG for this rhythm, you'll note that the atrial and ventricular rhythms are regular. The P and R waves can be "walked out" across the strip, meaning that they appear to march across the strip in rhythm. (See *Identifying third-degree AV block.*)

Some P waves may be buried in QRS complexes or T waves. The PR interval will vary with no pattern or regularity. If the resulting rhythm, called the *escape rhythm*, originates in the AV node, the QRS complex will be normal and the ventricular rate will be 40 to 60 beats/min. If the escape rhythm originates in the Purkinje system, the QRS complex will be wide, with a ventricular rate below 40 beats/min.

Escape!

The PR interval varies because the atria and ventricles beat independently of each other. The QRS complex is determined by the site of the escape rhythm. Usually, the duration and configuration are normal; however, with an idioventricular escape rhythm (an escape rhythm originating in the ventricles), the duration is greater than 0.12 second and the complex is distorted.

While atrial and ventricular rates can vary with third-degree block, they're nearly the same with complete AV dissociation, a similar rhythm. (See *Complete AV dissociation*, page 180.)

Serious signs and symptoms

Most patients with third-degree AV block experience significant symptoms, including severe fatigue, dyspnea, chest pain, light-headedness, changes in mental status, pulmonary edema, and loss of consciousness. You may note hypotension, pallor, diaphoresis, bradycardia, and a variation in the intensity of the pulse.

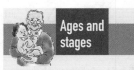

Ages and stages

Heart block after congenital heart repair

After repair of a ventricular septal defect, a child may require a permanent pacemaker if complete heart block develops. This arrhythmia may develop from interference with the bundle of His during surgery.

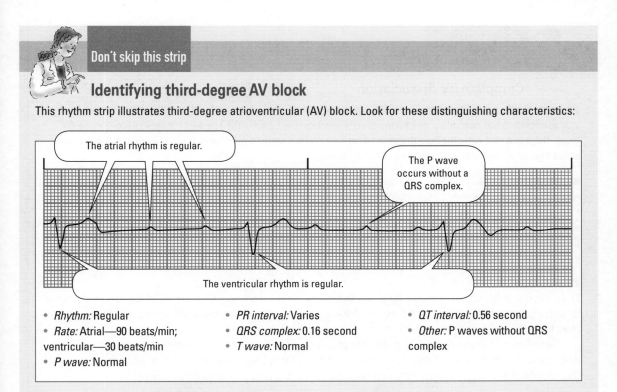

Don't skip this strip

Identifying third-degree AV block

This rhythm strip illustrates third-degree atrioventricular (AV) block. Look for these distinguishing characteristics:

The atrial rhythm is regular.

The P wave occurs without a QRS complex.

The ventricular rhythm is regular.

* *Rhythm:* Regular
* *Rate:* Atrial—90 beats/min; ventricular—30 beats/min
* *P wave:* Normal

* *PR interval:* Varies
* *QRS complex:* 0.16 second
* *T wave:* Normal

* *QT interval:* 0.56 second
* *Other:* P waves without QRS complex

A few patients will be relatively free from symptoms, complaining only that they can't tolerate exercise and that they're often tired for no apparent reason. The severity of symptoms depends to a great extent on the resulting ventricular rate.

How you intervene

If cardiac output isn't adequate or the patient's condition seems to be deteriorating, therapy aims to improve the ventricular rate. Atropine may be given, or a temporary pacemaker may be used to restore adequate cardiac output. Dopamine and epinephrine may also be indicated.

Temporary pacing may be required until the cause of the block resolves or until a permanent pacemaker can be inserted. A permanent block requires placement of a permanent pacemaker.

Don't skip this strip

Complete AV dissociation

With both third-degree atrioventricular (AV) block and complete AV dissociation, the atria and ventricles beat independently, each controlled by its own pacemaker. However, here's the key difference: In third-degree AV block, the atrial rate is faster than the ventricular rate. With complete AV dissociation, the two rates are usually about the same, with the ventricular rate slightly faster.

Rhythm disturbances

Never the primary problem, complete AV dissociation results from one of three underlying rhythm disturbances:

• slowed or impaired sinus impulse formation or sinoatrial conduction, as in sinus bradycardia or sinus arrest
• accelerated impulse formation in the AV junction or the ventricle, as in accelerated junctional or ventricular tachycardia
• AV conduction disturbance, as in complete AV block

When to treat

The clinical significance of complete AV dissociation—as well as treatment for the arrhythmia—depends on the underlying cause and its effect on the patient. If the underlying rhythm decreases cardiac output, the patient will need treatment to correct the arrhythmia.

Depending on the underlying cause, the patient may be treated with an antiarrhythmic, such as atropine and isoproterenol, to restore synchrony. Alternatively, the patient may be given a pacemaker to support a slow ventricular rate. If drug toxicity caused the original disturbance, the drug should be discontinued.

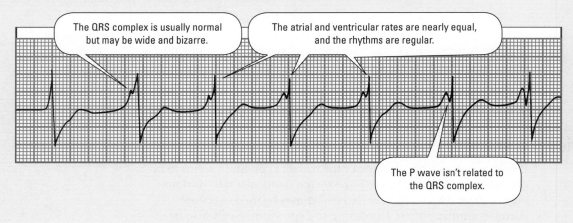

The QRS complex is usually normal but may be wide and bizarre.

The atrial and ventricular rates are nearly equal, and the rhythms are regular.

The P wave isn't related to the QRS complex.

Bundles of troubles

The patient with an anterior wall MI is more likely to have permanent third-degree AV block if the MI involved the bundle of His or the bundle branches than if it involved other areas of the myocardium. Those patients commonly require prompt placement of a permanent pacemaker.

An AV block in a patient with an inferior wall MI is more likely to be temporary, as a result of injury to the AV node. Placement of a permanent pacemaker is usually delayed in such cases to evaluate recovery of the conduction system.

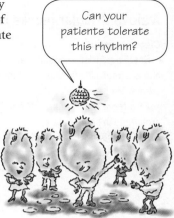

Can your patients tolerate this rhythm?

Check it out...

When caring for a patient with third-degree heart block, immediately assess the patient's tolerance of the rhythm and the need for treatment to support cardiac output and relieve symptoms. Make sure the patient has a patent I.V. catheter. Administer oxygen therapy as ordered. Evaluate for possible correctable causes of the arrhythmia, such as medications or ischemia. Minimize the patient's activity and maintain his bed rest.

That's a wrap!

Atrioventricular blocks review

AV blocks
• Result from an interruption in impulse conduction between the atria and ventricles
• Possibly occurring at the level of the AV node, the bundle of His, or the bundle branches
• Atrial rate commonly normal (60 to 100 beats/min) with slowed ventricular rate
• Classified according to severity, not location

First-degree AV block
• Occurs when impulses from the atria are consistently delayed during conduction through the AV node
• Can progress to a more severe block

Characteristics
• ECG shows normal sinus rhythm except for prolonged PR interval
• *Rhythms:* Regular
• *P wave:* Normal
• *PR interval:* Consistent for each beat; greater than 0.20 second
• *QRS complex:* Normal; occasionally widened due to bundle-branch block
• *QT interval:* Normal

Treatment
• Correction of the underlying cause

Type I second-degree AV block
• Also called *Mobitz type I block*

Characteristics
• *Rhythms:* Atrial—regular; ventricular—irregular
• *Rates:* Atrial rate exceeds ventricular rate
• *P wave:* Normal
• *PR interval:* Gradually gets longer with each beat until P wave fails to conduct to the ventricles
• *QRS complex:* Usually normal
• *T wave:* Normal

Treatment
• No treatment if asymptomatic
• Atropine to improve AV conduction
• Temporary pacemaker insertion

Type II second-degree AV block
• Also known as *Mobitz II block*
• Occasional impulses from the SA node fail to conduct to the ventricles

(continued)

Atrioventricular blocks review *(Continued)*

Characteristics

- *Rhythms:* Atrial—regular; ventricular—irregular if block is intermittent, regular if block is constant (such as 2:1 or 3:1)
- *PR interval:* Constant for all conducted beats, may be prolonged in some cases
- *QRS complex:* Usually wide
- *T wave:* Normal
- *Other:* PR and RR intervals constant before a dropped beat with no warning

Treatment

- Temporary or permanent pacemaker insertion
- Atropine, dopamine, or epinephrine for symptomatic bradycardia
- Discontinuation of digoxin if appropriate

Third-degree AV block

- Also known as *complete heart block*
- Impulses from the atria completely blocked at the AV node and not conducted to the ventricles

Characteristics

- *Rhythms:* Atrial—regular; ventricular—regular
- *Rates:* Atrial rate exceeds ventricular rate
- *P wave:* Normal
- *PR interval:* Variations with no regularity; no relation between P waves and QRS complexes

- *QRS complex:* Normal (junctional pacemaker) or wide and bizarre (ventricular pacemaker)
- *T wave:* Normal
- *Other:* P waves without QRS complex

Treatment

- Correction of the underlying cause
- Temporary or permanent pacemaker
- Atropine, dopamine, or epinephrine for symptomatic bradycardia

Complete AV dissociation

- Atria and ventricles beat independently, each controlled by its own pacemaker

Characteristics

- *Rates:* Atrial and ventricular rates are nearly equal with ventricular rate slightly faster
- *Rhythms:* Regular
- *P wave:* No relation to QRS
- *QRS complex:* Usually normal; may be wide and bizarre

Treatment

- Correction of the underlying cause
- Atropine or isoproterenol to restore synchrony
- Pacemaker insertion

Quick quiz

1. No treatment is necessary if the patient has the form of AV block known as:
- A. first-degree AV block.
- B. type II second-degree AV block.
- C. third-degree AV block.
- D. complete AV dissociation.

Answer: A. A patient with first-degree AV block rarely experiences symptoms and usually requires only monitoring for progression of the block.

2. In type I second-degree AV block, the PR interval:
    A. varies according to the ventricular response rate.
    B. progressively lengthens until a QRS complex is dropped.
    C. remains constant despite an irregular ventricular rhythm.
    D. is unmeasurable.

Answer: B. Progressive lengthening of the PR interval creates an irregular ventricular rhythm with a repeating pattern of groups of QRS complexes. Those groups are followed by a dropped beat in which the P wave isn't followed by a QRS complex.

3. Myocardial ischemia may cause cells in the AV node to repolarize:
    A. normally.
    B. more quickly than normal.
    C. more slowly than normal.
    D. in a retrograde fashion.

Answer: C. Injured cells conduct impulses slowly or inconsistently. Relief of the ischemia can restore normal function to the AV node.

4. Type II second-degree AV block is generally considered more serious than type I because in most cases of type II the:
    A. cardiac output is diminished.
    B. ventricular rate rises above 100 beats/min.
    C. peripheral vascular system shuts down almost as soon as the arrhythmia begins.
    D. atrial rate rises above 100 beats/min.

Answer: A. This form of AV block causes a decrease in cardiac output, particularly if the sinus rhythm is slow and the ratio of conducted beats to dropped beats is low such as 2:1.

5. AV block can be caused by inadvertent damage to the heart's conduction system during cardiac surgery. Damage is most likely to occur in surgery involving which area of the heart?
    A. Pulmonic or tricuspid valve
    B. Mitral or pulmonic valve
    C. Aortic or mitral valve
    D. Mitral or tricuspid valve

Answer: D. AV block can be caused by surgery involving the mitral or tricuspid valve or in the closure of a ventricular septal defect.

6. A main component of the treatment for third-degree AV block is:
    A. use of a pacemaker.
    B. administration of calcium channel blockers.
    C. administration of oxygen and antiarrhythmics.
    D. administration of beta-adrenergic blockers.

Answer: A. Temporary pacing may be required for this rhythm disturbance until the cause of the block resolves or until a permanent pacemaker can be implanted. Permanent third-degree AV block requires placement of a permanent pacemaker.

7. Treatment of first-degree AV block is aimed at correcting the underlying cause. Which of the following may cause first-degree AV block?

    A. Stress
    B. Digoxin
    C. Angiotensin-converting enzyme inhibitors
    D. Physical exertion

Answer: B. First-degree AV block may be caused by MI or ischemia, myocarditis, degenerative changes in the heart, and such medications as digoxin, calcium channel blockers, and beta-adrenergic blockers.

Test strips

Okay, try these test strips. Using the 8-step method for interpretation, fill in the blanks below with the particular characteristics of the strip. Then check your answers with ours.

Strip 1

Atrial rhythm: _____

Ventricular rhythm: _____

Atrial rate: _____

Ventricular rate: _____

P wave: _____

PR interval: _____

QRS complex: _____

T wave: _____

QT interval: _____

Other: _____

Interpretation: _____

Strip 2

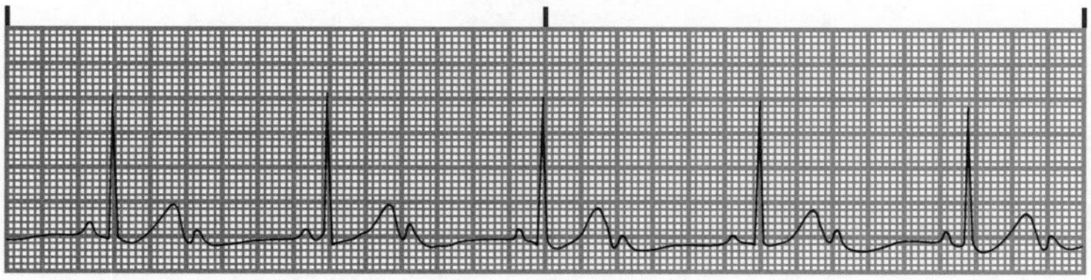

Atrial rhythm: _____

Ventricular rhythm: _____

Atrial rate: _____

Ventricular rate: _____

P wave: _____

PR interval: _____

QRS complex: _____

T wave: _____

QT interval: _____

Other: _____

Interpretation: _____

Strip 3

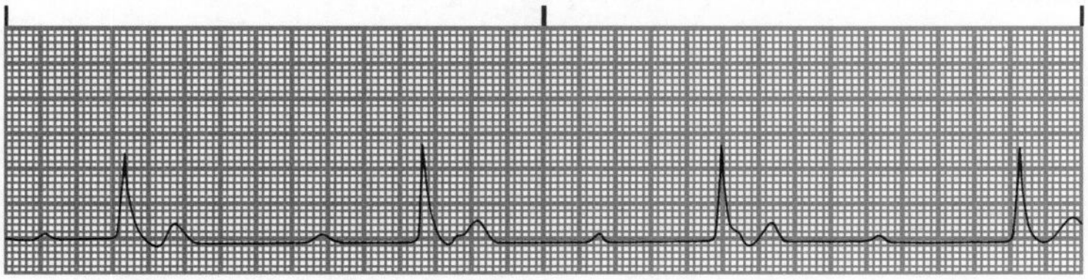

Atrial rhythm: _____

Ventricular rhythm: _____

Atrial rate: _____

Ventricular rate: _____

P wave: _____

PR interval: _____

QRS complex: _____

T wave: _____

QT interval: _____

Other: _____

Interpretation: _____

Answers to test strips

1. Rhythm: Regular atrial and ventricular rhythms
   Rate: 75 beats/min
   P wave: Normal size and configuration
   PR interval: 0.34 second
   QRS complex: 0.08 second
   T wave: Normal configuration
   QT interval: 0.42 second
   Other: None
   Interpretation: Normal sinus rhythm with first-degree AV block

2. Rhythm: Regular atrial and ventricular rhythms
   Rate: Atrial rates are 100 beats/min; ventricular rates are 50 beats/min
   P wave: Normal size and configuration
   PR interval: 0.14 second
   QRS complex: 0.06 second
   T wave: Normal configuration
   QT interval: 0.44 second
   Other: Two P waves for each QRS
   Interpretation: Type II second-degree AV block

3. Rhythm: Regular atrial and ventricular rhythms
   Rate: Atrial rates are 75 beats/min; ventricular rates are 36 beats/min
   P wave: Normal size; no constant relationship to QRS complex
   PR interval: N/A
   QRS complex: 0.16 second; wide and bizarre
   T wave: Normal except for second beat distorted by a P wave
   QT interval: 0.42 second
   Interpretation: Third-degree AV block

Scoring

★★★ If you correctly answered all seven questions and filled in all the blanks, way to go! We're willing to bet 2:1 that you're aces when it comes to AV block.

★★ If you answered six questions correctly and correctly filled in most of the blanks, good job! No real intervention is necessary; we'll just continue to monitor your progress.

★ If you answered fewer than six questions correctly and missed most of the blanks, give it another go. We certainly won't block your impulse to reread the chapter.

Recommended references

Brown, D. F. M., & Martindale, J. L. (2012). *Rapid interpretation of ECG's in emergency medicine.* Philadelphia, PA: Wolters Kluwer.

Crisel, R. K., Farzaneh-Far, R., Na, B., & Whooley, M. A. (2011). First-degree atrioventricular block is associated with heart failure and death in persons with stable coronary artery disease: Data from the Heart and Soul Study. *European Heart Journal, 32*(15), 1875–1880.

McLaughlin, M. A. (2014). *Cardiovascular care made incredibly easy* (3rd ed.). Philadelphia, PA: Wolters Kluwer.

Neumar, R. W., Otto, C. W., Link, M. S., Kronick, S. L., Shuster, M., Callaway, C. W., ... Morrison, L. J. (2010). American Heart Association Guidelines for Cardiovascular Resuscitation and Emergency Cardiovascular Care Science, Part 8.4: Management of Symptomatic Bradycardia and Tachycardia. *Circulation, 122,* S746–S757.

Wagner, G. S., & Strauss, D. G. (2013). *Marriott's practical electrocardiology* (12th ed.). Philadelphia, PA: Wolters Kluwer.

Part III

Treating arrhythmias

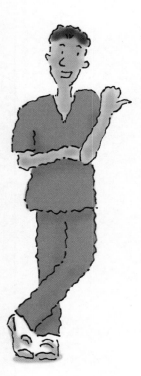

Chapter 9

Nonpharmacologic treatments

Just the facts

In this chapter, you'll learn:

♦ nonpharmacologic treatments of arrhythmias and how they work

♦ ways to identify and treat complications of nonpharmacologic treatments

♦ nursing care for patients receiving nonpharmacologic treatments

♦ patient teaching points for nonpharmacologic treatments.

A look at pacemakers

A pacemaker is an artificial device that electrically stimulates the myocardium to depolarize, which begins a contraction.

Pacemakers are usually used for (1) bradycardia caused by sinus node dysfunction, medications, or atrioventricular block, and (2) cardiac dyssynchrony due to advanced heart failure. The device may be temporary or permanent, depending on the patient's condition. Pacemakers are commonly necessary for the aging heart and following myocardial infarction or cardiac surgery.

And the beat goes on...

Pacemakers work by generating an impulse from a power source and transmitting that impulse to the heart muscle. The impulse flows throughout the heart and causes the heart muscle to depolarize. Pacemakers consist of three components: the pulse generator, the pacing leads, and the electrodes at the tips of the pacing leads.

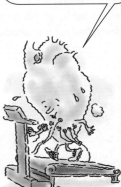

Keep up to pace with pacemaker information!

Making the pacer work

The pulse generator contains the pacemaker's power source and circuitry. The lithium batteries in a permanent or implanted pacemaker are its power source and last about 10 years. The circuitry of the pacemaker is a microchip that guides heart pacing.

A temporary pacemaker, which isn't implanted, is about the size of a small radio or a telemetry box and is powered by alkaline batteries. These units also contain a microchip and are programmed by a touch pad or dials.

A stimulus on the move

An electrical stimulus from the pulse generator moves through wires (referred to as pacing leads or leads) to the electrode tips. The leads for a pacemaker designed to stimulate a single heart chamber are

A look at pacing leads

Pacing leads have either one electrode (unipolar) or two (bipolar). These illustrations show the difference between the two leads.

Unipolar lead
In a unipolar system, electric current moves from the pulse generator through the pacing lead to the negative pole at the tip of the pacing lead. From there, it stimulates the heart and returns to the pulse generator's metal surface (the positive pole) to complete the circuit.

Bipolar lead
In a bipolar system, current flows from the pulse generator through the pacing lead to the negative pole at the tip. At that point, it stimulates the heart and then travels to the positive pole within the pacing lead to complete the circuit.

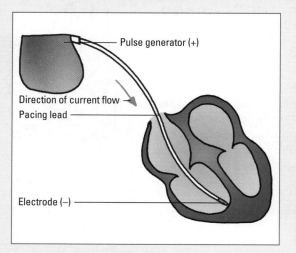

Pulse generator (+)

Direction of current flow
Pacing lead

Electrode (−)

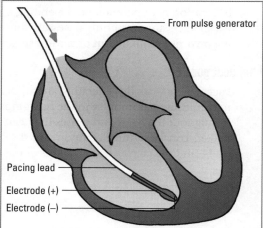

From pulse generator

Pacing lead
Electrode (+)
Electrode (−)

placed in either the atrium or the ventricle. For dual-chamber, or AV, pacing, the leads are placed in both chambers, usually on the right side of the heart.

One lead or two

The electrodes—one on a unipolar lead or two on a bipolar lead—send information about electrical impulses in the myocardium back to the pulse generator. The pulse generator senses the heart's electrical activity and responds according to how it has been programmed.

A unipolar lead system is more sensitive to the heart's intrinsic electrical activity than is a bipolar system. A bipolar system isn't as easily affected by electrical activity outside the heart and the generator (for example, from skeletal muscle contraction or magnetic fields). (See *A look at pacing leads.*)

Working with pacemakers

On an ECG, you'll notice the spike from a unipolar system right away. (See *Pacemaker spikes.*) It occurs when the pacemaker sends an electrical impulse to the heart muscle. That impulse appears as a vertical line or spike. The spike with a bipolar system can sometimes be difficult to see.

Depending on the position of the electrode, the spike appears in different locations on the waveform.
- When the atria are stimulated by the pacemaker, the spike is followed by a P wave and then the paced or patient's intrinsic QRS complex, then the T wave. This series of waveforms represents successful capture of the atrial myocardium. The P wave may look different from the patient's intrinsic P wave.
- When the ventricles are stimulated by a pacemaker, the spike is followed by a QRS complex and a T wave. The paced QRS complex appears wider than the patient's intrinsic QRS complex because of the longer time it takes the ventricles to depolarize when paced.
- When the pacemaker stimulates both the atria and the ventricles, the first spike is followed by a P wave, then another spike, and then a QRS complex. Be aware that the type of pacemaker used and the patient's condition may affect whether every beat is paced.

Permanent and temporary pacemakers

Depending on the patient's signs and symptoms, a permanent or a temporary pacemaker can be used to maintain heart rhythm. Pacing lead placement varies according to the patient's specific needs.

Pacemaker spikes

Pacemaker impulses—the stimuli that travel from the pacemaker to the heart—are visible on the patient's ECG tracing as spikes. Large or small, pacemaker spikes appear above or below the isoelectric line. This example shows an atrial and a ventricular pacemaker spike.

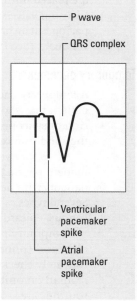

- P wave
- QRS complex
- Ventricular pacemaker spike
- Atrial pacemaker spike

Permanent pacemakers

A permanent pacemaker is used to treat chronic heart conditions such as sinus node dysfunction, AV block, or dyssynchrony. Sinus node dysfunction causing symptomatic bradycardia can be due to advanced age or drug therapy. AV block is commonly due to cardiomyopathy, cardiac surgery, or septal ablation. Dyssynchrony between all the chambers and within the left ventricle is caused by advanced cardiomyopathy. Permanent pacemakers are surgically implanted, usually under local anesthesia. (See *Placing a permanent pacemaker.*)

Pocket generator

The generator consists of a battery and microchip circuitry enclosed in a titanium case. It is implanted in a pocket made from subcutaneous tissue. The pocket is usually constructed under the clavicle. Permanent pacemakers are initially programmed during implantation. The programming sets the conditions under which the pacemaker functions and can be adjusted externally when necessary.

Permanent pacing leads

Permanent pacing leads are usually placed transvenously. They are positioned in the appropriate chambers and then anchored to the endocardium; or in the coronary sinus for left ventricular pacing. Some patients may require permanent epicardial pacing leads that are placed during cardiac surgery. This is common for patients with tricuspid valve surgery and for patients who require left ventricular pacing but a coronary sinus lead was unable to be placed transvenously. (See *Placing a permanent pacemaker.*)

Temporary pacemakers

A temporary pacemaker is commonly inserted in an emergency. The patient may show signs of decreased cardiac output, such as hypotension or syncope. The temporary pacemaker supports the patient until the condition resolves.

A temporary pacemaker can also serve as a bridge until a permanent pacemaker is inserted. Temporary pacemakers are used for patients with heart block, sinus bradycardia, or low cardiac output. Several types of temporary pacemakers are available, including transvenous, epicardial, and transcutaneous.

Temporary pacemakers should have the batteries, pacing thresholds, and connections between the pacing leads and generator routinely checked. The insertion sites should be kept sterile and be regularly monitored. Unit-based guidelines need to exist for this routine care.

Placing a permanent pacemaker

The doctor who implants the endocardial pacemaker usually selects a transvenous route and begins pacing lead placement by inserting a catheter percutaneously or by venous cutdown. Then, with a stylet and fluoroscopic guidance, the catheter is threaded through the vein until the tip reaches the endocardium.

Lead placement

For pacing lead placement in the atrium, the tip is usually anchored in the right atrium. For placement in the right ventricle, it is usually anchored within the right ventricular septum or in one of the interior muscular ridges, or *trabeculae* in the apex. Resynchronization therapy with a biventricular pacemaker requires a pacing lead to be placed in the coronary sinus which lies over the left ventricle. This enables capture of the left ventricular myocardium through the wall of the coronary sinus.

Implanting the generator

When the pacing lead is in the proper position, the pulse generator is secured in a subcutaneous pocket of tissue just below the clavicle. Changing the pacemaker's battery or microchip circuitry requires the whole generator to be changed. However, only a shallow incision over the previously made pocket and a quick generator exchange is done.

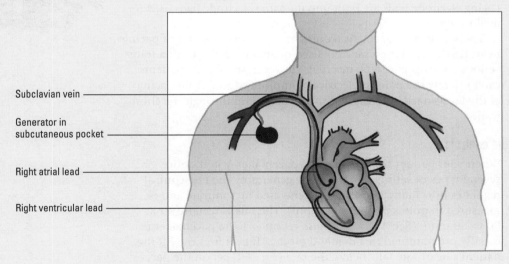

Subclavian vein

Generator in subcutaneous pocket

Right atrial lead

Right ventricular lead

Going the transvenous way

The transvenous approach may be used when inserting a temporary pacemaker in nonsurgical environments. In this method, the pacing leads are commonly inserted through the subclavian or internal jugular vein. The transvenous pacemaker is probably the most common and reliable type of temporary pacemaker. It's usually inserted at the bedside or in a fluoroscopy suite. The pacing leads are advanced through a catheter into the right ventricle or atrium and then connected to an external pulse generator.

Taking the epicardial route

Epicardial pacemakers are commonly used for patients undergoing cardiac surgery. The doctor attaches the tips of the pacing leads (thin wires) to the surface of the heart and then brings the wires through the chest wall, below the incision. They're then attached to an external pulse generator. The pacing wires are usually cut or removed several days after surgery or when the patient no longer requires them.

Following the transcutaneous path

Use of an external or transcutaneous pacemaker has become commonplace. In this non-invasive method, one electrode pad is placed over the heart on the patient's anterior chest wall, and a second is applied behind the heart on the back. An external pulse generator then emits pacing impulses that travel through the skin, muscle, and bone to the heart muscle. Transcutaneous pacing is also built into many external defibrillators for use in an emergency. In this case, the pacing electrode pads are built into the same electrode pads used for defibrillation.

Transcutaneous pacing is a quick and effective method of pacing heart rhythm and is commonly used in an emergency until a transvenous pacemaker can be inserted. However, some alert patients can't tolerate the painful electrical stimuli produced from pacing at the levels needed to capture the myocardium through the chest wall.

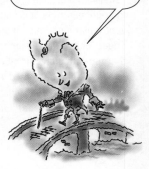

A temporary pacemaker can serve as a bridge until a permanent one can be placed. Types include transvenous, epicardial, and transcutaneous.

Setting the controls

When your patient has a temporary pacemaker, you'll notice several types of settings on the pulse generator. The rate control regulates how many impulses are generated in 1 minute and is measured in pulses per minute (ppm). The rate is usually set at 60 to 80 ppm. (See *A look at a pulse generator.*) The pacemaker is usually programmed in a demand mode. Thus, it fires only if the patient's heart rate falls below the rate (e.g., 60) set on the pacemaker. The rate may be set higher in an effort to increase cardiac output or if the patient has a tachyarrhythmia that's being treated with overdrive pacing.

Measuring the output

The electrical output of a temporary pacemaker is measured in milliamperes (mAs). First, the stimulation threshold, or the minimum amount of energy required to capture or stimulate the cardiac muscle to depolarize, is assessed. Then the pacemaker's output is set 10% higher than the stimulating threshold to ensure myocardial capture under various physiologic conditions, for example, hypokalemia.

A look at a pulse generator

This is an illustration of a single-chamber temporary pulse generator with brief descriptions of its various parts.

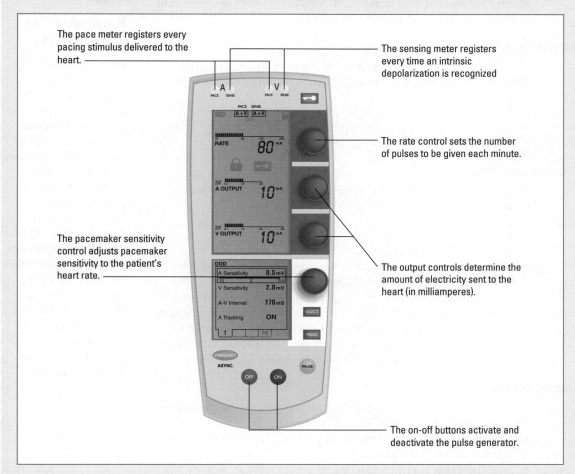

The pace meter registers every pacing stimulus delivered to the heart.

The sensing meter registers every time an intrinsic depolarization is recognized

The rate control sets the number of pulses to be given each minute.

The pacemaker sensitivity control adjusts pacemaker sensitivity to the patient's heart rate.

The output controls determine the amount of electricity sent to the heart (in milliamperes).

The on-off buttons activate and deactivate the pulse generator.

Sensing the norm

You can also program the pacemaker's sensing, or ability to sense electricity (e.g., P waves and QRS complexes). Sensing is measured and set in millivolts (mVs). Most pacemakers are programmed in a demand mode, therefore only pacing when the heart's own electrical activity is not sensed. Pacing is inhibited when the heart's own P waves and QRS complexes are sensed. This may be referred to as demand pacing. So many patients will at times have a paced rhythm and an intrinsic rhythm at other times.

Pacemaker codes

The capabilities of permanent pacemakers may be described by a generic five-letter coding system, although three letters are more commonly used. (See *Pacemaker coding system.*)

Introducing letter 1

The first letter of the code identifies the heart chambers being paced. These are the options and the letters used to signify those options:
- V = Ventricle
- A = Atrium
- D = Dual (ventricle and atrium)
- O = None

Learning about letter 2

The second letter of the code signifies the heart chamber in which the pacemaker senses the intrinsic activity:
- V = Ventricle
- A = Atrium
- D = Dual (ventricle and atrium)
- O = No sensing. When a pacemaker doesn't sense intrinsic electricity, it paces, even if intrinsic activity exists. This is referred to as asynchronous pacing. Although permanent pacemakers may be programmed this way if the patient is undergoing a procedure, temporary pacemakers should not be. Asynchronous pacing in the ventricle with a temporary pacemaker can lead to ventricular tachycardia, ventricular fibrillation, or torsades de pointes.

Looking at letter 3

The third letter indicates the pacemaker's response to the intrinsic electrical activity it senses in the atrium or ventricle:
- T = Triggers pacing (For instance, if atrial activity is sensed, ventricular pacing may be triggered.)
- I = Inhibits pacing (If the pacemaker senses intrinsic activity in a chamber, it won't fire in that chamber.)
- D = Dual (The pacemaker can be triggered or inhibited in the atrium, ventricle, or both.)
- O = None (The pacemaker doesn't respond to electrical activity.) If a pacemaker can't sense because the second letter is an *O*, then the third letter is usually also an *O*. A pacemaker that can't sense can't respond to an event.

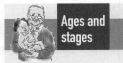

Ages and stages

Pacemakers in adult patients

Adult patients are more apt to have AV block. Therefore, they usually get a dual-chamber pacemaker. This allows for synchronous pacing and contraction between the atria and ventricles. Cardiac output and exercise tolerance are increased due to increased ventricular filling. Older adults are more prone to permanent atrial fibrillation. Since atrial pacing is not possible during atrial fibrillation, a single-chamber ventricular pacemaker is typical for these patients when they have bradycardia.

Don't be puzzled by pacemaker codes. Use a three or four-letter system.

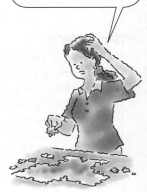

Pacemaker coding system

A coding system for pacemaker functions can provide a simple description of pacemaker capabilities. One commonly used coding system employs three letters to describe functions.

The first letter refers to the chamber paced by the pacemaker. The second refers to the chamber sensed by the pacemaker. The third refers to the pacemaker's response to the sensed event.

In the example shown here, both chambers can pace if necessary (represented in the code by the 1st *D*, for dual). Both chambers are sensed (represented in the code by the 2nd *D*, for dual). Since the 3rd letter is *D*, then pacing will be either inhibited or triggered. If intrinsic electrical activity is sensed in either the atrium or ventricle, the pacemaker will inhibit (or withhold) pacing in whichever chamber that the electricity is sensed. Sensed electricity in one chamber (e.g., the atrium) can also trigger pacing in the other chamber (e.g., the ventricle).

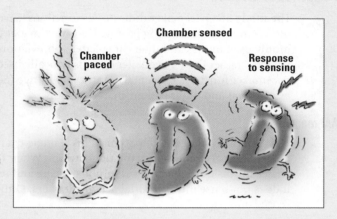

Chamber sensed

Chamber paced

Response to sensing

Figuring out letter 4

The fourth letter of the code describes rate modulation, also known as *rate responsiveness* or *rate adaptive pacing:*
- R = Rate modulation (A sensor adjusts the programmed paced heart rate in response to the patient's physiologic need. For example, increased movement or respiratory rate will increase the paced rate.) This is used for chronotropic incompetence, or when the patient's sinus node can't increase the sinus rate during increased physiologic demand.
- O = None (Rate modulation is unavailable or disabled.)

Finally, letter 5

The final letter of the code is rarely used but specifies the location or absence of multisite pacing:
- O = None (No multisite pacing is present.)
- A = Atrium or atria (Multisite pacing in the atrium or atria is present.)
- V = Ventricle or ventricles (Multisite pacing in the ventricle or ventricles is present.)
- D = Dual site (Dual site pacing in both the atrium and ventricles is present.)

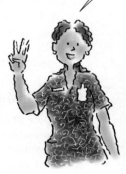

A three-letter code, rather than a five-letter code, is typically used to describe pacemaker function.

Pacemaker modes

The mode of a pacemaker indicates its functions. Several different modes may be used during pacing. Here are three of the more commonly used modes and their three-letter abbreviations. (A three-letter code, rather than a five-letter code, is typically used to describe pacemaker function.) Pacemaker rates vary by age (See *Pediatric pacemakers*) and other patient characteristics.

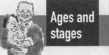

Ages and stages

Pediatric pacemakers

Many young children don't have AV block. Thus, they may get a single-chamber atrial pacemaker. The pulses per minute are initially set at an appropriate rate for the child's age. As the child grows, the heart rate can be adjusted to a lower rate.

AAI mode

The AAI, or atrial demand, pacemaker is a single-chambered pacemaker that paces and senses the right atrium. When the pacemaker senses intrinsic atrial activity, it inhibits pacing and resets itself. If it does not sense intrinsic atrial activity, it paces. Only the atria are sensed and paced.

Not in block

Because AAI pacemakers require a functioning AV node and ventricular conduction, they aren't used in AV block or ventricular bradycardia. An AAI pacemaker may be used in patients with sinus bradycardia, which may occur after cardiac surgery or with sick sinus syndrome as long as the His–Purkinje system isn't diseased.

VVI mode

The VVI, or ventricular demand, pacemaker paces and senses the ventricles. (See *AAI and VVI pacemakers.*) When it senses intrinsic ventricular activity, it inhibits pacing. This single-chambered pacemaker benefits patients with complete heart block and those needing intermittent pacing. Because it doesn't affect atrial activity, it may be used for patients with a temporary pacemaker (e.g., post cardiac surgery) who don't need an atrial kick. Atrial kick is the extra 15% to 30% of cardiac output that comes from atrial contraction. The VVI mode is also common for patients with a permanent pacemaker who have permanent atrial fibrillation.

Unsynchronized activity

If the patient has spontaneous atrial activity, the VVI pacemaker won't synchronize the ventricular activity with it. So there will be no relationship between the P waves and paced QRS complexes, and tricuspid and mitral regurgitation may develop. Sedentary patients who don't need the atrial kick, or patients with atrial fibrillation, may receive this pacemaker.

AAI and VVI pacemakers

AAI and VVI pacemakers are single-chamber pacemakers. Typically, the pacing electrode for an AAI is placed in the right atrium; and in a pacing lead in the right ventricle for a VVI pacemaker. These rhythm strips show how each pacemaker works.

AAI pacemaker

Note how the AAI pacemaker senses and paces the atria only. Each spike is immediately followed by a P-wave complex, depicting consistent capture. The QRS complex that follows occurs as a result of the heart's own AV conduction.

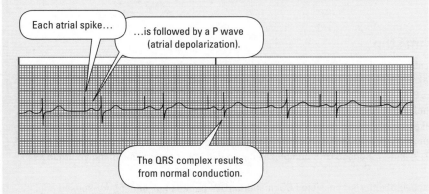

Each atrial spike…

…is followed by a P wave (atrial depolarization).

The QRS complex results from normal conduction.

VVI pacemaker

The VVI pacemaker senses and paces the ventricles. Each spike is immediately followed by a wide QRS complex, depicting consistent capture. When ALL QRS complexes are preceded by a spike, as shown here, the rhythm is said to reflect 100% pacing.

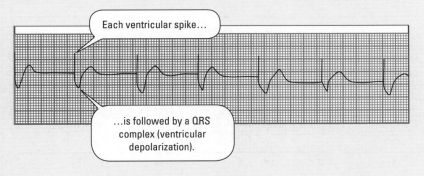

Each ventricular spike…

…is followed by a QRS complex (ventricular depolarization).

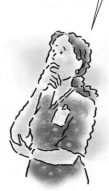

These rhythm strips show how AAI and VVI pacemakers work.

DDD mode

A DDD pacemaker is used with AV block. (See *DDD pacemaker rhythm strip*.) However, because the pacemaker possesses so many capabilities, it may be hard to troubleshoot problems. Its advantages include its

- versatility
- programmability
- ability to change modes automatically
- ability to mimic the normal physiologic cardiac cycle, maintaining AV synchrony
- ability to sense and pace the atria and ventricles at the same time according to the intrinsic atrial rate and the maximal rate limit.

DDD pacemaker rhythm strip

This DDD pacemaker rhythm strip reveals how this pacemaker ensures AV synchrony.

In the atrium: The pacemaker paces in the atrium if it does not sense an intrinsic P wave at a certain beats per minute (bpm) rate, as in beats 6, 9, 11, and 13. Therefore, a paced P wave should and does follow the atrial spike. Sensed P waves cause withholding of pacing in the atrium as in beats 1, 2, 3, 4, and 7. When the patient has an intrinsic P wave, the pacemaker serves only to make sure the ventricles respond.

In the ventricle: The pacemaker paces in the ventricle if it does not sense an intrinsic QRS complex in the ventricle, as in beats 1, 4, 6, 7, 9, and 11. Sensed QRS complexes cause withholding of pacing in the ventricle as in beats 2, 3, 5, 8, 10, and 12.

As you can see, there are several different possible ECG scenarios: AV-paced (e.g., beat 6), AV-sensed (e.g., beat 2), A-paced and V-sensed (e.g., beat 13), and A-sensed and V-paced (e.g., beat 4). This ECG strip has all four possibilities in one strip. However, patients typically have one or two scenarios in one strip. For example, a patient in sinus rhythm with only a very rare paced beat.

Also of note, these ventricularly paced beats have a QRS complex that is narrower than right ventricular paced beats. This may be due to pacing lead position (e.g., left ventricular pacing) or a QRS complex that is a result of fusion between ventricular pacing and an inherent beat.

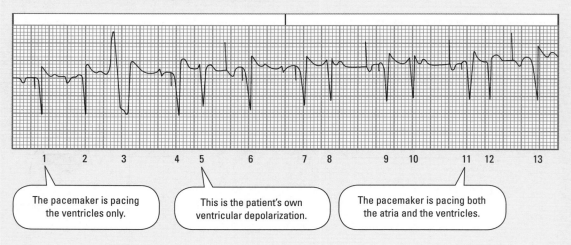

The pacemaker is pacing the ventricles only.

This is the patient's own ventricular depolarization.

The pacemaker is pacing both the atria and the ventricles.

Home, home on the rate range

Unlike other pacemakers, the DDD pacemaker is set with a rate range, rather than a single critical rate. It senses atrial activity and ensures that the ventricles track or respond to each atrial stimulation, thereby maintaining normal AV synchrony. A typical rate range is from 60 to 120 bpm. This causes pacing in the atrium once the atrial rate falls below 60. The ventricles will track (be paced after each P wave), if there is no sensed QRS complex, up to 120 bpm. A pacemaker can't stop a heart's intrinsic conduction. Therefore, even though a pacemaker's upper rate may be 120, the patient's heart rate may well exceed 120 bpm.

Taking the low road

The DDD pacemaker paces (sometimes referred to as 'fires') in the atria when the atrial rate falls below the lower set rate. If the ventricles don't respond to an atrial event, the pacemaker will pace the ventricles. (See *Evaluating a DDD pacemaker rhythm strip.*) You or the telemetry monitor may calculate the heart rate by averaging 6 or 10 seconds. However, the pacemaker calculates the heart rate between two consecutive beats. Therefore, although you or a monitor may average the heart rate as being 60 or higher, the pacemaker will pace if the patient's intrinsic rate is 59 between two consecutive beats.

Taking the high road

The upper set rate acts as a safety mechanism by preventing the pacemaker from following (or tracking) an atrial tachyarrhythmia such as atrial fibrillation, atrial tachycardia, or atrial flutter. That upper rate limit is usually set at 120 or 130 bpm. One's AV node would normally block the approximate 500 atrial bpm during atrial fibrillation from passing to the ventricle. The AF node is bypassed with a pacemaker, making the upper rate limit necessary with a DDD pacemaker.

Evaluating pacemakers

Now you're ready to find out if your patient's pacemaker is working correctly. To do this, follow the procedure described below.

1. Read the records

First, determine the pacemaker's mode and settings, particularly the rate setting. If your patient had a permanent pacemaker implanted before admission, ask him whether he has a wallet card from the

---

Evaluating a DDD pacemaker rhythm strip

Look for these possible events when examining a rhythm strip showing the activities of a DDD pacemaker:

- Intrinsic rhythm— No pacemaker activity occurs because none is needed.
- Intrinsic P wave followed by a ventricular pacemaker spike—The pacemaker is tracking the atrial rate and ensuring a ventricular response.
- Pacemaker spike before a P wave, then an intrinsic ventricular QRS complex—The atrial rate is falling below the lower rate limit, causing the atrial channel to fire. Normal conduction to the ventricles then ensues.
- Pacemaker spike before a P wave and a pacemaker spike before the QRS complex—No intrinsic activity above the lower rate limit occurs in either the atria or the ventricles.

manufacturer that notes which generator and pacing leads were implanted.

If the pacemaker was recently implanted, check the patient's records for information. Don't check only the ECG tracing—you might misinterpret it if you don't know the mode or which pacing leads the patient has.

2. Look at the 12-lead ECG

Next, review the patient's 12-lead ECG. If it isn't available, examine lead V_1 or MCL_1 on telemetry. If there is only one ventricular lead, it is usually in the right ventricle. Therefore, expect a negatively deflected paced QRS complex in V_1 or MCL_1, just as with a left bundle-branch block. An upright QRS complex in V_1 or MCL_1 may mean that the pacing lead is out of position, perhaps even perforating the septum and lodging in the left ventricle, or that there is a properly positioned pacing lead in the coronary sinus vein.

3. Scrutinize the spikes

Then select a monitoring lead that clearly shows the pacemaker spikes. Some monitors have a filter or bandwidth menu that allows adjustment for seeing larger pacemaker spikes. **Make sure to use the "paced mode" on the telemetry monitor.** If the monitor doesn't "know" it's looking at a rhythm that may have pacemaker spikes, it can interpret a pacemaker spike as a QRS complex. Therefore, a pacemaker spike that is not followed by a QRS complex without the "paced mode" on will NOT cause an important alarm.

4. Mull over the mode

When looking at the ECG tracing of a patient with a pacemaker, consider the pacemaker mode. Then interpret the paced rhythm. Does it match what you know about the pacemaker?

5. Unravel the rhythm

Look for information that tells you which chamber is paced. Is there capture? Is there a P wave or QRS complex after each atrial or ventricular spike? Or do the P waves and QRS complexes stem from intrinsic activity?

Look for information about the pacemaker's sensing ability. Do you see spikes where you wouldn't expect them? Like within or too close after a P wave or QRS complex? Remember if the pacemaker is sensing the electricity causing the P waves and QRS complexes, it should withhold a spike. Look at the rate. What's the pacing rate per minute? Is it appropriate given the pacemaker upper and lower rate

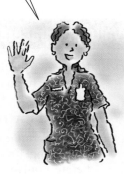

Check out these five procedure points to find out if your patient's pacemaker is working correctly.

setting? Although you can determine the rate quickly by counting the number of complexes in a 6-second ECG strip, a more accurate method is to count the number of small boxes between two complexes and divide this into 1,500.

Troubleshooting problems

Pacemaker malfunction can lead to arrhythmias and/or loss of AV synchrony. (See *When a temporary pacemaker malfunctions,* page 206.) If you see questionable pacemaker activity for a patient with a permanent pacemaker, call the cardiology or cardiac electrophysiology team. There are actions you should take for patients with temporary pacemakers who have questionable pacemaker activity. Pacemaker problems that can lead to low cardiac output, hypotension, syncope, and death include
- failure to capture
- failure to pace
- undersensing
- oversensing.

Failure to capture

Failure to capture is indicated on an ECG by a pacemaker spike without the appropriate atrial or ventricular response—a spike without a complex. Think of failure to capture as the pacemaker's inability to stimulate the chamber to contract.

Causes include hypoxia, acidosis, an electrolyte imbalance, fibrosis, an incorrect lead position, a low pacing output setting (milliampere with temporary pacemakers and volts with permanent pacemakers), depletion of the battery, a broken or cracked pacing lead, or perforation of the pacing lead through the myocardium. It can lead to asystole.

Failure to pace

Failure to pace is indicated by no pacemaker activity or spike at the set rate on an ECG. The problem is caused by battery or circuit failure, cracked or broken pacing leads, loose connections, oversensing, or the pacing output set too low. It can also lead to asystole.

Undersensing

Undersensing is demonstrated by a pacemaker spike when intrinsic cardiac activity is already present. When electricity is not sensed, the pacemaker paces even if intrinsic electricity is present. Think of it as help being given when none is needed. With undersensing, spikes occur on the ECG where they shouldn't. Although they may appear in any part of the cardiac cycle, the spikes are especially dangerous

Mixed signals

When a temporary pacemaker malfunctions

Occasionally, pacemakers fail to function properly. When that happens, you need to take immediate action to correct the problem. The strips shown below are examples of problems that can occur with a temporary pacemaker and corrective actions to take in response.

Failure to capture

- If the patient's condition has changed, notify the practitioner and ask for new settings. Be prepared to initiate cardiopulmonary resuscitation (CPR) if needed.
- If pacemaker settings have been altered by the patient or someone else, return them to their correct positions. If the pacemaker has dials, make sure the face of the pacemaker is covered with its plastic shield and remind the patient not to touch the dials.
- If the heart still doesn't respond, carefully check all connections. You can also increase the milliampere setting slowly (according to your facility's policy or the practitioner's orders), turn the patient from side to side, or change the battery. Keep in mind that the practitioner may order a chest X-ray to determine the position of the pacing lead.

Failure to pace

- If the pacing light is flashing, check the connections to the cable and the patient. The position of the pacing lead in the patient may need to be repositioned (usually under fluoroscopy).
- If the pulse generator is turned on but the indicators aren't flashing, change the battery. If that doesn't help, use a different pulse generator.
- Decrease the sensitivity by increasing the millivolts. The pacemaker may be inhibiting pacing due to oversensing electrical activity from another heart chamber, muscle, or external source.
- Make sure a transcutaneous pacemaker, isoproterenol, and atropine are available in case the patient's heart rate drops. Be prepared to initiate CPR if needed.

Failure to sense intrinsic beats

- If the pacemaker is undersensing (it fires but at the wrong times or for the wrong reasons), put the sensitivity control to a smaller number.
- Change the battery or pulse generator.
- Remove items in the room that might cause electromechanical interference. Check if the bed is grounded. Unplug each piece of equipment, and then check to see if the interference stops.
- If the pacemaker still fires on the T wave, turn off the pacemaker (per facility policy or practitioner's order). Make sure isoproterenol, atropine, and transcutaneous pacemaker are available in case the patient's heart rate drops, and be prepared to initiate CPR if needed.

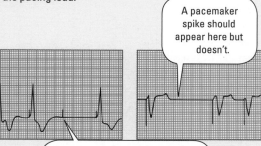

A pacemaker spike should appear here but doesn't.

There is a pacemaker spike but no response from the heart.

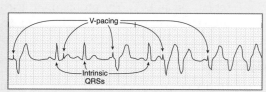

Undersensing causing inappropriate early pacing, R-on-T, and VT.

with a temporary pacemaker if they fall on the T wave. This can cause "R-on-T," resulting in ventricular tachycardia, ventricular fibrillation, or torsade de pointes. The output of a temporary pacemaker is much higher than that of a permanent pacemaker. Therefore, undersensing with a temporary pacemaker as opposed to a permanent pacemaker, can lead to a fatal arrhythmia. With a permanent pacemaker, the unneeded pacing would most likely result in early battery depletion.

The problem can be caused by millivoltage set too high, electrolyte imbalances, disconnection or dislodgment of a lead, improper pacing lead placement, edema or fibrosis at the electrode tip, drug interactions, or a depleted or dead pacemaker battery.

Oversensing

If the pacemaker is too sensitive, it can misinterpret other electricity as the heart's electricity and therefore withhold pacing. This extraneous electricity can be from myopotentials from nearby muscle movement, electrical events in a different chamber, electricity from nongrounded items, or certain equipment that has a strong magnetic or electrical field. You should wear rubber gloves when handling exposed temporary pacing wires. This will prevent you from transmitting electrical current from static or ungrounded equipment to the patient. Likewise, temporary pacing wires should be covered with something nonconductive, like the finger of a rubber glove. Oversensing causes inhibition of pacing when the patient actually needs it. The heart rate, AV synchrony, and cardiac output won't be maintained. This can cause asystole, hypotension, and/or syncope.

How you intervene

Make sure you're familiar with different types and modes of pacemakers and how they function. This will save you time and worry during an emergency. When caring for a patient with a pacemaker, follow these guidelines.

Checks and balances

Temporary pacemakers

- Assist with pacemaker insertion as appropriate.
- Regularly check the patient's pacemaker settings, connections, and functions.
- Reposition the patient carefully. Turning may dislodge the pacing wire.
- Avoid potential microshocks to the patient by ensuring that electrical equipment is grounded properly, including the patient's bed.

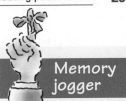

Memory jogger

Malfunction of a pacemaker can lead to fatal arrhythmias, hypotension, and syncope. To help you remember common pacemaker problems think "failure times two, under, over":

failure to capture—spike without a P wave or QRS complex following it

failure to pace—no spike on ECG at the rate set

undersensing—spike when intrinsic activity already present

oversensing—no spike when patient needs it.

Familiarize yourself with the various types and modes of pacemakers and how they work.

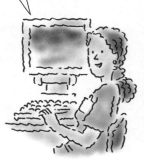

All pacemakers

- Remember that pacemaker spikes on the monitor don't mean there is capture or that your patient is stable. Be sure to check his vital signs and assess for signs and symptoms of decreased cardiac output, such as hypotension, chest pain, dyspnea, and syncope.
- Turn the telemetry monitor's "paced mode" on.
- Monitor the patient to see how well he tolerates the pacemaker.

On the alert

- Be alert for signs of infection.
- Look for pectoral or diaphragmatic muscle twitching or hiccups that occur in synchrony with the pacemaker. Both are signs of stimulation of a structure other than the heart, which may be serious. Notify the practitioner if you note either condition.
- Watch for a perforated ventricle and cardiac tamponade. Signs and symptoms include persistent hiccups, distant heart sounds, pulsus paradoxus (a drop in the strength of a pulse or a drop in systolic blood pressure greater than 10 mm Hg during inspiration), hypotension with narrowed pulse pressure, cyanosis, distended jugular veins, decreased urine output, restlessness, and complaints of fullness in the chest. Notify the practitioner immediately if you note any of these signs and symptoms.
- Watch for pneumothorax signs and symptoms, including shortness of breath, restlessness, and hypoxia. Mental status changes and arrhythmias may also occur. Palpate for subcutaneous air, which feels crunchy under your fingers, around the pacemaker insertion site. Auscultate for diminished breath sounds over the pneumothorax, usually at the apex of the lung on the side where the pacemaker was placed. Notify the practitioner if you suspect pneumothorax.
- Assess the area around the incision and report swelling, tenderness, drainage, redness, unusual warmth, or hematoma.

What to teach the patient and significant other(s)

Temporary pacemakers:

- Explain why a pacemaker is needed, how it works, and what they can expect.
- Warn the patient with a temporary pacemaker not to get out of bed without assistance.
- Explain that a transcutaneous pacemaker causes twitching of the pectoral muscles. Reassure that you will be asking the patient if medication is desired for the discomfort.

- Instruct the patient not to manipulate the temporary pacemaker wires or pulse generator; and not to "fiddle" with the implanted generator.

Permanent pacemakers: In addition to explaining need, function, and expectations, give patients with permanent pacemakers the following:

- Teach how to care for the incision. Advise the patient to avoid tight clothing or other direct pressure over the pulse generator. The patient should observe the incision daily, and notify the health-care practitioner of redness or other signs of infection.
- Give the patient the manufacturer's identification card, and tell him to carry it at all times. They should show it to airport or law enforcement personnel as to avoid walking through strong metal detectors used by these staff.
- Inform the patient that they may want to wear a medical identi-fication bracelet indicating that they have an implanted device in case they need medical attention and are unable to speak.
- Emphasize the importance of identifying pacemaker problems via of routine remote and in-office checks.
- Explain the signs and symptoms of pacemaker malfunction, how to take a pulse, and what to do if any signs or symptoms exist, including notification of the healthcare practitioner.
- Advise the patient to avoid moving the arm on the side of the pacemaker in an extreme, exaggerated, or repetitive manner for 6 to 8 weeks or per the healthcare provider who cares for the perma-nent pacemaker.
- Advise the patient to speak to the practitioner who manages the pacemaker before having magnetic resonance imaging, radiation therapy, surgery, or diagnostic studies. The practitioner should also be consulted before use of power-generating equipment, equip-ment with antennas, or strong magnets.
- Tell the patient to follow normal routines and to increase exercise as tolerated and as allowed by the practitioner.
- Stress the importance of follow-up care and regular check-ups.
- Explain that a remote monitor is frequently used in the patient's home to alert practitioners of rhythms and device function, and to reduce the need for some office visits.

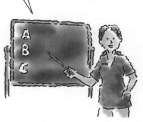

Teach your patient the ABCs of life with a pacemaker.

A look at biventricular pacemakers

Biventricular pacing is used in the treatment of some patients with class III and IV heart failure, with both systolic heart failure and intraventricular conduction delay. Also called *cardiac resynchronization therapy,* biventricular pacing reduces symptoms and improves the quality of life in patients with advanced heart failure. It also records heart failure parameters such as those indicating the amount of fluid in the chest.

Two ventricles, three leads

Unlike other pacemakers, a biventricular pacemaker usually has three leads rather than one or two: one to pace the right atrium, one to pace the right ventricle, and one to pace the left ventricle. Both ventricles are commonly either paced at the same time or the left ventricle is paced milliseconds before the right ventricle. This causes them to contract about the same time, increasing cardiac output.

An important tip

Unlike traditional lead placement, the pacing lead for the left ventricle is placed in the coronary sinus to a branch of the cardiac vein. Because this pacing lead isn't anchored in place, lead displacement may be more likely to occur. (See *Biventricular lead placement*.)

Improves symptoms and quality of life

Biventricular pacing produces an improvement in the patient's symptoms and activity tolerance. Moreover, biventricular pacing

Biventricular lead placement

The biventricular pacemaker uses three leads: one usually to pace the right atrium, one to pace the right ventricle, and one to pace the left ventricle. The left ventricular lead is placed in the coronary sinus. Both ventricles are paced at about the same time, causing them to contract almost simultaneously, improving cardiac output.

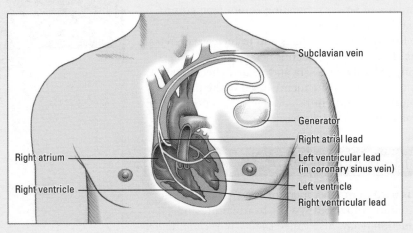

improves left ventricular remodeling and diastolic function and reduces sympathetic stimulation. As a result, in many patients, the progression of heart failure is slowed and quality of life is improved.

Different ventricles, different timing

Under normal conditions, the right and left ventricles contract simultaneously to pump blood to the lungs and body, respectively. However, in heart failure, the damaged ventricles can't pump as forcefully and the amount of blood ejected with each contraction is reduced. If the ventricular conduction pathways are also damaged, electrical impulses reach the ventricles at different times, producing asynchronous contractions. This condition, called *intraventricular conduction defect*, further reduces the amount of blood that the heart pumps, worsening the patient's symptoms.

Sympathetic response

To compensate for reduced cardiac output, the sympathetic nervous system releases neurohormones, such as aldosterone, norepinephrine, and vasopressin, to boost the amount of blood ejected with each contraction. The resultant tachycardia and vasoconstriction increases the heart's demand for oxygen, reduces diastolic filling time, promotes sodium and water retention, and increases the pressure that the heart must pump against. The effect on the patient is a worsening of symptoms.

Biventricular pacing produces an improvement in quality of life.

Who's a candidate?

Not all patients with heart failure benefit from biventricular pacing. Candidates should have both systolic heart failure and intraventricular conduction delay along with these characteristics:
- symptomatic heart failure despite maximal medical therapy
- moderate to severe heart failure (New York Heart Association class III or IV)
- QRS complex greater than 0.13 second
- left ventricular ejection fraction of 35% or less.

Many patients who meet criteria for biventricular pacing also meet criteria for a defibrillator. Therefore, patients having defibrillators with biventricular pacing (biventricular ICD) is very common.

Caring for the patient

Provide the same basic care for the patient with a biventricular pacemaker that you would for a patient with a standard permanent pacemaker. Specific care includes these guidelines:

- Before the procedure, ask the patient if he has an allergy to iodine or shellfish because contrast medium is used to visualize the coronary sinus and veins. Notify the practitioner if an allergy exists.
- Because of the position of the left ventricular lead, watch for stimulation of the diaphragm and left chest wall. Ask patients if they feel any thumping in or on their chest. Notify the practitioner if this occurs because the left ventricular pacing lead output or configuration may need to be reprogrammed, or the left ventricular lead may need repositioning.
- Observe the ECG for pacemaker spikes. Although both ventricles are paced, usually only one ventricular pacemaker spike is seen.
- Note the presence of positive R waves in lead V_1, and negative R waves I, and aV_L. Notify the practitioner if this isn't the case or if the R-wave direction changes at any time.

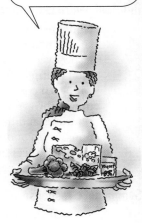

Ask the patient if he has a shellfish allergy before pacemaker insertion.

What to teach the patient

Provide the same basic teaching that you would for the patient receiving a permanent pacemaker. Additionally, when a patient gets a biventricular pacemaker, be sure to cover these points:

- Explain to the patient and his family why a biventricular pacemaker is needed, how it works, and what they can expect. Including that it can take 6 months for a patient to notice heart failure symptom improvement and that heart failure medications are still necessary.
- Tell the patient and his family that it's sometimes difficult to place the left ventricular lead and that the procedure can take 4 hours or more.
- Stress the importance of calling the practitioner immediately if the patient develops chest pain, shortness of breath, swelling of the hands or feet, or a weight gain of 3 lb (1.4 kg) in 24 hours or 5 lb (2.3 kg) in 72 hours.

A look at ICDs

An implantable cardioverter-defibrillator (ICD) is an electronic device implanted in the body to provide continuous monitoring of the heart for bradycardia, ventricular tachycardia, and ventricular fibrillation. The device then administers either over-ride pacing beats or shocks to treat the dangerous arrhythmia. Implanted defibrillators are indicated for patients who have had a myocardial infarction and have an EF of 30% or less, or who have had non-sustained VT and have an EF of 40% or less.

The procedure for ICD insertion is similar to that of a permanent pacemaker and is usually inserted in a electrophysiology laboratory. Occasionally, a patient who requires other cardiac surgery may have the device implanted in the operating room.

What it is

An ICD consists of a programmable pulse generator, a shocking lead, and one or more pacing leads. The pulse generator is a small battery-powered computer that monitors the heart's electrical signals and delivers electrical therapy when it identifies an abnormal rhythm. The leads are insulated wires that carry the heart's signal to the pulse generator and deliver the electrical energy from the pulse generator to the heart.

Storing and retrieving information

An ICD also stores information about the heart's activity before, during, and after an arrhythmia, along with tracking which treatment was delivered and the outcome of that treatment. Devices also store electrograms (electrical tracings similar to ECGs). With an interrogation programmer, a specially trained practitioner can retrieve information to evaluate ICD function, battery status, and to adjust ICD system settings. Biventricular ICDs, like biventricular pacemakers, store information that aid in heart failure assessment.

Automatic response

Today's advanced devices can detect a wide range of arrhythmias and automatically respond with the appropriate therapy, such as bradycardia pacing (both single- and dual-chamber), biventricular pacing, antitachycardia pacing, cardioversion, and defibrillation. ICDs that provide therapy for atrial arrhythmias, such as atrial fibrillation, are also available. (See *Types of ICD therapies*, page 214.) All ICD are also pacemakers.

How it's programmed

When caring for a patient with an ICD, it's important to know how the device is programmed. This information is available through a status report that can be obtained and printed when the specially trained practitioner interrogates the device. This involves placing a small piece of equipment on the skin, over the implanted pulse generator, to retrieve information. The stored information helps to

Types of ICD therapies

Implantable cardioverter-defibrillators (ICDs) can deliver a range of therapies depending on the arrhythmia detected and how the device is programmed. Therapies include antitachycardia pacing, cardioversion, defibrillation, biventricular pacing, and bradycardia pacing.

Therapy	Description
Antitachycardia pacing	A short series of rapid, electrical pacing pulses are used to interrupt ventricular tachycardia (VT) and return the heart to its normal rhythm. This pain-free therapy usually terminates VT.
Cardioversion	A low- or high-energy shock (up to 41 joules) is timed to the R wave to terminate VT and return the heart to its normal rhythm.
Defibrillation	A high-energy shock (up to 41 joules) to the heart is used to terminate ventricular fibrillation and return the heart to its normal rhythm.
Bradycardia pacing	Electrical pacing pulses are used when the heart's natural electrical signals are too slow. ICD systems can pace in any way that a pacemaker can pace, including biventricular pacing.

evaluate any arrhythmias that the device was programmed to store, any therapy delivered, and device function.

Program information includes
- type and model of the ICD
- status of the device arrhythmia detection and therapy (on or off)
- detection rates
- therapies that will be delivered: bradycardia pacing, antitachycardia pacing, cardioversion, and defibrillation.

Arresting developments

Follow these guidelines if your patient experiences an arrhythmia:
- If the patient experiences cardiac arrest, initiate CPR and advanced cardiac life support.
- If the ICD delivers a shock while you're performing chest compressions, you may also feel a slight shock. Wear gloves to prevent you feeling the shock.
- Externally defibrillating the patient is safe as long as the paddles aren't placed directly over the pulse generator. The anteroposterior pad position is preferred.

A tiny computer in the ICD tracks information before, during, and after an arrhythmia.

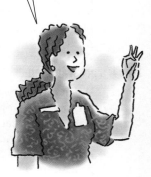

Be alert

Provide the same basic care for the patient with an ICD that you would for a patient with a permanent pacemaker. Frequently, patients who are biventricular paced also have an ICD. Specific care for patients with ICDs includes the following:

- Monitor the patient's rhythm for antitachycardia pacing or shocks.
- Patients post ICD implant may be more sedated than post pacemaker due to the anesthesia administered so the patient does not feel or remember any testing shocks.
- Put the telemetry monitor in "Paced Mode." All ICDs are programmed to pace once the patient's own heart rate gets below the programmed set heart rate, for example, 40 bpm.

What to teach the patient

- Explain to the patient and his family why an ICD is needed, how it works, potential complications, and what they can expect. Make sure they also understand ICD terminology.
- Discuss signs and symptoms to report to the practitioner immediately.
- Educate family members in emergency techniques (such as dialing 911 and performing CPR) in case the device fails to restore circulation.

A look at radiofrequency ablation

Radiofrequency ablation is an invasive procedure that may be used to treat arrhythmias in patients who haven't responded to antiarrhythmic drugs or cardioversion or can't tolerate antiarrhythmic drugs. In this procedure, bursts of radiofrequency energy are delivered through a catheter to the heart tissue to destroy the focus of the arrhythmia or block the conduction pathway.

Who's a candidate?

Radiofrequency ablation is commonly used in treating patients with atrial tachycardia, atrial fibrillation, atrial flutter, AV nodal re-entry tachycardia, inappropriate sinus tachycardia, bypass tracts like Wolff–Parkinson–White (WPW) syndrome, ventricular tachycardia (VT), and frequent premature ventricular contractions.

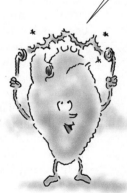

With radiofrequency ablation, a burst of energy is sent right to the part of me that's causing or supporting the arrhythmia.

Understanding the procedure

The patient first undergoes an electrophysiology study to identify and map the specific areas of the heart that causes or supports the arrhythmia. The ablation catheters are inserted into a vein, usually the femoral vein, and advanced into the heart where short bursts of radiofrequency waves destroy small targeted areas of heart tissue. The destroyed tissue can no longer conduct electrical impulses. Other types of energy may also be used, such as microwave, sonar, or cryo (freezing).

Hitting the target

Arrhythmias can be categorized by being either focal or re-entrant. Examples of focal arrhythmias include atrial tachycardia, inappropriate sinus tachycardia, premature atrial contractions, and right- or left-ventricular outflow tract ventricular tachycardia. The arrhythmia originates from one spot or foci. Re-entrant arrhythmias include ventricular tachycardia (other than outflow tract), atrial fibrillation, AV nodal re-entrant tachycardia (AVNRT), and accessory pathways like WPW syndrome. Re-entrant arrhythmias are supported by abnormal conduction that typically is in a continuous circular path or circuit. Radiofrequency ablation is used to either destroy the source of a focal tachycardia or block the abnormal pathway of the re-entrant conduction circuit. (See *Destroying the source or the circuit.*)

If a rapid arrhythmia originates above the atrioventricular (AV) node, the bundle of His in the AV node may be purposefully damaged with ablation to block impulses from reaching the ventricles. This may be done to control the ventricular rate for patients whose intolerable atrial rhythm can't be converted to sinus with chemical or electrical cardioversion or ablation. A permanent pacemaker would be necessary in tandem with this ablation. Also, anticoagulation therapy may be needed to reduce the risk of stroke.

If the patient has an accessory pathway as in WPW syndrome, electrophysiology studies are used to locate the accessory pathway and ablation can destroy the circuit.

After an ablation, one's heart rate and/or rhythm should return to normal. Thus, ablation can prevent tachycardia-mediated cardiomyopathy and may restore ventricular pumping function that has been damaged by the effects of prolonged tachycardia. Some ablations can be lifesaving, like ventricular tachycardia ablations.

Destroying the source or the circuit

In radiofrequency ablation, special catheters are inserted in a vein and advanced to the heart. After the type and source of the arrhythmia is identified, radiofrequency energy is used to either (1) ablate focal tissue, or (2) interrupt or isolate a re-entry path or circuit… These illustrations demonstrate two types of catheter ablation.

Sinus node modification

A focal arrhythmia, inappropriate sinus tachycardia, is characterized by a sinus rate out of proportion to physiologic need. It is treated with a Sinus Node Modification in which tissue in the sinus node is destroyed until the desired heart rate is achieved.

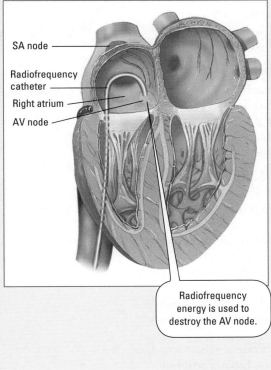

SA node

Radiofrequency catheter

Right atrium

AV node

Radiofrequency energy is used to destroy the AV node.

Atrial fibrillation ablation

In most patients with atrial fibrillation, the tissue inside the pulmonary veins is the source of the arrhythmia. Ablation within the pulmonary veins would cause pulmonary vein stenosis. Therefore, radiofrequency energy is used to destroy the tissue encircling the pulmonary veins to block the path of the abnormal impulses from exiting the pulmonary veins and traveling into the atria and ventricles. Hence, this procedure is commonly referred to as pulmonary vein isolation. Other sites within the right and left atria can also targeted. Although some believe that atrial fibrillation may be due to many re-entrant circuits, the mechanism is still not understood.

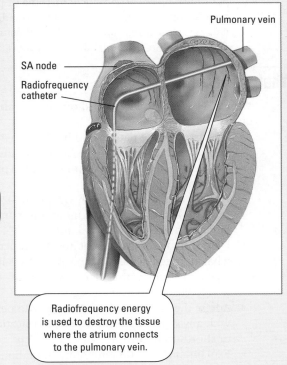

Pulmonary vein

SA node

Radiofrequency catheter

Radiofrequency energy is used to destroy the tissue where the atrium connects to the pulmonary vein.

How you intervene

When caring for a patient after radiofrequency ablation, follow these guidelines:

- Provide continuous cardiac monitoring, assessing for arrhythmias and ischemic changes.
- Place the patient on bed rest for 8 hours, or as ordered, and keep the affected extremity straight. Maintain the head of the bed between 15 and 30 degrees.
- Assess the patient's vital signs every 15 minutes for the first hour, then every 30 minutes for 4 hours, unless the patient's condition warrants more frequent checking.
- Assess peripheral pulses distal to the catheter insertion site as well as the color, sensation, temperature, and capillary refill of the affected extremity.
- Check the catheter insertion site for pain, bleeding, and hematoma formation.
- Medicate for pericardial discomfort.
- Monitor the patient for complications, such as hemorrhage, retroperitoneal bleed, access site hematoma or pseudoaneurism, stroke, perforation of the heart, cardiac tamponade, phrenic or vagus, nerve damage, pericarditis, atrial-esophageal fistula, pulmonic vein stenosis, heart failure, thrombosis, arrhythmias, and sudden death.

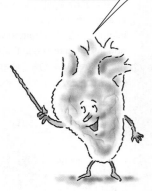

Caring for the patient after radiofrequency ablation requires specific guidelines as discussed here.

What to teach the patient

When a patient undergoes radiofrequency ablation, be sure to cover these points:

- Discuss with the patient and his family why radiofrequency ablation is needed, how it works, and what they can expect.
- Warn the patient and his family that the procedure can be lengthy; an average of 6 hours.
- Explain that the patient may be hospitalized for 24 to 48 hours to monitor his heart rhythm and monitor and/or remove intravascular and potential pericardial fluid.
- Demonstrate for the patient how to properly take a pulse. Describe what an irregular, fast, or slow pulse feels like. Explain actions to take if the pulse is irregular. Have the patient return the demonstration to ensure understanding.
- Advise the patient to call the team who performed the ablation with any signs or symptoms of complications, such as hemoptysis or shortness of breath.
- Explain rationale for temporary limitations per the cardiology team, such as in driving, upper endoscopy, or vigorous activity.
- Provide implanted device teaching if the patient had a pacemaker or ICD inserted. (For more information about pacemaker teaching, see *What to teach the patient*, pages 208 and 209.)

Nonpharmacologic treatments review

Pacemaker
- A device that electrically stimulates the myocardium to depolarize

Atrial and ventricular stimulation
- *Atrial only:* spike followed by a P wave and the patient's intrinsic QRS complex and T wave
- *Ventricular only:* patient's intrinsic atrial rhythm, then a spike followed by a QRS complex and T wave
- *Atrial and ventricular:* first spike followed by a P wave, then a second spike, followed by QRS complex

Pacemaker codes
- First letter identifies the heart chambers being paced.
- Second letter signifies the heart chamber sensed by the pacemaker.
- Third letter refers to the pacemaker's response to the intrinsic electrical activity of the heart.
- Fourth letter refers to the pacemaker's rate modulation.
- Fifth letter refers to the pacemaker's location or absence of multisite pacing.

Pacemaker modes
- AAI = single-chambered pacemaker; paces and senses the atria
- VVI = single-chamber pacemaker; paces and senses the ventricle(s)
- DDD = dual-chamber pacemaker; paces when the ventricle doesn't respond on its own; paces the atria when the atrial rate falls below the lower set rate; senses and paces both atria and ventricles

Evaluating pacemakers
- Determine the pacemaker's mode and settings.
- Review the patient's 12-lead ECG.
- Select a monitoring lead that clearly shows the pacemaker spikes. Adjust the ECG monitor filter or bandwidth if necessary and if possible.
- Select Paced Mode to prevent missed alarms for noncapture.
- Interpret the paced rhythm.
- Look for information that tells which chamber is paced and about the pacemaker's sensing ability.

Troubleshooting pacemakers
- Failure to capture: indicated by a spike without a complex
- Failure to pace: no spike
- Undersensing: spikes where they don't belong
- Oversensing: no spike when the patient actually needs it

Biventricular pacemaker
- Pacemaker usually has three leads: one to pace the right atrium, one to pace the right ventricle, and one to pace the left ventricle.
- Both ventricles contract simultaneously, increasing cardiac output.

Candidates
For treatment of patients with:
- class III and IV heart failure, with both systolic failure and ventricular dyssynchrony
- symptomatic heart failure despite maximal medical therapy

(continued)

Nonpharmacologic treatments review *(Continued)*

- QRS complex greater than 0.13 second
- left ventricular ejection fraction of 35% or less

Benefits of biventricular pacing

- Improves symptoms and activity tolerance
- Reverses left ventricular remodelling and diastolic function, and reduces sympathetic stimulation

Radiofrequency ablation

- Invasive procedure that uses radio frequency energy to destroy heart tissue or conduction pathway responsible for arrhythmia
- Useful for atrial tachycardia, atrial fibrillation and flutter; ventricular tachycardia; premature ventricular contractions, AV nodal re-entry tachycardia; inappropriate sinus tachycardia; and Wolff–Parkinson–White syndrome

Types of ablation

- Targeted ablation
- Pulmonary vein ablation
- His bundle ablation (with pacemaker insertion)
- Accessory pathway ablation

Implantable cardioverter-defibrillator

- Implanted device that monitors for bradycardia, ventricular tachycardia, and ventricular fibrillation
- Provides pacing for bradycardia, and pacing and shocks to break arrhythmias

Types of therapy

- *Antitachycardia pacing:* bursts of pacing to interrupt ventricular tachycardia
- *Cardioversion:* shock synchronized to the R wave to terminate ventricular tachycardia
- *Defibrillation:* asynchronized shock to terminate ventricular fibrillation
- *Bradycardia pacing:* pacing when the heart rate is below the rate set

Programming information

- Type and model
- Status of the device (on or off)
- Therapies to be delivered: antitachycardia pacing, bradycardia pacing, cardioversion, defibrillation

Quick quiz

1. When using a transcutaneous temporary pacemaker, the energy level should be set at:
    A. the highest milliampere setting the patient can tolerate.
    B. 10% above the milliampere needed for consistent capture of the myocardium.
    C. a milliampere setting midway between the setting that causes capture of the myocardium and the setting at which symptoms first appear.
    D. the milliampere setting that provides a heart rate of 80 beats per minute.

Answer: B. Determine the minimum amount of milliamperes required to capture the myocardium (threshold). Then set the milliampere output at 10% above the threshold. This should ensure capture under stressed physiologic conditions while keeping the possibly painful pacing stimuli at a minimum.

2. Failure to capture is represented on the ECG as:
    A. no pacemaker activity.
    B. spikes where they shouldn't be.
    C. a spike on a T wave.
    D. a spike without a complex.

Answer: D. A spike without a complex indicates the pacemaker's inability to capture or stimulate the chamber.

3. The first letter in the five-letter coding system for pacemakers identifies the:
    A. chamber in which the pacemaker senses intrinsic activity.
    B. heart chamber being paced.
    C. pacemaker's response to the intrinsic electrical activity.
    D. pacemaker's response to a tachyarrhythmia.

Answer: B. The first letter identifies the heart chamber being paced, the second letter signifies the heart chamber that senses intrinsic activity, the third letter shows the pacemaker's response to that activity, the fourth letter describes the rate modulation, and the fifth letter shows the location or absence of multisite pacing.

4. A patient with a biventricular pacemaker usually has which pacing leads?
    A. A lead for both ventricles only
    B. A lead for each atria and each ventricle
    C. A lead for the right atrium and each ventricle
    D. A lead for both atria and the left ventricle

Answer: C. A biventricular pacemaker usually has three leads: one to pace the right atrium, one to pace the right ventricle, and one to pace the left ventricle.

5. After ablation of the bundle of His, the patient may need a pacemaker because:
    A. impulses can no longer be conducted from the atria to the ventricles.
    B. the sinoatrial node no longer initiates an electrical impulse.
    C. accessory pathways now conduct impulses from the atria to the ventricles.
    D. the AV node begins to fire at its intrinsic rate.

Answer: A. After His bundle ablation, a pacemaker is needed because the electrical impulses from the atria are no longer conducted through the bundle of His in the AV node to the ventricles.

6. Which therapy is the patient with an ICD receiving when the device delivers a series of rapid electrical pacing pulses?
    A. Bradycardia pacing
    B. Defibrillation
    C. Cardioversion
    D. Antitachycardia pacing

Answer: D. Antitachycardia pacing consists of a series of, rapid electrical pacing pulses used to interrupt ventricular tachycardia and restore normal sinus rhythm.

Test strip

Time to try out a test strip. Ready? Go!

7. In the following ECG strip, the pacemaker is pacing and sensing the ventricles with 100% capture. The mode of response can't be evaluated because of lack of intrinsic activity. You would determine that the patient probably has:
    A. a VVI pacemaker.
    B. a DDD pacemaker.
    C. an AAI pacemaker.
    D. an AOO pacemaker.

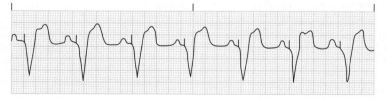

Answer: B. The patient has a DDD pacemaker. It senses atrial activity and therefore inhibits atrial pacing. The P wave then triggers the pacemaker to try to sense a QRS complex. Since there is no intrinsic QRS complex after the P wave, the pacemaker paces the ventricle.

Scoring

☆☆☆ If you answered all seven questions correctly, all right! You've taken the lead when it comes to nonpharmacologic treatment methods.

☆☆ If you answered six questions correctly, terrific! Keep up the good pace.

☆ If you answered fewer than six questions correctly, no sweat. Go with your impulse to reread the chapter and you're sure to do better next time.

Recommended references

Brown, D. F. M., & Martindale, J. L. (2012). *Rapid interpretation of ECG's in emergency medicine*. Philadelphia, PA: Wolters Kluwer.

Brown, D. F. M., & Borczuk, P. (2014). Emergent management of atrial flutter. Retrieved from http://emedicine.medscape.com/article/151066-overview

Budzikowski, A. S., & Rottman, J. (2014). Atrial tachycardia practice essentials. Retrieved from http://emedicine.medscape.com/article/151456-overview

Cohen, B. J., & Taylor, J. J. (2013). *Memmler's structure and function of the human body* (10th ed.). Philadelphia, PA: Wolters Kluwer.

Ellenbough, K. A., & Kaszala, K. (2014). *Cardiac pacing and ICDs*. Chichester: John Wiley & Sons.

Katritsis, D. G., Gersch, B. J., & Camm, A. J. (2013). *Clinical Cardiology: Current Practice Guidelines*. Oxford, United Kingdom: Oxford University Press.

Mann, D. L., Zipes, D. P., Libby, P., & Bonow, R. D. (2014). *Braunwald's heart disease: A textbook of cardiovascular medicine* (10th ed.). St. Louis, MO: Saunders | Elsevier.

McLaughlin, M. A. (clinical ed.) (2014). *Cardiovascular care made incredibly easy* (3rd ed.). Philadelphia, PA: Wolters Kluwer.

Urden, L., & Stacy, K. (2013). *Critical care nursing* (7th ed.). St Louis, MO: Mosby | Elsevier.

Wagner, G. S., & Strauss, D. G. (2013). *Marriott's practical electrocardiology* (12th ed.). Philadelphia, PA: Wolters Kluwer.

Chapter 10

Pharmacologic treatments

Just the facts

In this chapter, you'll learn:

◆ basic details about the antiarrhythmic drug classification system (also known as the Vaughn Williams classification system)

◆ the effects antiarrhythmics have on the cardiovascular system and other body systems

◆ administration techniques and adverse effects of antiarrhythmic drugs

◆ nursing interventions for patients on antiarrhythmic drugs

◆ patient teaching related to antiarrhythmic administration.

A look at antiarrhythmics

Almost half a million Americans die each year from cardiac arrhythmias; countless others suffer symptoms or lifestyle limitations. Along with other treatments, antiarrhythmic drugs can help alleviate symptoms and prolong life. It is important to keep in mind that all of these drugs have potential adverse effects, possibly life-threatening in nature, and must be prescribed with caution and the patients carefully monitored.

Antiarrhythmic drugs affect the movement of ions across the cell membrane and alter the electrophysiology of the cardiac cell. They're classified according to their effect on the cell's electrical activity (action potential) and their mechanism of action. (See *Antiarrhythmics and the action potential,* page 226.)

Drugs in the same class are similar in action and adverse effects. When you know where a particular drug fits in the classification system, you'll be better able to remember its actions and adverse effects.

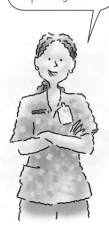

Antiarrhythmic drugs can help prolong life.

Antiarrhythmics and the action potential

Each class of antiarrhythmic drugs acts, primarily, on a particular phase of the heart's action potential. Here's a rundown of the four classes of antiarrhythmics and how they affect action potential.

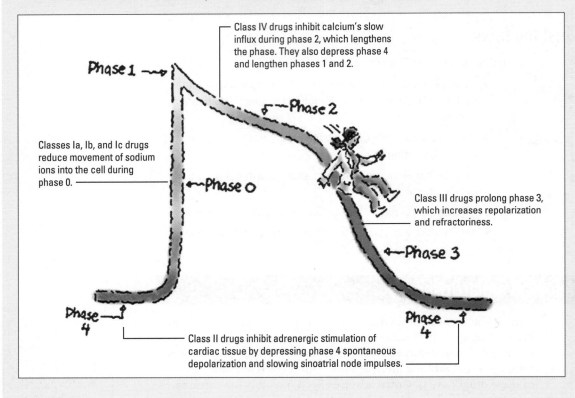

Class IV drugs inhibit calcium's slow influx during phase 2, which lengthens the phase. They also depress phase 4 and lengthen phases 1 and 2.

Phase 1

Phase 2

Classes Ia, Ib, and Ic drugs reduce movement of sodium ions into the cell during phase 0.

Phase 0

Class III drugs prolong phase 3, which increases repolarization and refractoriness.

Phase 3

Phase 4

Phase 4

Class II drugs inhibit adrenergic stimulation of cardiac tissue by depressing phase 4 spontaneous depolarization and slowing sinoatrial node impulses.

Classifying antiarrhythmics

The classification system divides antiarrhythmic drugs into four major classes. Let's take a look at each one.

Class I blocks sodium

Class I drugs block the influx of sodium into the cell during phase 0 (rapid depolarization) of the action potential, which minimizes the chance of sodium reaching its threshold potential and causing cells to depolarize. Because phase 0 is also referred to as the *sodium channel* or *fast channel*, these drugs may also be called *sodium channel blockers* or *fast channel blockers*. Drugs in this class are potentially proarrhythmic, meaning they can cause or worsen arrhythmias.

Antiarrhythmic drugs in this class are further categorized as:
- Class Ia, which prolong conduction and repolarization
- Class Ib, which slow phase 0 depolarization, don't affect conduction, and shorten phase 3 repolarization
- Class Ic, which markedly slow phase 0 depolarization and prolong conduction, with little effect on repolarization.

Class II blocks beta receptors

Class II drugs block sympathetic nervous system beta-adrenergic receptors and thereby decrease heart rate. Phase 4 depolarization is diminished resulting in depressed sinoatrial (SA) node automaticity and increased atrial and atrioventricular (AV) nodal refractoriness, or resistance to stimulation.

Class III blocks potassium

Class III drugs are called *potassium channel blockers* because they block the movement of potassium during phase 3 of the action potential and prolong repolarization and the refractory period.

Class IV blocks calcium

Class IV drugs block the movement of calcium during phase 2 of the action potential. Because phase 2 is also called the *calcium channel* or the *slow channel*, drugs that affect phase 2 are also known as *calcium channel blockers* or *slow channel blockers*. They prolong conductivity and increase the refractory period at the AV node.

Some drugs don't fit

Not all drugs fit neatly into these classifications. For example, sotalol possesses characteristics of both class II and class III drugs. Some drugs used to treat arrhythmias don't fit into the classification system at all, including adenosine (Adenocard), atropine, digoxin (Lanoxin), epinephrine, and magnesium sulfate. Despite these limitations, the classification system helps nurses understand how antiarrhythmic drugs prevent and treat arrhythmias.

Drug distribution and clearance

Many patients receive antiarrhythmic drugs by I.V. bolus or infusion because they're more readily available that way than orally. The cardiovascular system then distributes the drugs throughout the body, specifically to the site of action.

Most drugs are changed, or *biotransformed,* into active or inactive metabolites in the liver. The kidneys are the primary sites for the excretion of those metabolites. When administering these drugs, remember that patients with impaired heart, liver, or kidney function

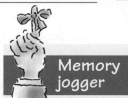

Some antiarrhythmic drugs possess characteristics that don't fit into the classification system.

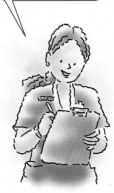

may suffer from inadequate drug effect or toxicity. (See *Drug metabolism and elimination across the life span.*)

Antiarrhythmics by class

Broken down by classes, the following section describes commonly used antiarrhythmic drugs. It highlights their dosages, adverse effects, and recommendations for patient care.

Class Ia antiarrhythmics

Class Ia antiarrhythmic drugs are called *sodium channel blockers*. They include quinidine (the prototype drug), procainamide, and disopyramide. These drugs reduce the excitability of the cardiac cell, have an anticholinergic effect, and decrease cardiac contractility. Because these drugs prolong the QT interval, the patient is prone to polymorphic ventricular tachycardia (VT). (See *Effects of class Ia antiarrhythmics.*)

Quinidine

Quinidine is effective against supraventricular and ventricular arrhythmias. It is no longer commonly prescribed, but was used to treat atrial fibrillation, atrial flutter, paroxysmal supraventricular tachycardia (PSVT), AV node re-entrant tachycardia (AVNRT), and Wolff–Parkinson–White (WPW) syndrome. The drug comes in several forms, including quinidine sulfate and quinidine gluconate.

How to give it

Here's how to administer quinidine:

- To convert atrial flutter or fibrillation—Give 200 mg of quinidine sulfate orally every 2 to 3 hours for five to eight doses, with subsequent daily increases until sinus rhythm is restored or toxic effects develop. NOTE: It is critical to control AV node conduction before administering quinidine, as the drug can slow the atrial rate and increase conduction over the AV node, causing rapid 1:1 conduction of atrial arrhythmias. Class II or class IV medications are used for this purpose.
- Initial dosage for PSVT—Give 400 to 600 mg of quinidine sulfate orally every 6 hours.
- Initial dosage for premature atrial and ventricular contractions, paroxysmal AV junctional rhythm, paroxysmal atrial tachycardia (PAT), paroxysmal VT, or maintenance after cardioversion of atrial fibrillation or flutter—Give 200 mg of quinidine sulfate orally, then 200 to 300 mg orally every 4 to 6 hours, or 300 to 600 mg

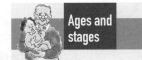

Ages and stages

Drug metabolism and elimination across the life span

Neonates have a reduced ability to metabolize drugs because of the limited activity of liver enzymes at the time of birth. As the infant grows, drug metabolism improves. The glomerular filtration rate is also reduced at birth, causing neonates to eliminate drugs more slowly than adults.

In older patients, advancing age usually reduces the blood supply to the liver and certain liver enzymes become less active. Consequently, the liver loses some of its ability to metabolize drugs. With reduced liver function, higher drug levels remain in circulation, causing more intense drug effects and increasing the risk of drug toxicity. Because kidney function also diminishes with age, drug elimination may be impaired, resulting in increased drug levels.

Effects of class Ia antiarrhythmics

Class Ia antiarrhythmic drugs—including drugs such as quinidine, procainamide, and disopyramide—affect the cardiac cycle in specific ways and lead to specific ECG changes, as shown on the rhythm strip below. Class Ia antiarrhythmics

- block sodium influx during phase 0, which depresses the rate of depolarization.

- prolong repolarization and the duration of the action potential.

- lengthen the refractory period (in accessory pathways, as well).
- decrease contractility.

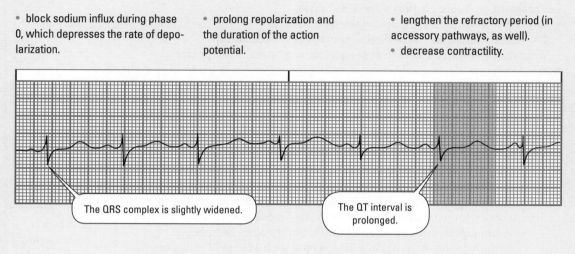

The QRS complex is slightly widened.

The QT interval is prolonged.

of extended-release quinidine sulfate every 8 to 12 hours. For I.V. administration, give 800 mg of quinidine gluconate added to 40 mL of dextrose 5% in water (D_5W), infused at 1 mL/min.

What can happen

Adverse cardiovascular effects of quinidine include hypotension, cardiotoxicity, VT, ECG changes (widening of the QRS complex, widened QT and PR intervals), torsades de pointes, AV block, and exacerbation of heart failure. (See *Noncardiac adverse effects of quinidine,* page 230.)

How you intervene

Keep the following points in mind when caring for a patient taking quinidine:

- Monitor the patient's ECG, heart rate, and blood pressure closely. Don't give more than 4 g/day. Adjust dosages in patients with heart failure and liver disease.
- Obtain a baseline QT-interval measurement before the patient begins therapy. Watch for and notify the practitioner if the patient develops prolongation of the QT interval, a sign that the patient is predisposed to developing polymorphic VT. Also notify the practitioner if the QRS complex widens by 25% or more.

Noncardiac adverse effects of quinidine

In addition to adverse cardiovascular effects of quinidine, other adverse effects include:
* *Central nervous system*—vertigo, confusion, light-headedness, depression, delirium, headache, tinnitus, hearing loss, vision disturbances
* *Respiratory*—acute asthmatic attack, respiratory arrest
* *GI*—nausea, vomiting, diarrhea, abdominal pain, anorexia, hepatotoxicity
* *Hematologic*—hemolytic anemia, thrombocytopenia, anaphylaxis, or allergic reactions including rash
* *Other*—photosensitivity, angioedema.

* Remember that quinidine should be avoided in patients with second- or third-degree AV block who don't have pacemakers. It should also be avoided in patients with profound hypotension, myasthenia gravis, intraventricular conduction defects, or hypersensitivity to the drug. Use it cautiously in elderly patients and in those with renal disease, hepatic disease, or asthma.
* Avoid rapidly conducted atrial fibrillation or atrial flutter by administering AV nodal blocking agents, such as beta blockers or calcium channel blockers, before giving quinidine.
* Closely monitor patients receiving quinidine and digoxin for signs and symptoms of digoxin toxicity, such as nausea, vision changes, or arrhythmias. Digoxin levels will be increased.
* Monitor serum drug levels. The therapeutic level for arrhythmia control is 2 to 5 mcg/mL.
* Ask the patient about herb use. Concomitant use with jimsonweed may adversely affect cardiovascular function. Licorice combined with quinidine use may prolong the patient's QT interval.

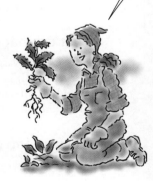

Herbs can affect the way quinidine works. Ask your patient about herb use.

Procainamide

Procainamide is indicated for supraventricular and ventricular arrhythmias. It is used intravenously to acutely convert atrial fibrillation, atrial flutter, or ventricular tachycardia. It is the drug of choice for atrial fibrillation with conduction over an accessory pathway. It is also used for AVNRT.

How to give it

Here's how to administer procainamide:
* Orally—Initial dosage is 50 mg/kg/day of conventional formulation in divided doses every 3 hours until a therapeutic level is reached. For maintenance, an extended-release form is substituted to deliver the total daily dose divided every 6 hours.

An extended-release form may be used to deliver the dose divided every 12 hours.

- I.M.—Initial daily dosage is 50 mg/kg divided into equal doses every 3 to 6 hours.
- I.V.—Slow injection of 100 mg is given with the patient in a supine position, no faster than 25 to 50 mg/min until the arrhythmia is suppressed, adverse effects develop, or 500 mg has been given. The usual loading dose is 500 to 600 mg.
- I.V. infusion—Infuse at 1 to 6 mg/min for a maintenance dosage.

What can happen

Adverse cardiovascular effects of procainamide include bradycardia, hypotension, worsening heart failure, AV block, ventricular fibrillation, and asystole. (See *Noncardiac adverse effects of procainamide.*)

How you intervene

Keep the following points in mind when caring for a patient taking procainamide:

- Monitor the patient's heart rate, blood pressure, and ECG. Notify the practitioner if the patient has hypotension or if you notice widening of the QRS complex by 50% or more. Also report a prolonged QT interval if it's more than one-half of the R-R interval—a sign that the patient is predisposed to developing polymorphic VT.
- Warn the patient taking procainamide orally not to chew it, which might cause him to get too much of the drug at once.
- Monitor serum drug levels. (See *Monitoring procainamide.*)
- Remember that procainamide should be avoided in patients with second- or third-degree AV block who don't have pacemakers and in patients with blood dyscrasias, myasthenia gravis, profound hypotension, or known hypersensitivity to the drug. Procainamide may also aggravate digoxin toxicity.

Noncardiac adverse effects of procainamide

In addition to adverse cardiovascular effects of procainamide, other dose-related adverse effects include:

- *Central nervous system*—mental depression, hallucinations, seizures, confusion, dizziness
- *GI*—anorexia, nausea, vomiting, diarrhea, bitter taste
- *Hematologic*—agranulocytosis, hemolytic anemia, neutropenia
- *Skin*—rash, urticaria
- *Other*—fever, lupus-like syndrome in long-term therapy, Raynaud's phenomenon.

Monitoring procainamide

For patients taking procainamide, you'll need to monitor serum drug levels and the active metabolite *N*-acetylprocainamide (NAPA) to prevent toxic reactions. To suppress ventricular arrhythmias, the therapeutic serum concentration of procainamide should range between 4 and 12 mcg/mL. Therapeutic levels of NAPA should average between 9 and 20 mcg/mL.

Disopyramide

Disopyramide (Norpace) is effective in digitalis-induced arrhythmias, atrial arrhythmias, AVNRT, supraventricular tachycardia (SVT) due to accessory pathways, and ventricular tachyarrhythmias. The negative inotropic action of disopyramide can be useful in neurocardiogenic (vasodepressor) syncope and hypertrophic cardiomyopathy.

How to give it

Here's how to give disopyramide:
- Orally, 100 mg to 150 mg every 6 hours or 200 mg to 300 mg every 12 hours (controlled release formula)

What can happen

Adverse cardiovascular effects include sinus bradycardia in patients with sick sinus syndrome (SSS), QRS and QT prolongation by 10% to 15%, variable AV conduction changes, and proarrhythmia including VF and torsades de pointes.

How you intervene

Keep the following points in mind when caring for a patient taking disopyramide:
- Monitor ECG and HR closely.
- Obtain 12-lead ECG for baseline and periodically, for accurate interval measurements.
- Give AVN blocking agents prior to disopyramide, when treating atrial fibrillation or atrial flutter.
- Reduce dose in renal and hepatic dysfunction.
- Do not use in patients with systolic CHF.
- Check K^+ and magnesium levels before initiating Norpace and replete if necessary.
- Avoid use of erythromycin with Norpace as it can increase levels and lead to torsades de pointes.

Class Ib antiarrhythmics

Class Ib antiarrhythmics in use include such drugs as lidocaine and mexiletine. Because of their actions on ventricular muscle and Purkinje fibers, these drugs are effective in suppressing ventricular ectopy but do not affect atrial muscle. (See *Effects of class Ib antiarrhythmics.*) These drugs slow phase 0 depolarization and shorten phase 3 repolarization and the action potential. Sinus node automaticity and AV node automaticity and conductivity are not affected by lidocaine.

Effects of class Ib antiarrhythmics

Class Ib antiarrhythmic drugs—such as lidocaine, tocainide, and mexiletine—may affect the QRS complexes, as shown on the rhythm strip below. These drugs

- block sodium influx during phase 0, which depresses the rate of depolarization.
- shorten repolarization and the duration of the action potential.
- suppress ventricular automaticity in ischemic tissue.

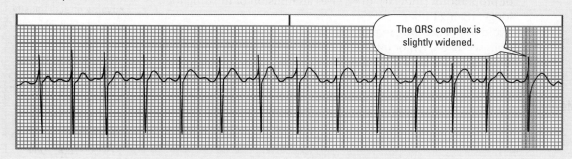

The QRS complex is slightly widened.

Lidocaine

Lidocaine was once the drug of choice for suppressing ventricular arrhythmias; however, amiodarone is now favored. When lidocaine is used, a patient is generally first given a loading dose and then an infusion.

How to give it

Here's how to administer lidocaine:
- I.V. bolus injection—Administer 1 to 1.5 mg/kg (usually 50 to 100 mg) at 25 to 50 mg/min and repeat every 3 to 5 minutes to a maximum of 300 mg total bolus during a 1-hour period.
- I.V. infusion immediately following the bolus dose—Infuse at 1 to 4 mg/min.

What can happen

Cardiovascular adverse effects of lidocaine include hypotension, bradycardia, and cardiac arrest. (See *Noncardiac adverse effects of lidocaine*, page 234.)

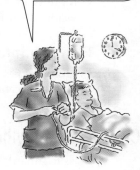

As ordered, administer an antiarrhythmic such as lidocaine to help suppress ventricular ectopy.

How you intervene

Keep the following points in mind when caring for a patient receiving lidocaine:

- Monitor the patient's heart rate, blood pressure, and ECG.
- Watch for signs and symptoms of drug toxicity. Seizures may be the first sign of toxicity. The potential for toxicity is increased if the patient has liver disease, is elderly, is taking cimetidine (Tagamet) or propranolol (Inderal), or receives an infusion of the drug for longer than 24 hours.
- Avoid use of the drug in patients known to be hypersensitive to it or in severe SA, AV, or intraventricular block in the absence of an artificial pacemaker.
- Administer cautiously with other antiarrhythmics.

Mexiletine

Mexiletine is an oral congener of lidocaine, used in the treatment of ventricular arrhythmias. It has no activity against atrial arrhythmias.

How to give it

- 150 to 200 mg every 8 hours to a maximum dose of 400 mg every 8 hours. Decrease dose in hepatic disease. No adjustment required in renal disease or with CHF.

What can happen

- Proarrhythmia is very rare, about 1.3%.
- Very little effect on HR, BP, or cardiac output.
- Exacerbation of CHF is rare, about 2%.
- Monitor for GI side effects and CNS effects of tremor, blurred vision, dysarthria, ataxia, and confusion.

How you intervene

- Monitor ECG for efficacy in controlling ventricular arrhythmias.
- Give medication with food to avoid GI effects.

Class Ic antiarrhythmics

Class Ic antiarrhythmic drugs include flecainide (Tambocor) and propafenone (Rythmol). These drugs slow conduction without affecting the duration of the action potential. (See *Effects of class Ic antiarrhythmics.*) These drugs are primarily used for supraventricular arrhythmias. Due to their proarrhythmic potential, they are avoided in patients with structural heart disease.

Noncardiac adverse effects of lidocaine

In addition to adverse cardiovascular effects of lidocaine, other adverse effects (mostly dose-related) include:

- *Central nervous system*—seizures, confusion, drowsiness, dizziness, tremors, restlessness, light-headedness, paresthesia, tinnitus, double vision
- *Respiratory*—respiratory arrest, status asthmaticus
- *GI*—nausea, vomiting
- *Other*—anaphylaxis.

Effects of class Ic antiarrhythmics

Class Ic antiarrhythmic drugs—including flecainide and propafenone—cause the effects shown below on an ECG by exerting particular actions on the cardiac cycle. Class Ic antiarrhythmics block sodium influx during phase 0, which depresses the rate of depolarization. Repolarization is not affected.

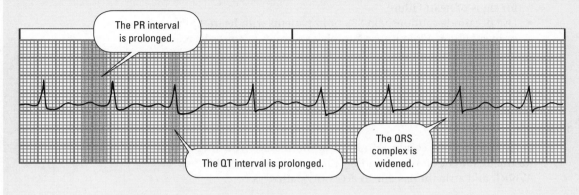

The PR interval is prolonged.

The QT interval is prolonged.

The QRS complex is widened.

Flecainide

Flecainide is used to treat paroxysmal atrial fibrillation or flutter in patients without structural heart disease. It is also used to prevent PSVT.

How to give it

The dosage for flecainide is 50 to 200 mg orally every 12 hours, to a maximum of 400 mg/day.

What can happen

Adverse cardiovascular effects of flecainide include bradycardia (in the presence of sinus node disease), chest pain, palpitations, heart failure, new or worsened arrhythmias, and cardiac arrest. (See *Noncardiac adverse effects of flecainide.*)

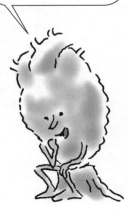

Flecainide helps me take it easy. It slows conduction without affecting the duration of the action potential.

Noncardiac adverse effects of flecainide

In addition to adverse cardiovascular effects of flecainide, other adverse effects include:
- *Central nervous system*—headache, drowsiness, dizziness, syncope, fatigue, blurred vision, tremor, ataxia, vertigo, light-headedness, paresthesia, flushing
- *Respiratory*—dyspnea
- *GI*—nausea, vomiting, constipation, abdominal pain, diarrhea, anorexia
- *Hematologic*—neutropenia.

How you intervene

Keep the following points in mind when caring for a patient taking flecainide:

- Monitor the patient's heart rate, blood pressure, and ECG. Report widening of the QRS complex by 25% or more, and watch closely for signs of heart failure.
- Use flecainide cautiously in SSS or in patients with heart, kidney, or liver failure. Avoid its use entirely in second- or third-degree AV block, and use caution in bifascicular block.
- Administer flecainide cautiously in patients receiving cimetidine, digoxin, or propranolol.
- Correct electrolyte imbalances before starting flecainide therapy.

Propafenone

Propafenone slows conduction in all cardiac tissues. The drug is used for the treatment of SVT, including atrial fibrillation, atrial flutter, AVNRT, and arrhythmias due to accessory pathways.

How to give it

The usual dosage of propafenone is 150 to 300 mg orally every 8 hours, to a maximum dosage of 900 mg/day.

What can happen

Propafenone's adverse effects on the cardiovascular system include exacerbation of heart failure, AV block, and such proarrhythmias as VT, ventricular fibrillation, and PVCs. However, proarrhythmia is rare in patients treated for SVT, with a structurally normal heart. (See *Noncardiac adverse effects of propafenone.*)

Noncardiac adverse effects of propafenone

In addition to adverse cardiovascular effects of propafenone, other adverse effects include:

- *Central nervous system*—dizziness, blurred vision, fatigue, headache, paresthesia, anxiety, ataxia, drowsiness, insomnia, syncope, tremors
- *Respiratory*—dyspnea, exacerbation of asthma
- *GI*—unusual taste, nausea, vomiting, dyspepsia, constipation, diarrhea, abdominal pain, dry mouth, flatulence.

How you intervene

Keep the following points in mind when caring for a patient taking propafenone:

- Monitor the patient's heart rate, blood pressure, and ECG. Report widening of the QRS complex greater than 25%. If widening occurs, the dosage may need to be reduced. Monitor the patient closely for exacerbation of heart failure.
- Correct electrolyte imbalances before starting propafenone therapy.
- Remember that propafenone should be avoided in patients with a structurally abnormal heart (low ejection fraction, previous myocardial infarction, cardiomyopathy or significant left ventricular hypertrophy), bronchospastic disorders, hypotension, or SA, AV, or bifascicular blocks.
- Administer propafenone cautiously in patients also receiving cimetidine, propranolol, or metoprolol.
- Be aware that patients receiving digoxin along with propafenone may have increased plasma concentration of digoxin, leading to digoxin toxicity.
- Use cautiously in patients also taking warfarin (Coumadin); propafenone can increase the plasma concentration of the anticoagulant.

Class II antiarrhythmics

Class II antiarrhythmic drugs are used to treat supraventricular and ventricular arrhythmias, especially those caused by excess catecholamines. The drugs are called *beta-adrenergic blockers* because they block beta-adrenergic receptors in the sympathetic nervous system. (See *Effects of class II antiarrhythmics,* page 238.)

Two types of beta-adrenergic receptors exist: $beta_1$ and $beta_2$. $Beta_1$-adrenergic receptors increase heart rate, contractility, and conductivity. Blocking those receptors decreases the actions listed above.

$Beta_2$-adrenergic receptors relax smooth muscle in the bronchi and blood vessels. Keep in mind that blocking these receptors may result in vasoconstriction and bronchospasm.

Beta-adrenergic blockers that block only $beta_1$-adrenergic receptors are referred to as *cardioselective.* Those that block both $beta_1$-adrenergic and $beta_2$-adrenergic receptors are referred to as *noncardioselective.*

Beta blockers depress the slope of phase 4 depolarization, suppress automaticity, and prolong AV node conduction. These drugs are used to control ventricular rate in atrial fibrillation and atrial flutter, reduce the risk of sudden cardiac death (SCD) in patients with nonsustained VT and structural heart disease, reduce SCD in patients post

> Smooth muscle in the bronchi and blood vessels are relaxed by $beta_2$-adrenergic receptors. I choose a good book to relax!

Effects of class II antiarrhythmics

Class II antiarrhythmic drugs—including such beta-adrenergic blockers as propranolol, esmolol, acebutolol, and sotalol—cause certain effects on an ECG (as shown here) by exerting particular actions on the cardiac cycle. Class II antiarrhythmics

- depress sinoatrial node automaticity.
- shorten the duration of the action potential.

- increase the refractory period of atrial and atrioventricular junctional tissues, which slows conduction.

- inhibit sympathetic activity.

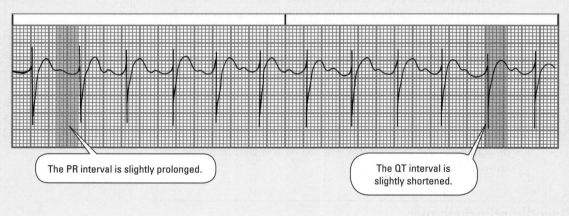

The PR interval is slightly prolonged.

The QT interval is slightly shortened.

MI, prevent SCD in long QT interval syndrome, prevent recurrence of SVT, and to slow HR in PAT.

Beta-adrenergic blockers

The following beta-adrenergic blockers are approved by the U.S. Food and Drug Administration for use as antiarrhythmics:

- Acebutolol (Sectral), which is classified as cardioselective and decreases contractility, heart rate, and blood pressure
- Propranolol (Inderal), which is classified as noncardioselective; decreases heart rate, contractility, and blood pressure; and reduces the incidence of SCD after myocardial infarction (MI)
- Esmolol (Brevibloc), which is a short-acting, cardioselective drug administered by I.V. titration, that decreases heart rate, contractility, and blood pressure
- Sotalol (Betapace), which is a noncardioselective drug that also has class III characteristics, decreases heart rate, slows AV conduction, decreases cardiac output, and has proarrhythmic effects and increases the QT interval. It has little effect on blood pressure. It is used primarily to maintain SR with atrial fibrillation or atrial flutter.

Other beta blockers often used to treat arrhythmias include metoprolol, atenolol, nadolol, and bisoprolol.

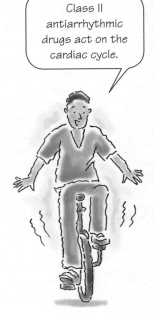

Class II antiarrhythmic drugs act on the cardiac cycle.

How to give it

These four beta-adrenergic blockers should be administered as follows:
- Acebutolol—The normal dosage is 200 mg orally twice daily, increased as needed to a usual dosage of 600 to 1,200 mg daily.
- Propranolol—It may be given orally or I.V. The oral dosage is 10 to 30 mg three or four times daily. The I.V. dose is 0.5 to 3.0 mg, at a rate not to exceed 1 mg/min. If necessary, a second I.V. dose may be administered after 2 minutes; subsequent doses may be given no sooner than every 4 hours.
- Esmolol—The loading dose is 500 mcg/kg over 1 minute, then 50 mcg/kg/min for 4 minutes. If an adequate response doesn't occur within 5 minutes, repeat the loading dose and infuse 100 mcg/kg/min for 4 minutes. If needed, increase infusion to a maximum of 200 mcg/kg/min.
- Sotalol—The initial dosage is 80 mg orally twice daily. Most patients respond to a daily dose of 160 to 320 mg.

What can happen

The adverse effects of beta-adrenergic blockers on the cardiovascular system may vary, but they include bradycardia, hypotension, and AV block. (See *Noncardiac adverse effects of class II beta-adrenergic blockers.*)

How you intervene

Keep the following points in mind when caring for a patient taking a beta-adrenergic blocker:
- Monitor the patient's heart rate, blood pressure, and ECG.
- Remember that beta-adrenergic blockers should be avoided in patients with symptomatic bradycardia, second- or third-degree

Noncardiac adverse effects of class II beta-adrenergic blockers

In addition to adverse cardiovascular effects of class II beta-adrenergic blockers, other adverse effects include:
- *Central nervous system*—insomnia, syncope, mental depression, emotional lability, fatigue, headache, dizziness, lethargy, vivid dreams, hallucinations, light-headedness
- *Respiratory*—dyspnea, bronchospasm, especially in patients with asthma or other bronchospastic disease.

AV block without a pacemaker, and shock. Use them cautiously in patients with diabetes mellitus (they mask the signs of hypoglycemia), heart failure, kidney disease, liver disease, myasthenia gravis, peripheral vascular disease, and hypotension.
- Keep in mind that noncardioselective beta-adrenergic blockers are contraindicated in patients with asthma or other bronchospastic disease.
- Correct electrolyte imbalances before starting therapy with a beta-adrenergic blocker.
- Remember that beta-adrenergic blockers diminish the patient's ability to withstand exercise because the heart rate can't increase. These drugs also block sympathetic response to shock.

Class III antiarrhythmics

Class III antiarrhythmics are called *potassium channel blockers.* (See *Effects of class III antiarrhythmics.*) They include amiodarone hydrochloride (Cordarone), ibutilide (Corvert), and dofetilide (Tikosyn). Sotalol has qualities of both class II and class III antiarrhythmics. All class III antiarrhythmics have proarrhythmic potential.

Amiodarone

Amiodarone is used to treat supraventricular arrhythmias, including atrial fibrillation and atrial flutter, as well as ventricular arrhythmias.

Effects of class III antiarrhythmics

Class III antiarrhythmic drugs—including amiodarone, sotalol, and ibutilide—cause the effects shown below on an ECG by exerting particular actions on the cardiac cycle. Class III antiarrhythmics

- block potassium movement during phase 3.
- increase duration of the action potential.
- prolong the effective refractory period.

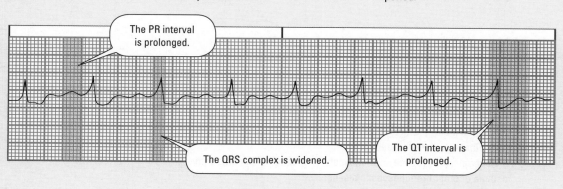

The PR interval is prolonged.

The QRS complex is widened.

The QT interval is prolonged.

How to give it

Here's how to administer amiodarone:

- Orally—Give 800 to 1,600 mg daily in divided doses for 1 to 3 weeks, followed by 400 to 800 mg/day for 4 weeks, followed by 200 to 400 mg/day as a maintenance dosage.
- I.V. infusion—Infuse 150 mg over 10 minutes (15 mg/min); then infuse 360 mg over the next 6 hours (1 mg/min), followed by 540 mg infused over 18 hours (0.5 mg/min). After the first 24 hours, a maintenance I.V. infusion of 720 mg per 24 hours (0.5 mg/min) should be continued.

What can happen

Adverse cardiovascular effects of amiodarone given by I.V. infusion include bradycardia, hypotension, AV block, heart failure, asystole, and pulseless electrical activity.

Long-term oral therapy can be associated with bradycardia, pulmonary fibrosis, thyroid dysfunction, elevated liver function tests, and corneal deposits, not usually leading to visual disturbances. (See *Noncardiac adverse effects of amiodarone.*)

How you intervene

Keep the following points in mind when caring for a patient taking amiodarone:

- Monitor the patient's vital signs, ECG, and respiratory status.
- Monitor laboratory test results, such as electrolyte levels, liver function studies, thyroid function studies, pulmonary function studies, and chest X-rays.
- Check for signs of digoxin toxicity or increased prothrombin time. Amiodarone can increase the serum levels of digoxin and warfarin.

Noncardiac adverse effects of amiodarone

In addition to adverse cardiovascular effects of amiodarone, other adverse effects include:

- *Central nervous system*—malaise, fatigue, dizziness, peripheral neuropathy, ataxia, paresthesia, tremors, headache, vision disturbances
- *Respiratory*—pulmonary toxicity (progressive dyspnea, cough, fever, pleuritic chest pain)
- *GI*—nausea, vomiting, constipation, anorexia, elevated liver function tests
- *Other*—photosensitivity, abnormal taste and smell, hypothyroidism or hyperthyroidism, bleeding disorders, muscle weakness.

- Remember that amiodarone should be avoided in patients with hypersensitivity to the drug, cardiogenic shock, marked sinus bradycardia, and second- or third-degree AV block without a pacemaker. Use the drug cautiously in patients with cardiomegaly, pre-existing bradycardia or sinus node disease, conduction disturbances, or depressed ventricular function.
- Be aware that the drug has a long half-life (56 days, with a range from 13 to 103 days) and therefore takes weeks to reach therapeutic levels and possibly up to 3 months to be cleared by the body.
- Know that amiodarone may increase theophylline levels in patients taking theophylline. Monitor the patient for signs of theophylline toxicity.
- Be aware that amiodarone may increase phenytoin (Dilantin) levels. Monitor phenytoin levels closely.
- Instruct the patient to wear sunscreen and protective clothing to avoid photosensitivity reactions. A blue-gray discoloration of exposed skin may occur.
- Recommend that the patient have yearly ophthalmic examinations. Within 1 to 4 months after beginning amiodarone therapy, most patients show corneal microdeposits upon slit-lamp ophthalmic examination. Instillation of methylcellulose ophthalmic solution minimizes corneal microdeposits.
- Administer the I.V. drug through a central venous access device to avoid phlebitis.
- The lowest possible effective maintenance dose should be used to avoid toxicity.

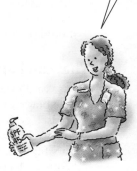

Tell the patient taking amiodarone to wear sunscreen and protective clothing to avoid photosensitivity reactions.

Ibutilide

Ibutilide is used for the rapid conversion of recent-onset atrial fibrillation or flutter to sinus rhythm. The drug increases atrial and ventricular refractoriness.

How to give it

If your adult patient weighs greater than 132 lb (60 kg) or more, he or she will receive 1 mg of ibutilide I.V. over 10 minutes. If he weighs less than 132 lb, the dose is 0.01 mg/kg.

If the arrhythmia is still present 10 minutes after the infusion is complete, the dose may be repeated.

What can happen

Adverse cardiovascular effects of ibutilide include PVCs, nonsustained VT, sustained polymorphic VT, hypotension, bundle-branch block, AV block, hypertension, bradycardia, tachycardia, palpitations, heart failure, and lengthening of the QT interval. Noncardiac adverse effects include headache, nausea, and renal failure.

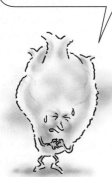

Adverse effects of ibutilide include PVCs, VT, hypotension (gulp), AV block (gulp)...Is it getting hot in here?

How you intervene

Keep these points in mind when giving ibutilide:

- Correct electrolyte abnormalities before administering ibutilide.
- Monitor the patient's vital signs and ECG continuously during the infusion and for at least 4 hours afterward. The infusion will be stopped if the arrhythmia terminates or if the patient develops VT or marked prolongation of the QT interval, which signals the risk of polymorphic VT.
- Have emergency equipment and medication nearby for the treatment of sustained VT.
- Don't give ibutilide to patients with a history of polymorphic VT.
- Give the drug cautiously in patients receiving digoxin (Lanoxin) because it can mask signs and symptoms of cardiotoxicity associated with excessive digoxin levels.
- Don't administer ibutilide at the same time or within 4 hours of class Ia or other class III antiarrhythmics.
- Don't give ibutilide with other drugs that prolong the QT interval, such as phenothiazines and tricyclic or tetracyclic antidepressants.
- Be aware that patients with atrial fibrillation that has lasted longer than 24 to 48 hours must receive anticoagulants for at least 3 weeks before the initiation of ibutilide therapy, unless atrial thrombosis is confirmed negative by transesophageal echocardiogram.

Dofetilide (Tikosyn)

Dofetilide is used to maintain normal sinus rhythm in patients with symptomatic atrial fibrillation or atrial flutter. It is also used to convert atrial fibrillation and atrial flutter to normal sinus rhythm.

How to give it

Dosage is based on creatinine clearance and QTc interval, which must be determined before the first dose (QT interval should be used if the heart rate is less than 60 beats/min). The usual recommended dosage is 500 mcg orally twice per day for patients with a creatinine clearance greater than 60 mL/min. The dose is 250 mcg twice daily if the creatinine clearance is 40 to 60 mL/min and 125 mcg twice daily if the creatinine clearance is 20 to 40 mL/min. QTc should be <440 ms before administration of the first dose of Tikosyn.

What can happen

Adverse cardiovascular effects of dofetilide include ventricular fibrillation, VT, torsades de pointes, AV block, bundle-branch block, heart block, bradycardia, chest pain, edema, cardiac arrest, and MI. (See *Noncardiac adverse effects of dofetilide,* page 244.)

Noncardiac adverse effects of dofetilide

In addition to adverse cardiovascular effects of dofetilide, other adverse effects include:
- *Central nervous system*—headache, dizziness, insomnia, migraine, paresthesia
- *GI*—nausea, diarrhea, abdominal pain
- *Respiratory*—respiratory tract infection, dyspnea
- *Skin*—rash
- *Other*—angioedema.

How you intervene

Remember these facts when giving dofetilide:
- Use cautiously in patients with severe hepatic impairment.
- Provide continuous ECG monitoring for at least 3 days.
- Avoid discharging the patient within 12 hours of conversion to normal sinus rhythm.
- Monitor the patient for prolonged diarrhea, sweating, and vomiting. Report these signs to the practitioner because electrolyte imbalance may increase the potential for arrhythmia development.
- Assess for hypokalemia and hypomagnesemia if the patient is receiving potassium-depleting diuretics, which increase the risk of torsades de pointes. Potassium level should be within normal range before giving dofetilide and kept in normal range.
- Stop antiarrhythmic therapy under careful monitoring for a minimum of three plasma half-lives before starting dofetilide.
- Don't give dofetilide after amiodarone therapy until the amiodarone level is below 0.3 mcg/mL or until amiodarone has been stopped for at least 3 months.
- Provide a wash-out period of at least 2 days before starting other drug therapy if dofetilide is stopped to allow treatment with other drugs (such as those that interact with dofetilide).
- Don't give dofetilide with grapefruit juice; it may decrease hepatic metabolism and increase the drug level.
- Don't give with drugs that prolong the QT interval, such as phenothiazines, tricyclic or tetracyclic antidepressants, and erythromycin.
- Avoid using with cimetidine (Tagamet), ketoconazole (Nizoral), co-trimoxazole (Bactrim), verapamil (Calan), and inhibitors of CYP3A4, such as amiodarone (Cordarone), diltiazem (Cardizem), norfloxacin (Noroxin), and selective serotonin reuptake inhibitors.
- Avoid using with inhibitors of renal cationic secretion, such as megestrol (Megace), amiloride (Midamor), metformin (Glucophage), and triamterene (Dyrenium).

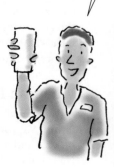

When giving dofetilide, skip the grapefruit juice and go for water instead. Grapefruit juice can affect metabolism of this drug.

Effects of class IV antiarrhythmics

Class IV antiarrhythmic drugs—including such calcium channel blockers as verapamil and diltiazem—affect the cardiac cycle in specific ways and may lead to the ECG change shown here. Class IV antiarrhythmics

- block calcium movement during phase 2.

- prolong the conduction time and increase the refractory period in the atrioventricular node.

- decrease contractility.

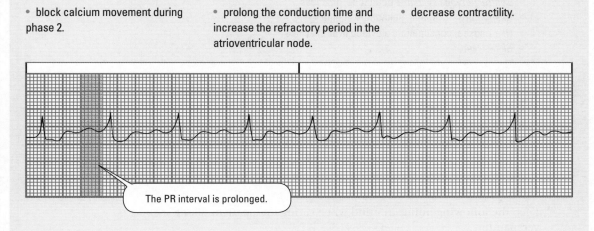

The PR interval is prolonged.

Class IV antiarrhythmics

Class IV antiarrhythmic drugs are called *calcium channel blockers*. They include verapamil and diltiazem. These drugs prolong conduction time and the refractory period in the AV node. (See *Effects of class IV antiarrhythmics.*)

Other calcium channel blockers, including nifedipine (Procardia) and amlodipine (Norvasc), don't cause electrophysiologic changes and aren't used as antiarrhythmics. They're used primarily to treat hypertension.

Verapamil

Verapamil is used for PSVT because of its effect on the AV node. It also slows the ventricular response in atrial fibrillation and flutter.

How to give it

Here's how to administer verapamil:

- Orally for chronic atrial fibrillation—Give 80 to 120 mg three or four times per day to a maximum of 480 mg/day.
- I.V. injection for supraventricular arrhythmias—Give 0.075 to 0.15 mg/kg (usually 5 to 10 mg) over 2 minutes; you can repeat in 30 minutes if no response occurs.

> ## Noncardiac adverse effects of verapamil
>
> In addition to adverse cardiovascular effects of verapamil, other adverse effects include:
> * *Central nervous system*—headache, dizziness
> * *Respiratory*—dyspnea, pulmonary edema
> * *GI*—nausea, constipation, elevated liver enzymes
> * *Skin*—rash.

What can happen

Cardiovascular adverse effects of verapamil include bradycardia, AV block, hypotension, heart failure, edema, and ventricular fibrillation. (See *Noncardiac adverse effects of verapamil.*)

How you intervene

Keep the following points in mind when caring for a patient taking verapamil:
* Monitor the patient's heart rate, blood pressure, and ECG. Also monitor liver function studies.
* Note that calcium may be given before verapamil to prevent hypotension.
* Advise the patient to change position slowly to avoid orthostatic hypotension.
* Remember that verapamil should be avoided in SSS or second- or third-degree AV block without a pacemaker and in atrial fibrillation or flutter caused by WPW syndrome. It also should be avoided in patients with hypersensitivity to the drug, advanced heart failure, cardiogenic shock, profound hypotension, acute MI, or pulmonary edema.
* Give the drug cautiously to patients receiving digoxin or oral beta-adrenergic blockers, elderly patients, and patients with heart failure, hypotension, liver disease, or kidney disease. Don't give verapamil to patients receiving I.V. beta-adrenergic blockers.

Diltiazem

Diltiazem is administered I.V. to treat PSVT and atrial fibrillation or flutter. Diltiazem is also used to treat angina and hypertension, but those uses aren't discussed here.

Noncardiac adverse effects of diltiazem

In addition to adverse cardiovascular effects of diltiazem, other adverse effects include:
* *Central nervous system*—headache, dizziness
* *GI*—nausea, transient elevation of liver enzymes, constipation, abdominal discomfort, acute hepatic injury
* *Skin*—rash.

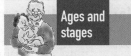

Ages and stages

Prolonged effects in elderly patients

Administer diltiazem cautiously to an older adult because the half-life of the drug may be prolonged. Be especially careful if the older adult also has heart failure or impaired hepatic or renal function.

How to give it

Here's how to give diltiazem:
* I.V. injection—Give 0.25 mg/kg (usually 20 mg) over 2 minutes; you can repeat in 15 minutes at 0.35 mg/kg (usually 25 mg) over 2 minutes.
* I.V. infusion—Infuse at a rate of 5 to 15 mg/hr (usually 10 mg/hr).

What can happen

Adverse cardiovascular effects of diltiazem include edema, flushing, bradycardia, hypotension, heart failure, arrhythmias, conduction abnormalities, sinus node dysfunction, and AV block. (See *Noncardiac adverse effects of diltiazem.*)

How you intervene

Keep the following points in mind when caring for a patient receiving diltiazem:
* Monitor the patient's heart rate, blood pressure, and ECG.
* Diltiazem should be avoided in patients with SSS or second- or third-degree AV block without a pacemaker, atrial fibrillation or flutter due to WPW syndrome, advanced heart failure, cardiogenic shock, profound hypotension, acute MI, pulmonary edema, or sensitivity to the drug.
* Use cautiously in elderly patients; in patients with heart failure, hypotension, or liver or kidney disease; and in those receiving digoxin or beta-adrenergic blockers. (See *Prolonged effects in elderly patients.*)
* Give cautiously to patients receiving I.V. beta-adrenergic blockers. I.V. diltiazem and I.V. beta-adrenergic blocker shouldn't be given within a few hours of each other.
* Advise the patient to change position slowly to avoid orthostatic hypotension.

Patients taking diltiazem should change position slowly.

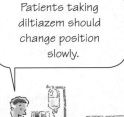

Unclassified antiarrhythmics

Some antiarrhythmic drugs defy categorization. Let's look at some of those drugs, which are called unclassified or miscellaneous antiarrhythmic drugs.

Adenosine

Adenosine is a naturally occurring nucleoside used to treat PSVT. It acts on the AV node to slow conduction and inhibit re-entry pathways. It's also useful in treating PSVT associated with WPW syndrome.

Although adenosine isn't effective for atrial fibrillation or atrial flutter, it does slow the rate in PSVT enough to determine the rhythm so that a more appropriate agent, such as verapamil, can be used.

How to give it

Administer 6 mg of adenosine I.V. over 1 to 2 seconds, immediately followed by a rapid flush with 20 mL of normal saline solution. Because the drug's half-life is less than 10 seconds, it needs to reach the circulation quickly. The intravenous line should be placed at the antecubital space, rather than more distal to the heart. Repeat with an I.V. injection of 12 mg of adenosine if the rhythm doesn't convert within 1 to 2 minutes.

What can happen

Adverse cardiovascular effects of adenosine include transient arrhythmias such as a short asystolic pause at the time of conversion. Other adverse effects include hypotension (if large doses are used), facial flushing, diaphoresis, chest pressure, and recurrence of the arrhythmia. (See *Noncardiac adverse effects of adenosine.*)

How you intervene

Keep the following points in mind when caring for a patient receiving adenosine:

Noncardiac adverse effects of adenosine

In addition to adverse cardiovascular effects of adenosine, other adverse effects include:
- *Central nervous system*—anxiety, light-headedness, burning sensation, headache, numbness and tingling in arms
- *Respiratory*—dyspnea
- *GI*—nausea.

- Monitor the patient's heart rate, blood pressure, ECG, ventilatory rate and depth, and breath sounds for wheezes.
- Remember that adenosine should be avoided in patients with hypersensitivity to the drug, second- or third-degree AV block, or SSS without a pacemaker. Use cautiously in older adults and in patients with asthma or those receiving dipyridamole (Persantine) or carbamazepine (Tegretol).
- Store adenosine at room temperature.
- Be aware that the patient may require a higher dose or may not respond to therapy at all if he or she is also taking aminophylline or another xanthine derivative.

Atropine

Atropine is an anticholinergic drug that blocks vagal effects on the SA and AV nodes. This enhances conduction through the AV node and speeds the heart rate. Atropine is used to treat symptomatic bradycardia and asystole. However, atropine is ineffective in patients following dissection of the vagus nerve during heart transplant surgery. Isoproterenol (Isuprel) can be used to treat symptomatic bradycardia in these patients.

How to give it

Administer atropine by a 0.5- to 1-mg I.V. injection repeated as needed at 3- to 5-minute intervals, to a maximum dose of 2 mg. The initial dose for asystole is 1 mg. The maximum dose is 3 mg.

What can happen

Adverse cardiovascular effects of atropine include tachycardia (with high doses), palpitations, bradycardia if given slowly or in a dose of less than 0.5 mg, hypotension, and chest pain and increased myocardial oxygen consumption in patients with coronary artery disease. (See *Noncardiac adverse effects of atropine.*)

Noncardiac adverse effects of atropine

In addition to cardiovascular effects of atropine, other adverse effects include:
- *Central nervous system*—ataxia, disorientation, delirium, agitation, confusion, headache, restlessness, insomnia, dizziness, blurred vision, dilated pupils, photophobia
- *GI*—dry mouth, constipation, paralytic ileus, nausea, vomiting
- *Genitourinary*—urine retention
- *Other*—increased intraocular pressure, anaphylaxis, urticaria.

How you intervene

Keep the following points in mind when caring for a patient receiving atropine:

- Monitor the patient's heart rate, blood pressure, ECG, urine output, and bowel sounds.
- Remember that atropine should be avoided in patients with hypersensitivity to belladonna, acute angle–closure glaucoma, GI obstruction, obstructive uropathy, myasthenia gravis, and tachyarrhythmias.
- Use atropine cautiously in patients with renal disease, heart failure, hyperthyroidism, hepatic disease, hypertension, and acute MI. Don't give atropine for bradycardia unless the patient is symptomatic. Increasing the heart rate in these patients can lead to increased myocardial oxygen consumption and a worsening of the infarction.

Digoxin

Digoxin (Lanoxin) is used to treat PSVT and atrial fibrillation and flutter, especially in patients with heart failure. It provides antiarrhythmic effects by enhancing vagal tone and slowing conduction through the SA and AV nodes. It also strengthens myocardial contraction. Digoxin has visible effects on the patient's ECG. (See *Effects of digoxin*.)

Effects of digoxin

Digoxin affects the cardiac cycle in various ways and may lead to the ECG changes shown here.

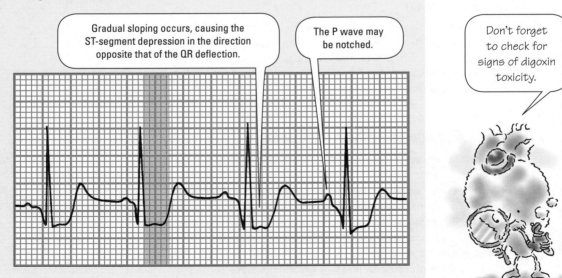

Gradual sloping occurs, causing the ST-segment depression in the direction opposite that of the QR deflection.

The P wave may be notched.

Don't forget to check for signs of digoxin toxicity.

How to give it

To administer digoxin rapidly and orally or I.V., give a digitalizing dose of 0.5 to 1 mg divided into two or more doses every 6 to 8 hours. The usual maintenance dosage is 0.125 to 0.5 mg daily.

What can happen

Too much digoxin in the body causes toxicity. Toxic cardiac effects include SA and AV blocks and junctional and ventricular arrhythmias. Digoxin toxicity is treated by discontinuing digoxin; correcting oxygenation and electrolyte imbalances; treating arrhythmias with phenytoin, lidocaine, atropine, or a pacemaker; giving digoxin immune fab (Digibind) to reverse life-threatening arrhythmias or blocks (occurs within 30 to 60 minutes); and correcting the potassium level before giving digoxin immune fab. (See *Noncardiac adverse effects of digoxin.*)

How you intervene

Keep the following points in mind when caring for a patient receiving digoxin:
- Check for signs of digoxin toxicity, especially in patients with hypokalemia, hypocalcemia, hypercalcemia, or hypomagnesemia. Monitor serum electrolyte levels as ordered.
- Monitor the patient's apical heart rate and ECG. A heart rate below 60 beats/min or a change in rhythm can signal digoxin toxicity. If this occurs, withhold digoxin and notify the practitioner.
- Remember that digoxin should be avoided in patients with known hypersensitivity to the drug; SSS, SA, or AV block (without an implanted cardiac pacemaker); VT; hypertrophic cardiomyopathy; or WPW syndrome. Use cautiously in older adults and in patients with acute MI, liver or kidney disease, or hypothyroidism.
- Withhold digoxin for 1 to 2 days before performing electrical cardioversion.
- Be sure to question the patient about herbal preparation use because digoxin reacts with many preparations. Fumitory, lily of the valley, goldenseal, motherwort, shepherd's purse, and rue may enhance the cardiac effects of digoxin. Licorice, oleander, Siberian ginseng, foxglove, and squill may increase the risk of digoxin toxicity.

Noncardiac adverse effects of digoxin

In addition to adverse cardiovascular effects of digoxin, other adverse effects resulting from toxicity include:
- *Central nervous system*—headache, vision disturbances, hallucinations, fatigue, muscle weakness, agitation, malaise, dizziness, stupor, paresthesia
- *GI*—anorexia, nausea, vomiting, diarrhea
- *Other*—yellow-green halos around visual images, blurred vision, light flashes, photophobia, diplopia.

Epinephrine

Epinephrine is a naturally occurring catecholamine. It acts directly on alpha-adrenergic and beta-adrenergic receptor sites of the sympathetic nervous system, and it's used to help restore cardiac rhythm in cardiac arrest and to treat symptomatic bradycardia. Its actions include increasing the systolic blood pressure and slightly decreasing diastolic blood pressure, heart rate, and cardiac output.

How to give it

To restore sinus rhythm in cardiac arrest in adults, administer epinephrine by I.V. injection as a 1-mg dose (10 mL of 1:10,000 solution). Each dose given by peripheral I.V. injection should be followed by a 20-mL flush of I.V. fluid to ensure quick delivery of the drug. Doses may be repeated every 3 to 5 minutes as needed. (Some practitioners advocate doses of up to 5 mg, especially for patients who don't respond to the usual I.V. dose.) After initial I.V. administration, an infusion may be given at 1 to 4 mcg/min.

What can happen

Adverse cardiovascular effects include palpitations, hypertension, tachycardia, ventricular fibrillation, anginal pain, shock, and ECG changes, including a decreased T-wave amplitude. (See *Noncardiac adverse effects of epinephrine.*)

How you intervene

Keep these points in mind when administering epinephrine:
* Be sure to document the concentration of the epinephrine solution used. (Remember that 1 mg equals 1 mL of 1:1,000 or 10 mL of 1:10,000 concentration.)
* When administering I.V. epinephrine, monitor the patient's heart rate, ECG rhythm, and blood pressure throughout therapy.
* Don't mix the drug with alkaline solutions. Use D_5W, lactated Ringer's solution, or normal saline solution or a combination of dextrose and saline solution.
* Remember that some epinephrine products contain sulfites. Use of those products usually should be avoided in patients with sulfite allergies. The only exception is when epinephrine is being used in an emergency.
* Know that the use of epinephrine with digoxin (Lanoxin) or such general anesthetics as cyclopropane or a halogenated hydrocarbon like halothane (Fluothane) may increase the risk of ventricular arrhythmias.
* Avoid giving epinephrine with other drugs that exert a similar effect. Doing so can cause severe adverse cardiovascular effects.

Magnesium sulfate

Magnesium sulfate is used to treat ventricular arrhythmias, especially polymorphic VT and paroxysmal atrial tachycardia. It's also used as a preventive measure in acute MI. Magnesium sulfate acts similarly

---

Noncardiac adverse effects of epinephrine

In addition to adverse cardiovascular effects of epinephrine, other adverse effects include:
* *Central nervous system*—nervousness, tremor, dizziness, vertigo, headache, disorientation, agitation, fear, pallor, weakness, cerebral hemorrhage, increased rigidity and tremor (in patients with Parkinson's disease)
* *Respiratory*—dyspnea
* *GI*—nausea, vomiting
* *Other*—tissue necrosis.

to class III antiarrhythmic drugs because it decreases myocardial cell excitability and conduction. It slows conduction through the AV node and prolongs the refractory period in the atria and ventricles.

How to give it

For life-threatening arrhythmias, administer 1 to 2 g magnesium sulfate over 5 to 60 minutes. Follow with an infusion of 0.5 to 1 g/hr. The dosage and duration of therapy depend on the patient's response and serum magnesium levels. The optimum dosage is still under study.

What can happen

Adverse cardiovascular effects of magnesium sulfate include diaphoresis, flushing, depressed cardiac function, bradycardia, hypotension, and circulatory collapse. (See *Noncardiac adverse effects of magnesium sulfate.*)

How you intervene

Keep the following points in mind when caring for a patient receiving magnesium sulfate:
- Monitor the patient's heart rate, blood pressure, ventilatory rate, ECG, urine output, deep tendon reflexes, and mental status.
- Remember that magnesium sulfate should be avoided in patients with renal disease. Use it cautiously in patients with renal insufficiency and in those taking digoxin.
- Monitor closely for signs and symptoms of hypermagnesemia, such as hypotension, AV block, central nervous system depression, depressed or absent deep tendon reflexes, muscle weakness or paralysis, and respiratory arrest.
- Have I.V. calcium available to counteract the effects of hypermagnesemia.
- Have intubation equipment and a mechanical ventilator available.
- Magnesium sulfate is contraindicated in heart block and in patients with myocardial damage.

Teaching about antiarrhythmics

Here are some important points to emphasize when teaching your patient about antiarrhythmic drugs:
- Take the drug exactly as prescribed. Don't stop taking the drug without consulting your practitioner.
- Call the practitioner if you experience chest pain, shortness of breath, cough, palpitations, dizziness, fatigue, a weight gain of

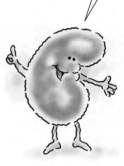

Avoid administering magnesium sulfate to patients with renal disease.

Noncardiac adverse effects of magnesium sulfate

In addition to adverse cardiovascular effects of magnesium sulfate, other adverse effects include:
- *Central nervous system*—drowsiness, depressed reflexes, flaccid paralysis, hypothermia
- *Respiratory*—respiratory paralysis
- *Other*—hypocalcemia.

more than 2 lb (0.9 kg) per day, a very fast or slow heart rate, or a change in the regularity of the heartbeat or if you notice persistent changes you feel might be related to drug therapy.

• See your practitioner for regular checkups, as scheduled. Periodic physical examinations, ECGs, chest X-rays, and laboratory studies will help evaluate the effectiveness of therapy.

• Use herbal preparations with care. Some preparations can cause life-threatening interactions.

That's a wrap!

Pharmacologic treatments review

Antiarrhythmic drugs
• Classified according to effect on the cell's electrical activity (action potential) and mechanism of action

Class Ia antiarrhythmics
• Are called sodium channel blockers
• Reduce excitability of cardiac cells and decrease contractility
• Have anticholinergic and proarrhythmic effects
• Show widened QRS complex and prolonged QT intervals on ECG

Quinidine
• Used for supraventricular and ventricular arrhythmias

Procainamide hydrochloride
• Used for supraventricular and ventricular arrhythmias

Class Ib antiarrhythmics
• Suppress ventricular ectopy
• Slow phase 0 depolarization
• Shorten phase 3 repolarization and action potential

Lidocaine hydrochloride
• Former drug of choice for suppressing ventricular arrhythmias

Mexiletine
• Oral congener of lidocaine, used to treat ventricular arrhythmias

Class Ic antiarrhythmics
• Slow conduction

Flecainide acetate
• Used for paroxysmal atrial fibrillation or flutter in patients without structural heart disease; prevents supraventricular tachycardia

Propafenone hydrochloride
• Used for paroxysmal atrial fibrillation or flutter in patients without structural heart disease; prevents supraventricular tachycardia

Class II antiarrhythmics
• Are called beta-adrenergic blockers
• Block sympathetic nervous system beta receptors and decrease heart rate
• Used to treat supraventricular and ventricular arrhythmias
• Include acebutolol, propranolol, esmolol, and sotalol

Class III antiarrhythmics
• Are called potassium channel blockers

Pharmacologic treatments review *(Continued)*

- Block potassium movement during phase 3
- Increase the duration of the action potential
- Prolong the effective refractory period
- Show prolonged PR and QT intervals and widened QRS complex on ECG

Amiodarone
- Used for supraventricular arrhythmias, atrial fibrillation, and atrial flutter; PSVT caused by accessory pathway conduction (as in WPW syndrome); and ventricular arrhythmias

Ibutilide fumarate
- Rapidly converts recent-onset atrial fibrillation or flutter

Dofetilide
- Used for maintenance of normal sinus rhythm in patients with atrial fibrillation or flutter
- Used to convert atrial fibrillation and flutter to normal sinus rhythm

Class IV antiarrhythmics
- Are called calcium channel blockers
- Prolong conduction time and refractory period in the AV node
- Decrease contractility
- Show PR interval prolonged on ECG

Verapamil
- Used for PSVT and to slow ventricular response in atrial fibrillation and flutter

Diltiazem
- Used for PSVT and atrial fibrillation or flutter

Unclassified antiarrhythmics
- Also called miscellaneous antiarrhythmics

Adenosine
- Slows AV node conduction and inhibits re-entry pathways
- Used to treat PSVT

Atropine
- Anticholinergic drug that blocks vagal effects on the SA and AV nodes
- Used to treat symptomatic bradycardia and asystole

Digoxin
- Enhances vagal tone and slows conduction through the SA and AV nodes
- Shows ST-segment depression opposite the QRS deflection on ECG; P wave may be notched
- Used to treat PSVT and atrial fibrillation and flutter

Epinephrine
- Catecholamine that acts on alpha-adrenergic and beta-adrenergic receptor sites of the sympathetic nervous system
- Used for symptomatic bradycardia and to restore cardiac rhythm in cardiac arrest

Magnesium sulfate
- Decreases cardiac cell excitability and conduction; slows conduction through the AV node, and prolongs the refractory period
- Used to treat ventricular arrhythmias

Quick quiz

1. Antiarrhythmic drugs that depress the rate of depolarization belong to class:
    A. I.
    B. II.
    C. III.
    D. IV.

Answer: A. Class I antiarrhythmic drugs block sodium influx during phase 0, depressing the rate of depolarization.

2. The drug that blocks vagal stimulation and increases the heart rate is:
    A. magnesium sulfate.
    B. diltiazem.
    C. verapamil.
    D. atropine.

Answer: D. Atropine blocks vagal effects on the SA node, enhances conduction through the node, and speeds the heart rate. The drug is used to treat symptomatic bradycardia.

3. The class III antiarrhythmic drug used for the rapid conversion of recent-onset atrial fibrillation or flutter to sinus rhythm is:
    A. digoxin.
    B. ibutilide fumarate.
    C. procainamide.
    D. verapamil.

Answer: B. Ibutilide fumarate increases atrial and ventricular refractoriness and is used for the rapid conversion of recent-onset atrial fibrillation or flutter.

4. A drug known for lowering the resting heart rate is:
    A. quinidine.
    B. amiodarone.
    C. propranolol.
    D. lidocaine.

Answer: C. Beta-adrenergic blockers, such as propranolol, block sympathetic nervous system beta-adrenergic receptors and lower heart rate, contractility, and conduction.

Scoring

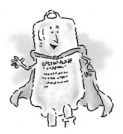

☆☆☆ If you answered all four questions correctly, just say "wow"! You're
the antiarrhythmic drug czar.

☆☆ If you answered three questions correctly, great job! You're the dep-
uty antiarrhythmic drug czar.

☆ If you answered fewer than three questions correctly, don't fret. Get
into the rhythm of antiarrhythmics by reviewing this chapter again.

Recommended references

Brown, D. F. M., & Martindale, J. L. (2012). *Rapid interpretation of ECG's in emergency medicine: A visual guide.* Philadelphia, PA: Wolters Kluwer.

Brown, D. F. M., & Borczuk, P. (2014). Emergent management of atrial flutter. Retrieved from http://emedicine.medscape.com/article/151066-overview

Budzikowski, A. S., & Rottman, J. (2014). Atrial tachycardia practice essentials. Retrieved from http://emedicine.medscape.com/article/151456-overview

Cohen, B. J., & Taylor, J. J. (2013). *Memmler's structure and function of the human body* (10th ed.). Philadelphia, PA: Wolters Kluwer.

Ganjehei, L., Massumi, A., Nazeri, A., & Razavi, M. (2011). Pharmacologic management of arrhythmias. *Texas Heart Institute Journal, 38*(4), 344–349.

Katritsis, D. G., Gersh, B. J., & Camm, A. J. (2013). *Clinical cardiology: Current practice guidelines.* Oxford, United Kingdom: Oxford University Press.

Libby, P., & Bonow, R. D. (2014). *Braunwald's heart disease: A textbook of cardiovascular medicine* (10th ed.). St. Louis, MO: Saunders | Elsevier.

Mann, D. L., Zipes, D. P., Nazeri, A., & Razavi, M. (2011). Pharmacologic management of arrhythmias. *Texas Heart Institute Journal, 38*(4), 344–349.

McLaughlin, M. A. (clinical ed.). (2014). *Cardiovascular care made incredibly easy* (3rd ed.). Philadelphia, PA: Wolters Kluwer.

Urden, L., & Stacy, K. (2013). *Critical care nursing* (7th ed.). St Louis: Mosby | Elsevier.

Wagner, G. S., & Strauss, D. G. (2013). *Marriott's practical electrocardiology* (12th ed.). Philadelphia, PA: Wolters Kluwer.

Part IV

The 12–lead ECG

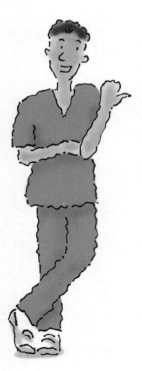

Chapter 11

Obtaining a 12-lead ECG

Just the facts

In this chapter, you'll learn about the:

♦ role of the 12-lead ECG in diagnosing pathologic conditions

♦ relationship between the heart's electrical axis and the 12-lead ECG

♦ proper technique for preparing your patient, placing the electrodes, and recording the ECG

♦ diagnostic purposes of the posterior-lead ECG and the right chest–lead ECG

♦ function of a signal-averaged ECG.

A look at the 12–lead ECG

The 12-lead ECG is a diagnostic test that helps identify pathologic conditions, especially angina and acute myocardial infarction (AMI). It gives a more complete view of the heart's electrical activity than a rhythm strip and can be used to assess left ventricular function. Patients with other conditions that affect the heart's electrical system may also benefit from a 12-lead ECG. (See *Why a 12-lead ECG?*)

Interdependent evidence

Like other diagnostic tests, a 12-lead ECG must be viewed alongside other clinical evidence. Always correlate the patient's ECG results with his history, physical assessment findings, laboratory results, and medication regimen.

Remember, too, that an ECG can be done in various ways, including over a telephone line. (See *Transtelephonic cardiac monitoring*, page 262.) Transtelephonic monitoring, in fact, has become increasingly important as a tool for assessing patients at home and in other nonclinical settings.

Why a 12-lead ECG?

A 12-lead ECG is performed on patients having a myocardial infarction. It may also be ordered for patients with other conditions that affect the heart, including:

• angina
• arrhythmias
• heart chamber enlargement
• digoxin or other drug toxicity
• electrolyte imbalances
• pulmonary embolism
• pericarditis
• hypothermia.

Transtelephonic cardiac monitoring

Using a special recorder-transmitter, patients at home can transmit ECGs by telephone to a central monitoring center for immediate interpretation. This technique, called transtelephonic cardiac monitoring (TTM), reduces healthcare costs and is widely used.

Nurses play an important role in TTM. Besides performing extensive patient and family teaching, they may run the central monitoring center and help interpret ECGs sent by patients.

TTM allows the practitioner to assess transient conditions that cause such symptoms as palpitations, dizziness, syncope, confusion, paroxysmal dyspnea, and chest pain. Such conditions commonly aren't apparent while the patient is in the presence of a practitioner, which can make diagnosis difficult and costly.

With TTM, the patient can transmit an ECG recording from his home when symptoms appear, avoiding the need to go to the hospital for diagnosis and offering a greater opportunity for early diagnosis. Even if symptoms don't appear often, the patient can keep the equipment for long periods of time, which further aids in the diagnosis of the patient's condition.

Home care

TTM can also be used by patients having cardiac rehabilitation at home. The patient is called regularly during this period to receive transmissions and assess progress. This monitoring can help reduce the anxiety felt by many patients and their families after discharge, especially if the patient suffered a myocardial infarction.

TTM is especially valuable for assessing the effects of drugs and for diagnosing and managing paroxysmal arrhythmias. In both cases, TTM can eliminate the need for admitting the patient for evaluation and a potentially lengthy hospital stay.

Understanding TTM equipment

TTM requires three main pieces of equipment: an ECG recorder-transmitter, a standard telephone line, and a receiver. The ECG recorder-transmitter converts electrical activity picked up from the patient's heart into acoustic waves. Some models contain built-in memory that stores a recording of the activity so the patient can transmit it later.

A standard telephone line is used to transmit information. The receiver converts the acoustic waves transmitted over the telephone line into ECG activity, which is then recorded on ECG paper for interpretation and documentation in the patient's chart. The recorder-transmitter uses an electrode applied to the finger, chest, or a wrist bracelet. These electrodes produce ECG tracings similar to those of a standard 12-lead ECG.

Credit card–size recorder

One type of recorder operates on a battery and is about the size of a credit card. When a patient becomes symptomatic, he holds the back of the card firmly to the center of his chest and pushes the start button. Four electrodes located on the back of the card sense electrical activity and record it. The card can store 30 seconds of activity and can later transmit the recording across phone lines for evaluation by a practitioner.

Other transtelephonic monitors are approximately the size of a beeper and store lengths of ECGs on a digital chip which can then be transmitted over the phone line and recorded on paper.

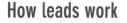

Now that's one heck of a charge card!

How leads work

The 12-lead ECG records the heart's electrical activity using a series of electrodes placed on the patient's extremities and chest wall. The 12 leads include three bipolar limb leads (I, II, and III), three unipolar augmented limb leads (aV_R, aV_L, and aV_F), and six unipolar precordial, or chest, leads (V_1, V_2, V_3, V_4, V_5, and V_6). These leads provide 12 different views of the heart's electrical activity. (See *A look at the leads.*)

A look at the leads

Each of the 12 leads views the heart from a different angle. These illustrations show the direction of each lead relative to the wave of depolarization (shown in color) and list the 12 views of the heart.

Views reflected on a 12-lead ECG	Leads	View of the heart
	Standard limb leads (bipolar)	
	I	Lateral wall
	II	Inferior wall
	III	Inferior wall
	Augmented limb leads (unipolar)	
	aV_R	No specific view
	aV_L	Lateral wall
	aV_F	Inferior wall
	Precordial, or chest, leads (unipolar)	
	V_1	Septal wall
	V_2	Septal wall
	V_3	Anterior wall
	V_4	Anterior wall
	V_5	Lateral wall
	V_6	Lateral wall

Up, down, and across

Scanning up, down, and across the heart, each lead transmits information about a different area. The waveforms obtained from each lead vary depending on the location of the lead in relation to the wave of depolarization, or electrical stimulus, passing through the myocardium.

Limb leads

The six limb leads record electrical activity in the heart's frontal plane. This plane is a view through the middle of the heart from top to bottom. Electrical activity is recorded from the anterior to the posterior axis.

Precordial leads

The six precordial leads provide information on electrical activity in the heart's horizontal plane, a transverse view through the middle of the heart, dividing it into upper and lower portions. Electrical activity is recorded from either a superior or an inferior approach.

The electrical axis

Besides assessing 12 different leads, a 12-lead ECG records the heart's electrical axis. The axis is a measurement of electrical impulses flowing through the heart.

As impulses travel through the heart, they generate small electrical forces called *instantaneous vectors*. The mean of these vectors represents the force and direction of the wave of depolarization through the heart. That mean is called the *electrical axis*. It's also called the *mean instantaneous vector* and the *mean QRS vector*.

Havin' a heart wave

In a healthy heart, impulses originate in the sinoatrial node, travel through the atria to the atrioventricular node, and then to the ventricles. Most of the movement of the impulses is downward and to the left, the direction of a normal axis.

Swingin' on an axis

In an unhealthy heart, axis direction varies. That's because the direction of electrical activity swings away from areas of damage or necrosis and toward areas of hypertrophy. Knowing the normal deflection of each lead will help you evaluate whether the electrical axis is normal or abnormal.

Obtaining a 12-lead ECG

To obtain an ECG, you'll need to:
- gather the appropriate supplies
- explain the procedure to the patient
- attach the electrodes properly
- know how to use the ECG machine.

Let's take a closer look at obtaining an ECG:

1. Explain the procedure

Tell the patient that the practitioner has ordered an ECG, and explain the procedure. Emphasize that the test takes only a few minutes and that it's a safe, painless, and risk-free way to evaluate cardiac function.

Answer the patient's questions, and offer reassurance. Preparing him well helps alleviate anxiety and promote cooperation.

2. Prepare the patient

Ask the patient to lie in a supine or semi-Fowlers position with his arms at his sides. Ensure privacy, and expose the patient's arms, legs, and chest, draping him for comfort. Make sure the patient's legs are uncrossed. Remove electrical devices, including cell phones, from the area due to the interference they may cause. (See *Obtaining a pediatric ECG.*)

3. Skin preparation

Select the areas where you'll attach the electrodes. Choose spots that are flat and fleshy, avoid areas that are muscular or bony. Dry the skin if it is wet or diaphoretic. Clip the area if it's excessively hairy. Clean excess oil or other substances from the skin to enhance electrode contact. Follow your hospital policy for any additional skin preparation such as the use of a nonalcohol wipe or abrasive skin prep pad. Remember—the better the electrode contact, the better the recording.

4. Make the recording

The 12-lead ECG offers 12 different views of the heart, just as 12 photographers snapping the same picture would produce 12 different snapshots. To help ensure an accurate recording—or set of "pictures"—the electrodes must be applied correctly. Inaccurate placement of an electrode by greater than ⅝" (1.5 cm) from its standardized position may lead to inaccurate waveforms and an incorrect ECG interpretation.

The 12-lead ECG requires four electrodes on the limbs and six across the front of the chest wall.

Ages and stages

Obtaining a pediatric ECG

You'll need patience when obtaining a pediatric ECG. With the help of the parents, if possible, try distracting the attention of a young child. If artifact from arm and leg movement is a problem, place the electrodes in a more proximal position on the extremity.

Going out on a limb lead

To record the bipolar limb leads I, II, and III and the unipolar limb leads aV_R, aV_L, and aV_F, place electrodes on both of the patient's arms and on his left leg. The right leg also receives an electrode, but that electrode acts as a ground and doesn't contribute to the waveform.

Where the wires go

Finding where to place the electrodes on the patient is easy because each leadwire is labeled or color coded. (See *Monitoring the limb leads*.) For example, a wire—usually white—might be labeled "RA"

Monitoring the limb leads

These diagrams show electrode placement for the six limb leads. RA indicates right arm; LA, left arm; RL, right leg; and LL, left leg. The plus sign (+) indicates the positive pole, the minus sign (–) indicates the negative pole, and G indicates the ground. Below each diagram is a sample ECG recording for that lead.

Lead I	Lead II	Lead III
This lead connects the right arm (negative pole) with the left arm (positive pole).	This lead connects the right arm (negative pole) with the left leg (positive pole).	This lead connects the left arm (negative pole) with the left leg (positive pole).

for right arm. Another wire—usually red—might be labeled "LL" for left leg. Precordial leads are also labeled or color coded according to which wire corresponds to which lead.

No low leads allowed

To record the six precordial leads (V_1 through V_6), position the electrodes on specific areas of the anterior chest wall. It is vital that the practitioner knows the exact placement of each electrode on the patient as incorrect placement can lead to a false diagnosis of infarction or negative changes on the ECG. (See *Positioning precordial electrodes,* page 268.)

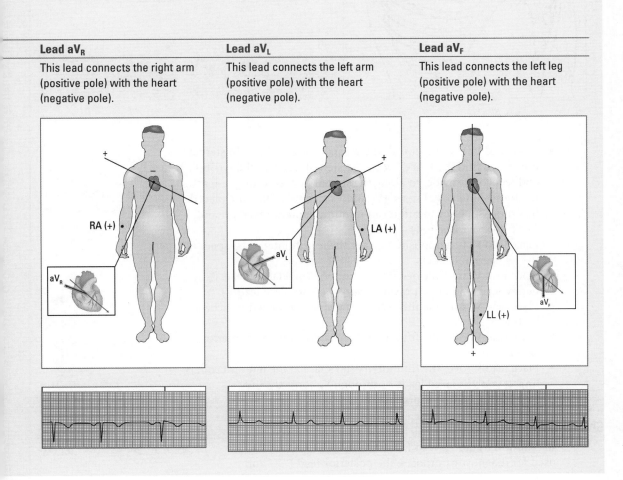

Lead aV$_R$

This lead connects the right arm (positive pole) with the heart (negative pole).

Lead aV$_L$

This lead connects the left arm (positive pole) with the heart (negative pole).

Lead aV$_F$

This lead connects the left leg (positive pole) with the heart (negative pole).

Positioning precordial electrodes

The precordial leads complement the limb leads to provide a complete view of the heart. To record the precordial leads, place the electrodes as shown below.

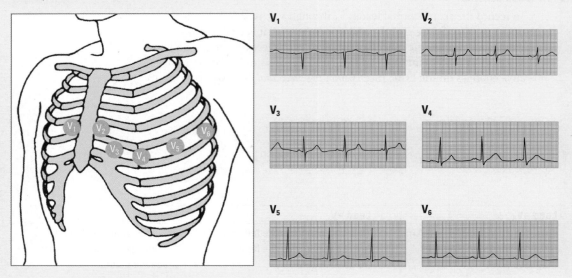

- Place lead V_1 over the fourth intercostal space at the right sternal border. To find the space, locate the sternal notch at the second rib and feel your way down along the sternal border until you reach the fourth intercostal space (V_1 and V_2 electrodes that are placed in a more superior location can mimic an anterior wall MI and cause T wave inversion).
- Place lead V_2 just opposite V_1, over the fourth intercostal space at the left sternal border.
- Place lead V_3 midway between V_2 and V_4. *Tip:* Placing lead V_4 before lead V_3 makes it easier to see where to place lead V_3.
- Place lead V_4 over the fifth intercostal space at the left midclavicular line.
- Place lead V_5 over the fifth intercostal space at the left anterior axillary line.
- Place lead V_6 over the fifth intercostal space at the left midaxillary line. If you've placed leads V_4 through V_6 correctly, they should line up horizontally.

Precordial leads (V_1 through V_6) that are misplaced inferiorly or laterally can alter the amplitude and lead to a misdiagnosis.

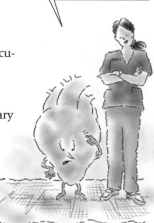

Give me more electrodes!

In addition to the 12-lead ECG, two other ECGs may be used for diagnostic purposes: the posterior-lead ECG and the right chest–lead ECG. These ECGs use chest leads to assess areas standard 12-lead ECGs can't.

Seeing behind your back

Because of lung and muscle barriers, the usual chest leads can't "see" the heart's posterior surface to record myocardial damage there. Some practitioners add three posterior leads to the 12-lead ECG: leads V_7, V_8, and V_9. These leads are placed opposite anterior leads V_4, V_5, and V_6, on the left side of the patient's back, following the same horizontal line.

On rare occasions, a practitioner may request right-sided posterior leads. These leads are labeled V_{7R}, V_{8R}, and V_{9R} and are placed on the right side of the patient's back. Their placement is a mirror image of the electrodes on the left side of the back. This type of ECG provides information on the right posterior area of the heart.

Checking out the right chest

The usual 12-lead ECG evaluates only the left ventricle. If the right ventricle needs to be assessed for damage or dysfunction, the practitioner may order a right chest–lead ECG. For example, a patient with an inferior wall MI might have a right chest–lead ECG to rule out right ventricular involvement.

With this type of ECG, the six leads are placed on the right side of the chest in a mirror image of the standard precordial lead placement. Electrodes start at the left sternal border and swing down under the right breast area.

Know your machine

After you understand how to position the electrodes, familiarize yourself with the ECG machine. Machines come in two types: multichannel recorders and single-channel recorders. Because single-channel recorders are rarely used, we'll only discuss a multichannel recorder.

With a multichannel recorder, you'll attach all electrodes to the patient at once and the machine prints a simultaneous view of all leads. To begin recording the patient's ECG, follow these steps:

- Plug the cord of the ECG machine into a grounded outlet. If the machine operates on a charged battery, it may not need to be plugged in.
- Enter the patient's identification data as prompted by the ECG machine.
- Prepare the patient's skin, and then place the electrodes on the patient's chest, arms, and legs.
- Make sure all leads are securely attached.

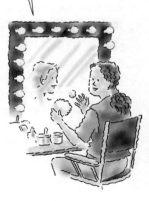

With a right chest lead ECG, the leads are placed in a mirror image of the standard placement.

- Instruct the patient to relax, lie still, and breathe normally. Ask him not to talk during the recording to prevent distortion of the ECG tracing.
- Verify that the ECG paper speed selector is set to 25 mm/sec. If necessary, calibrate or standardize the machine according to the manufacturer's instructions.
- Press the appropriate button to record the ECG. If you're performing a right chest–lead ECG, select the appropriate button for recording or note it on the ECG hardcopy.
- Observe the quality of the tracing. When the machine finishes the recording, turn it off.
- Remove the electrodes and, if necessary, clean the patient's skin. If the ECG machine you're using also transmits a copy to a central monitoring area, make sure the copy has been transmitted.

Interpreting the recording

ECG tracings from multichannel machines will all look the same. (See *Multichannel ECG recording.*) The printout will show the

Multichannel ECG recording

The top of a 12-lead ECG recording usually shows patient identification information along with the interpretation done by the machine. A rhythm strip is usually included at the bottom of the recording.

Standardization marks
Look for the standardization marks on the recording, normally 10 small squares high. If the patient has high voltage complexes, the marks will be half as high. You'll also notice that lead markers separate the lead recordings on the paper and that each lead is labeled.

ECG tracing layout
Also familiarize yourself with the order in which the leads are arranged on the ECG tracing. Getting accustomed to the layout of the tracing will help you interpret the ECG more quickly and accurately.

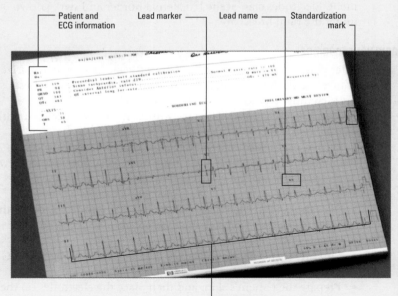

patient's name and identification number. At the top of the print-out, you'll see the patient's heart rate and wave durations, measured in seconds.

Some machines can also record ST-segment elevation and depression. The name of the lead appears next to each 6-second strip.

Remember, ECGs are legal documents. They belong on the patient's chart and must be saved for future reference and comparison with baseline strips.

Signal-averaged ECG

Although most patients will be tested with a 12-lead ECG, some may benefit from being tested with a signal-averaged ECG (SAECG). This simple, noninvasive test helps identify patients at risk for sudden death from sustained ventricular tachycardia.

The test uses a computer to identify late electrical potentials—tiny impulses that follow normal depolarization. Late electrical potentials can't be detected by a 12-lead ECG.

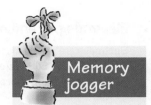

Memory jogger

To help you remember the electrodes for the signal-averaged ECG, think of the phrase "XYZ times 2 and G." The electrodes are X^-, X^+, Y^-, Y^+, Z^-, Z^+, and G (ground).

Who gets the signal?

Patients prone to ventricular tachycardia—those who have had a recent MI, coronary heart disease, cardiomyopathy, or unexplained syncope, for example—are good candidates for an SAECG. Keep in mind that a 12-lead ECG should be done when the patient is free from arrhythmias.

Noise free

An SAECG is a noise-free, surface ECG recording taken from three specialized leads for several hundred heartbeats. (See *Electrode placement for a signal-averaged ECG*, page 272.) The test takes approximately 7 to 10 minutes. The machine's computer detects late electrical potentials and then enlarges them so they're recognizable. The electrodes for an SAECG are labeled X^-, X^+, Y^-, Y^+, Z^-, Z^+, and G.

The machine averages signals from these leads to produce one representative QRS complex without artifacts. This process cancels noise, electrical impulses that don't occur as a repetitious pattern or with the same consistent timing as the QRS complex. Multiple electric signals from the heart are averaged to remove interference and reveal small variations in the QRS complex, usually called "late potentials." These late potentials may represent a predisposition towards potentially dangerous ventricular arrhythmias. Muscle noise can't be filtered, however, so the patient must lie still for the test.

Electrode placement for a signal-averaged ECG

Electrodes are placed much differently for a signal-averaged ECG than they are for a 12-lead ECG. Here's one method:

1. Place the positive X electrode at the left fourth intercostal space, midaxillary line.
2. Place the negative X electrode at the right fourth intercostal space, midaxillary line.
3. Place the positive Y electrode at the left iliac crest.
4. Place the negative Y electrode at the superior aspect of the manubrium of the sternum.
5. Place the positive Z electrode at the fourth intercostal space left of the sternum.
6. Place the ground (G) on the lower right at the eighth rib.
7. Reposition the patient on his side, or have him sit forward. Then place the negative Z electrode on his back, directly posterior to the positive Z electrode.
8. Attach all the leads to the electrodes, being careful not to dislodge the posterior lead.

Now, you can obtain the tracing.

Anterior chest

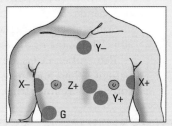

Posterior chest

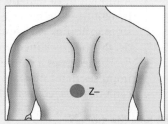

That's a wrap!

Obtaining a 12-lead ECG

12-lead ECG basics
- Provides 12 different views of the heart's electrical activity
- Record electrical activity in the heart's horizontal plane, providing a transverse view through the middle of the heart, dividing it into upper and lower portions

The limb leads
- Three bipolar limb leads: I, II, and III
- Three unipolar limb leads: aV_R, aV_L, and aV_F
- Record electrical activity in the heart's frontal plane, providing a view through the middle of the heart from top to bottom

The precordial leads
- Six unipolar precordial (chest) leads: V_1 through V_6

Electrical axis
- Measurement of the electrical impulses flowing through the heart
- Normal axis downward and to the left
- Direction of electrical activity swings away from areas of damage or necrosis and toward areas of hypertrophy

Placing the leads
- Bipolar and unipolar limb leads: electrodes on both arms and the left leg, ground on right leg

Obtaining a 12-lead ECG *(Continued)*

- V_1: Over fourth intercostal space at the right sternal border
- V_2: Over fourth intercostal space at the left sternal border
- V_3: Midway between leads V_2 and V_4
- V_4: Over fifth intercostal space at left midclavicular line
- V_5: Over fifth intercostal space at left anterior axillary line
- V_6: Over fifth intercostal space at left midaxillary line

Views of the heart walls
- Lead I: Lateral wall
- Lead II: Inferior wall
- Lead III: Inferior wall
- Lead aV_R: No specific view
- Lead aV_L: Lateral wall
- Lead aV_F: Inferior wall
- Lead V_1: Septal wall
- Lead V_2: Septal wall
- Lead V_3: Anterior wall
- Lead V_4: Anterior wall

- Lead V_5: Lateral wall
- Lead V_6: Lateral wall

Other lead placements
- Posterior leads: V_7, V_8, and V_9 are placed opposite V_4, V_5, and V_6 on the left side of the back to view posterior surface of the heart
- Right chest leads: placed on right chest in mirror image of standard precordial leads to view right ventricle

Types of ECGs
- Multichannel ECG: all electrodes attached at one time to provide simultaneous views of all leads
- Signal-averaged ECG: use of computer to identify late electrical potentials from three specialized leads over hundreds of beats; identifies patients at risk for sudden cardiac death from ventricular tachycardia

Quick quiz

1. The precordial leads are placed on the:
   A. anterior chest starting with the fourth intercostal space at the right sternal border.
   B. lateral chest starting with the fourth intercostal space at the left midaxillary line.
   C. posterior chest wall starting with the fourth intercostal space at the midscapular line.
   D. left leg and both arms.

   Answer: A. Lead V_1 is placed anteriorly between the fourth and fifth ribs at the right sternal border. Leads V_2 to V_6 are then placed accordingly.

2. A 12-lead ECG is used to assess function of the:
    A. right ventricle.
    B. left ventricle.
    C. right and left ventricle simultaneously.
    D. right and left atria simultaneously.

Answer: B. A 12-lead ECG gives a more complete view of the heart's electrical activity than a rhythm strip and is used to assess left ventricular function.

3. A posterior-lead ECG is used to assess:
    A. posterior myocardial damage.
    B. inferior myocardial damage.
    C. damage to the interventricular septum.
    D. damage to the base of the heart.

Answer: A. The posterior-lead ECG assesses damage to the posterior surface of the heart, an area a standard 12-lead ECG can't detect.

4. When recording a 12-lead ECG, the paper speed should be set at:
    A. 10 mm/sec.
    B. 20 mm/sec.
    C. 25 mm/sec.
    D. 50 mm/sec.

Answer: C. The correct paper speed for a 12-lead ECG is 25 mm/sec.

5. A signal-averaged ECG measures:
    A. electrical impulses from the sinoatrial node.
    B. electrical impulses arriving at the atrioventricular node.
    C. action potentials of individual cardiac cells.
    D. late electrical potentials throughout the heart.

Answer: D. Signal-averaged ECGs measure late electrical potentials, tiny electrical impulses that occur after depolarization and can cause ventricular tachycardia.

6. To record the bipolar limb leads I, II, and III and the unipolar limb leads aV_R, aV_L, and aV_F, place electrodes on:
    A. both of the patient's arms and left leg, with a ground on his right leg.
    B. the patient's right arm and left leg, with a ground on his left arm.
    C. both of the patient's legs and his left arm, with a ground on his right arm.
    D. both of the patient's arms and his right leg, with a ground on his left leg.

Answer: A. To record these bipolar and unipolar limb leads, place electrodes on both of the patient's arms and left leg, with a ground on his right leg.

7. Transtelephonic cardiac monitoring:
    A. is a process whereby the patient can transmit his own ECG from home to a central monitoring center for interpretation.
    B. is a costly procedure.
    C. utilizes a special telephone line.
    D. is not as accurate as a standard 12-lead ECG.

Answer: A. It is a process whereby the patient can transmit his own ECG from home to a central monitoring center for interpretation.

Scoring

☆☆☆   If you answered all seven questions correctly, great job! You're the new leader of the 12-lead ECG pack.

☆☆   If you answered six questions correctly, we're impressed! Your leadership qualities are obvious, and you should be next in line for a top job.

☆   If you answered fewer than six questions correctly, that's okay! You'll be sure to take the lead in the next chapter.

Recommended references

Brown, D. F. M., & Martindale, J. L. (2012). *Rapid interpretation of ECG's in emergency medicine.* Philadelphia, PA: Wolters Kluwer.

Cohen, B. J., & Taylor, J. J. (2013). *Memmler's structure and function of the human body* (10th ed.). Philadelphia, PA: Wolters Kluwer.

García-Niebla, J. (2009). Comparison of P-wave patterns derived from correct and incorrect placement of V1-V2 electrodes. *Journal of Cardiovascular Nursing 24*(2), 156–161.

Katritsis, D. G., Gersch, B. J., & Camm, A. J. (2013). *Clinical cardiology: Current practice guidelines.* Oxford, United Kingdom: Oxford University Press.

Mann, D. L., Zipes, D. P., Libby, P., & Bonow, R. D. (2014). *Braunwald's heart disease: A textbook of cardiovascular medicine* (10th ed.). St. Louis, MO: Saunders | Elsevier.

McLaughlin, M. A. (clinical ed.) (2014). *Cardiovascular care made incredibly easy* (3rd ed.). Philadelphia, PA: Wolters Kluwer.

Rosen, A. V., Koppikan, S., Shaw, C., & Baranchuk, A. (2014). Common ECG lead placement errors. Part 1: Limb lead reversals. *International Journal of Medical Students, 2*(3), 92–98.

Urden, L., & Stacy, K. (2013). *Critical care nursing* (7th ed.). St Louis, MO: Mosby | Elsevier.

Wagner, G. S., & Strauss, D. G. (2013). *Marriott's practical electrocardiology* (12th ed.). Philadelphia, PA: Wolters Kluwer.

Chapter 12

Interpreting a 12-lead ECG

Just the facts

In this chapter, you'll learn:

♦ to examine each lead's waveforms for abnormalities

♦ to determine techniques that evaluate the heart's electrical axis

♦ ECG changes in patients with angina

♦ ECG characteristics to differentiate types of acute myocardial infarction

♦ 12-lead ECG changes that occur with a bundle-branch block.

A look at 12-lead ECG interpretation

To interpret a 12-lead ECG, use the systematic approach outlined here. Compare the patient's previous ECG, if available, with the current one to help you identify changes.

1. Check the ECG tracing to ensure the baseline is free from electrical interference and drift.
2. Lead aV_R is typically negative. If it isn't, the leads may be placed incorrectly.
3. Locate the lead markers on the waveform. Lead markers are the points where one lead changes to another.
4. Check the standardization markings to make sure all leads were recorded with the ECG machine's amplitude at the same setting. Standardization markings are usually located at the beginning of the strip.
5. Assess the heart rate and rhythm as you learned in earlier chapters.
6. Determine the heart's electrical axis. Use either the quadrant method or the degree method, described later in this chapter.
7. Examine the limb leads: I, II, and III. The R wave in leads I and II should be dominant with upright P and T waves. The R wave in lead III may be dominant or absent, with upright, flat, or inverted P and T waves. Each lead should have flat ST segments and pathologic Q waves should be absent.

R-wave progression

These waveforms show normal R-wave progression through the precordial leads. Note that the R wave is the first positive deflection in the QRS complex. Also note that the S wave gets smaller, or regresses, from lead V_1 to V_6 until it finally disappears.

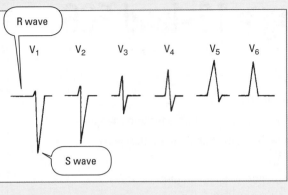

R wave

V_1 V_2 V_3 V_4 V_5 V_6

S wave

That's progress!

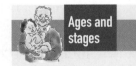

8. Examine the augmented leads: aV_L, aV_F, and aV_R. The tracings from leads aV_L and aV_F should be similar, but lead aV_F should have taller P and R waves. Lead aV_R has little diagnostic value. Its P wave, QRS complex, and T wave should be deflected downward.

9. Examine the R wave in the precordial leads, V_1 to V_6. Normally, the R wave—the first positive deflection of the QRS complex—gets progressively taller from lead V_1 to lead V_5, then it gets slightly smaller in lead V_6. (See *R-wave progression.*)

10. Examine the S wave—the negative deflection after an R wave—in the precordial leads. It appears extremely deep in lead V_1 and becomes progressively more shallow, usually disappearing at lead V_5 or V_6.

All about waves

As you examine each lead, note where changes occur so you can identify the area of the heart that's affected. Remember that P waves should be upright; however, they may be inverted in lead aV_R or biphasic or inverted in leads III, aV_L, and V_1.

PR intervals should always be constant, just like QRS-complex durations. QRS-complex deflections will vary in different leads. Observe for pathologic Q waves. (See *Normal findings in pediatric ECGs.*)

Ages and stages

Normal findings in pediatric ECGs

In a neonate, dominant R waves in the chest leads and upright T waves are normal findings. By the end of the first week of life, the T wave in lead V_1 becomes inverted and remains inverted through age 7.

Elevated one minute, depressed the next

ST segments should be isoelectric or have minimal deviation. ST-segment elevation greater than 1 mm above the baseline and ST-segment depression greater than 0.5 mm below the baseline are considered abnormal. Leads facing an injured area will have ST-segment elevations, and leads facing away will display ST-segment depressions.

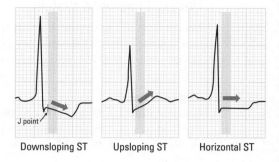

J point

Downsloping ST   Upsloping ST   Horizontal ST

That old, changeable T wave

The T wave should be slightly rounded and upright. It normally deflects upward in leads I, II, and V_3 through V_6. It may also be inverted in leads III, aV_R, aV_F, aV_L, and V_1. T waves shouldn't be tall, peaked, or notched. There are numerous reasons for T-wave changes and these are not always cause for alarm. However, excessively tall, flat, or inverted T waves in the presence of symptoms, such as chest pain indicate myocardial ischemia.

Split-second duration

A normal Q wave generally has a duration of less than 0.04 second. An abnormal Q wave has either a duration of 0.04 second or more, a depth greater than 4 mm, or a height one-fourth of the R wave.

Abnormal Q waves indicate myocardial necrosis. These waves develop when depolarization does not take its normal path because of damaged tissue in the area. Remember that lead aV_R normally has a large Q wave, so disregard this lead when searching for abnormal Q waves.

Finding the electrical axis

The electrical axis is the average direction of the heart's electrical activity during ventricular depolarization. Leads placed on the body sense the sum of the heart's electrical activity and record it as waveforms.

Cross my heart

You can determine your patient's electrical axis by examining the waveforms recorded from the six frontal plane leads: I, II, III, aV_R, aV_L, and aV_F. Imaginary lines drawn from each of the leads intersect the center of the heart and form a diagram known as the hexaxial reference system. (See *Hexaxial reference system*, page 280.)

Hexaxial reference system

The hexaxial reference system consists of six bisecting lines, each representing one of the six limb leads, and a circle, representing the heart. The intersection of all lines divides the circle into equal, 30-degree segments.

Shifting degrees

Note that +0 degree appears at the 3 o'clock position (positive pole lead I). Moving counterclockwise, the degrees become increasingly negative, until reaching ±180 degrees, at the 9 o'clock position (negative pole lead I).

The bottom half of the circle contains the corresponding positive degrees. However, a positive-degree designation doesn't necessarily mean that the pole is positive.

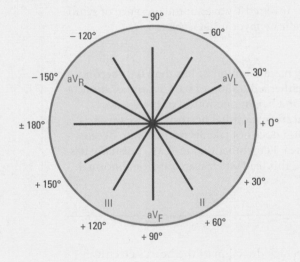

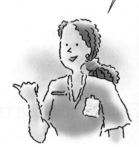

This diagram is called the hexaxial reference system. Use it to determine your patient's electrical axis.

Where the axis falls

An axis that falls between 0 and +90 degrees (some references concede −30 to +90) is considered normal. An axis between +90 and +180 degrees indicates right axis deviation, and one between 0 and −90 degrees indicates left axis deviation. An axis between +180 and −90 degrees indicates extreme axis deviation and is called an *indeterminate axis*.

To determine your patient's electrical axis, use one of the two methods described here, the quadrant method or the degree method. (See *Axis deviation across the life span.*)

Quadrant method

The quadrant method, a fast, easy way to plot the heart's axis, involves observing the main deflection of the QRS complex in leads I and aV$_F$. (See *Quadrant method.*) Lead I indicates whether impulses are moving to the right or left, and lead aV$_F$ indicates whether they're moving up or down.

If the QRS-complex deflection is positive or upright in both leads, the electrical axis is normal. If lead I is upright and lead aV$_F$ points down, left axis deviation exists.

Quadrant method

This chart will help you quickly determine the direction of a patient's electrical axis. Just observe the deflections of the QRS complexes in leads I and aV$_F$. Then check the chart to determine whether the patient's axis is normal or has a left, right, or extreme axis deviation.

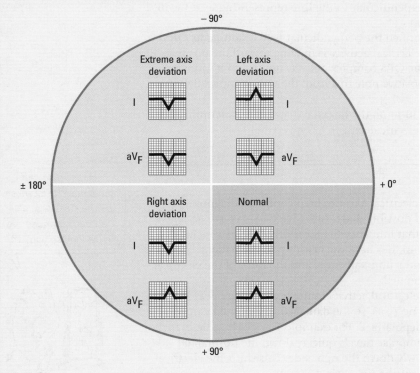

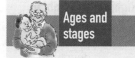

Ages and stages

Axis deviation across the life span

Right axis deviation, between +60 degrees and +160 degrees, is normal in a neonate due to dominance of the right ventricle. By age 1, the axis shifts to fall between +10 degrees and +100 degrees as the left ventricle becomes dominant.

Left axis deviation commonly occurs in elderly people. This axis shift may result from fibrosis of the anterior fascicle of the left bundle branch or thickness of the left ventricular wall, which increases by 25% between ages 30 and 80.

Right on and right in

When lead I points downward and lead aV$_F$ is upright, right axis deviation exists. Both waves pointing down signal extreme axis deviation.

Degree method

A more precise axis calculation, the degree method gives an exact degree measurement of the electrical axis. (See *Degree method.*) It also allows you to determine the axis even if the QRS complex isn't clearly positive or negative in leads I and aV$_F$. To use this method, follow these steps.

1. Review all six leads, and identify the one that contains either the smallest QRS complex or the complex with an equal deflection above and below the baseline.
2. Use the hexaxial diagram to identify the lead perpendicular to this lead. For example, if lead I has the smallest QRS complex, then the lead perpendicular to the line representing lead I would be lead aV$_F$.
3. After you've identified the perpendicular lead, examine its QRS complex. If the electrical activity is moving toward the positive pole of a lead, the QRS complex deflects upward. If it's moving away from the positive pole of a lead, the QRS complex deflects downward.
4. Plot this information on the hexaxial diagram to determine the direction of the electrical axis.

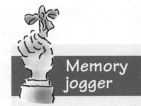

Memory jogger

Think of the QRS-complex deflections in leads I and aV$_F$ as thumbs pointing up or down. Two thumbs up is normal; anything else is abnormal.

Axis deviation

Finding a patient's electrical axis can help confirm a diagnosis or narrow the range of possible diagnoses. (See *Causes of axis deviation,* page 284.) Factors that influence the location of the axis include the heart's position in the chest, the heart's size, the patient's body size or type, the conduction pathways, and the force of the electrical impulses being generated.

Remember that electrical activity in the heart swings away from areas of damage or necrosis, so the damaged part of the heart will be the last area to be depolarized. For example, in right bundle-branch block (RBBB), the impulse travels quickly down the normal left side and then moves slowly down the right side. This shifts the electrical forces to the right, causing right axis deviation.

Heart size can influence the location of the electrical axis. Tell me, how does my size look to you...?

Degree method

The degree method of determining axis deviation allows you to identify a patient's electrical axis by degrees on the hexaxial system, not just by quadrant. To use this method, follow these steps.

Step 1
Identify the lead with the smallest QRS complex or the equiphasic QRS complex. In this example, it's lead III.

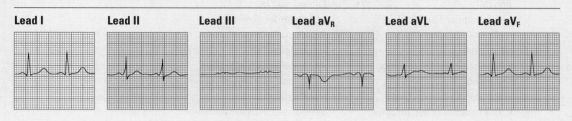

Lead I	Lead II	Lead III	Lead aV$_R$	Lead aVL	Lead aV$_F$

Step 2
Locate the axis for lead III on the hexaxial diagram. Then find the axis perpendicular to it, which is the axis for lead aV$_R$.

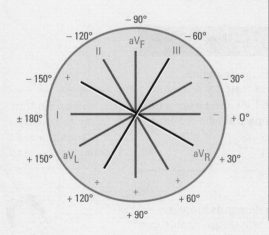

Step 3
Now, examine the QRS complex in lead aV$_R$, noting whether the deflection is positive or negative. As you can see, the QRS complex for this lead is negative. This tells you that the electric current is moving toward the negative pole of aV$_R$, which, on the hexaxial diagram, is in the right lower quadrant at +30 degrees. So the electrical axis here is normal at +30 degrees.

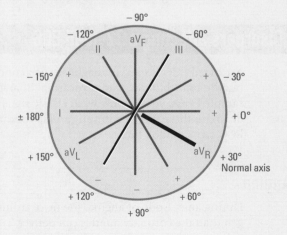

Causes of axis deviation

This list covers common causes of right and left axis deviation.

Left
- Normal variation
- Inferior wall myocardial infarction (MI)
- Left anterior hemiblock
- Wolff–Parkinson–White syndrome
- Mechanical shifts (ascites, pregnancy, tumors)
- Left bundle-branch block
- Left ventricular hypertrophy
- Aging

Right
- Normal variation
- Dextrocardia
- Lateral wall MI
- Left posterior hemiblock
- Right bundle-branch block
- Emphysema/COPD
- Acute pulmonary embolism
- Right ventricular hypertrophy
- Hyperkalemia
- Ventricular rhythm disturbances (ventricular tachycardia, accelerated idioventricular)

No worries

Axis deviation isn't always cause for alarm, and it isn't always cardiac in origin. For example, infants and children normally have right axis deviation. Pregnant women normally have left axis deviation.

Disorders affecting a 12-lead ECG

A 12-lead ECG is used to diagnose such conditions as angina, bundle-branch block, and myocardial infarction (MI). By reviewing sample ECGs, you'll know what classic signs to look for. Here's a rundown on these three common cardiac conditions and what 12-lead ECG signs to look for.

Angina

During an episode of angina, the myocardium demands more oxygen than the coronary arteries can deliver. The arteries are unable to deliver enough oxygenated blood to the heart, commonly as a result of atherosclerosis seen in coronary artery disease (CAD), whereby arteries narrow over time due to plaque deposition and calcification. The pathophysiologic process of this condition is further complicated by platelet aggregation, thrombus formation, or vasospasm.

An episode of angina usually lasts a few minutes and may be a precursor to myocardial infarction.

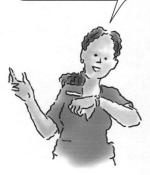

Angina pain that lasts close to 30 minutes most likely signals an MI.

Stable, unstable, variant?

You may hear the term stable, unstable, or variant angina applied to certain conditions. In stable angina, an episode of pain is triggered by exertion or stress and is usually relieved by rest or with medicine. Each episode follows the same pattern and may be associated with chest pain that radiates to the arms, back, or another area.

Unstable angina, which is one of the components of acute coronary syndrome (ACS), is more easily provoked, usually waking the patient. It is also unpredictable, worsens over time, and may last for a longer period of time than stable angina. Chest pain associated with unstable angina may radiate. The patient with unstable angina is treated as a medical emergency as the onset is a common precursor to MI.

Prinzmetal or variant angina usually arises at rest, frequently during the night to early morning. Younger patients experience this type of angina caused by coronary artery spasm triggered by cold weather, stress, smoking, cocaine use, or medicine.

Fleeting change of heart

Ischemic changes are evident on the ECG during the episodes of angina and may resolve to some degree when the angina subsides. (See *ECG changes associated with angina.*) Because these changes may be fleeting, always obtain an order for, and perform, a 12-lead ECG as soon as the patient reports chest pain.

The ECG will allow you to analyze the electrical activity associated with the myocardium, which allows us to determine the culprit coronary artery(ies) involved. By recognizing danger early, you may be able to prevent morbidity or mortality associated with MI.

ECG changes associated with angina

Here are some classic ECG changes involving the T wave and ST segment that you may see when monitoring a patient with angina.

Peaked T wave	**Flattened T wave**	**T-wave inversion**	**ST-segment depression with T-wave inversion**	**ST-segment depression without T-wave inversion**

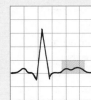 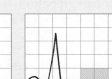 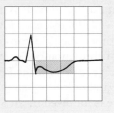 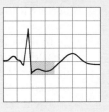

Pharmacologic agents are a key component of anginal treatment and may include nitrates, beta-adrenergic blockers, calcium channel blockers, and aspirin or glycoprotein IIb/IIIa inhibitors to reduce platelet aggregation.

Bundle-branch block

One potential complication of an MI is a bundle-branch block. In this disorder, either the left or the right bundle branch fails to conduct impulses. A bundle-branch block that occurs farther down the left bundle, in the posterior or anterior fasciculus, is called a *hemiblock*.

Some blocks require treatment with a temporary pacemaker. In other cases, blocks are monitored to detect whether they progress to a more complete heart block.

Impulsive behavior

In a bundle-branch block, the impulse travels down the unaffected bundle branch and then from one myocardial cell to the next to depolarize the ventricle.

Because this cell-to-cell conduction progresses much more slowly than the conduction along the specialized cells of the conduction system, ventricular depolarization is prolonged.

Wide world of complexes

Prolonged ventricular depolarization means that the QRS complex is widened. The normal width of the complex is 0.06 to 0.12 second. If the width increases to greater than 0.12 second, a bundle-branch block is present.

After you identify a bundle-branch block, examine lead V_1, which lies to the right of the heart, and lead V_6, which lies to the left of the heart. You'll use these leads to determine whether the block is in the right or left bundle.

Right bundle-branch block

RBBB occurs with such conditions as anterior wall MI, CAD, cardiomyopathy, cor pulmonale, and pulmonary embolism. It may also occur without cardiac disease. If this block develops as the heart rate increases, it's called *rate-related RBBB*. (See *How RBBB occurs*.)

In this disorder, the QRS complex is greater than 0.12 second and has a different configuration, sometimes resembling rabbit ears or the letter "M." (See *Recognizing RBBB*, page 288.) Septal depolarization isn't affected in lead V_1, so the initial small R wave remains.

The R wave is followed by an S wave, which represents left ventricular depolarization, and a tall R wave (called *R prime*, or *R'*), which

How RBBB occurs

In right bundle-branch block (RBBB), the initial impulse activates the interventricular septum from left to right, just as in normal activation. Next, the left bundle branch activates the left ventricle. The impulse then crosses the interventricular septum to activate the right ventricle.

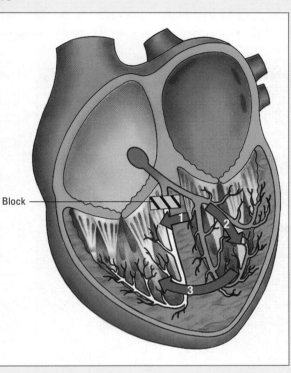

Block

represents late right ventricular depolarization. The T wave is negative in this lead. However, that deflection is called a *secondary T-wave change* and is of no clinical significance.

Opposing moves

The opposite occurs in lead V_6. A small Q wave is followed by depolarization of the left ventricle, which produces a tall R wave. Depolarization of the right ventricle then causes a broad S wave. In lead V_6, the T wave should be positive.

Left bundle-branch block

Left bundle-branch block (LBBB) develops from underlying pathology often caused by hypertensive heart disease, aortic stenosis, degenerative changes of the conduction system, or CAD. (See *How LBBB occurs*, page 289.) When it occurs in conjunction with an anterior wall MI, it usually signals complete heart block requiring insertion of a pacemaker.

Recognizing RBBB

This 12-lead ECG shows the characteristic changes of right bundle-branch block (RBBB). In lead V₁, note the rsR′ pattern and T-wave inversion. In lead V₆, see the widened S wave and the upright T wave. Also note the prolonged QRS complexes.

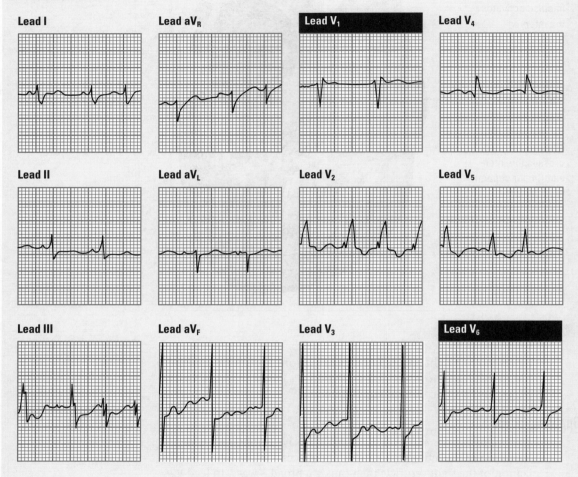

One ventricle after another

In LBBB, the QRS complex will be greater than 0.12 second because the ventricles are activated sequentially, not simultaneously. (See *Recognizing LBBB*, page 290.) As the wave of depolarization spreads from the right ventricle to the left, a wide S wave is produced in lead

How LBBB occurs

In left bundle-branch block (LBBB), the impulse first travels down the right bundle branch. Then the impulse activates the interventricular septum from right to left, the opposite of normal activation. Finally, the impulse activates the left ventricle.

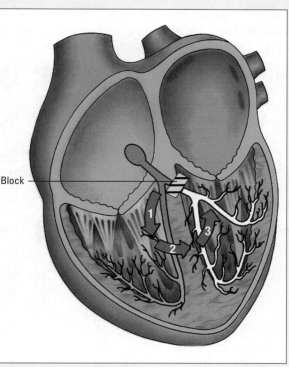

Block

V_1, with a positive T wave. The S wave may be preceded by a Q wave or a small R wave.

Slurring your R waves

In lead V_6, no initial Q wave occurs. A tall, notched R wave, or a slurred one, is produced as the impulse spreads from right to left. This initial positive deflection is a sign of LBBB. The T wave is negative.

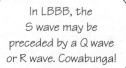

In LBBB, the S wave may be preceded by a Q wave or R wave. Cowabunga!

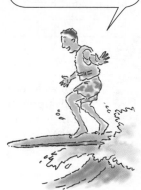

Myocardial infarction

Unlike angina, pain from an MI lasts from several minutes up to several hours and is unrelieved by rest. The location of the MI varies depending on the culprit coronary artery.

Recognizing LBBB

This 12-lead ECG shows characteristic changes of left bundle-branch block (LBBB). All leads have prolonged QRS complexes. In lead V$_1$, note the QS-wave pattern. In lead V$_6$, you'll see the slurred R-wave and T-wave inversion. The elevated ST segments and upright T waves in leads V$_1$ to V$_4$ are also common in LBBB.

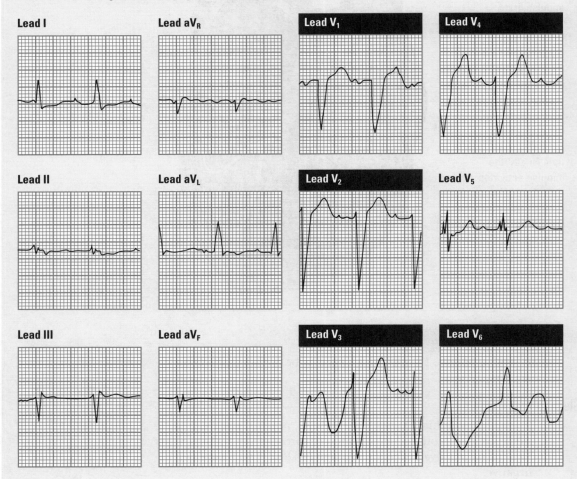

For as long as the myocardium is deprived of an oxygen-rich blood supply, an ECG will reflect the three pathologic changes of an MI: ischemia, injury, and infarction. (See *Reciprocal changes in an MI.*)

Reciprocal changes in an MI

Ischemia, injury, and infarction—the three I's of a myocardial infarction (MI)—produce characteristic ECG changes. Changes shown by the leads that reflect electrical activity in damaged areas are shown on the right of the illustration.

Reciprocal leads, those opposite the damaged area, will show opposite ECG changes, as shown to the left of the illustration.

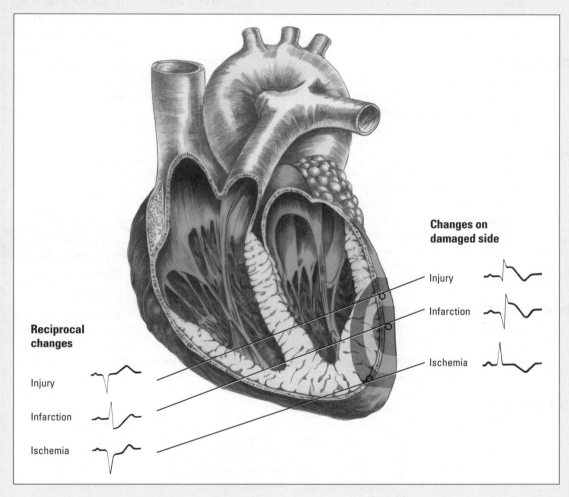

Changes on damaged side

Injury

Infarction

Ischemia

Reciprocal changes

Injury

Infarction

Ischemia

Zone of infarction

The area of myocardial necrosis is called the zone of infarction. Scar tissue eventually replaces the dead tissue, and the damage caused is irreversible.

The ECG change associated with a necrotic area is a pathologic Q wave, which results from lack of depolarization. Such Q waves are permanent. MIs that don't produce Q waves are called *non–Q-wave MIs.* (See *Q waves in children.*)

Zone of injury

The zone of infarction is surrounded by the zone of injury, which appears on an ECG as an elevated ST segment. ST-segment elevation results from a prolonged lack of oxygenated blood supplied to the myocardium.

Zone of ischemia

The outermost area is called the *zone of ischemia* and results from an interrupted supply of oxygenated blood. This zone is represented on an ECG by T-wave inversion. Changes in the zones of ischemia or injury are reversible.

From ischemia to injury

Generally, as an MI occurs, the patient experiences chest pain and an ECG shows changes, such as ST-segment elevation, which indicates that myocardial injury is in process. Accompanying changes include flattened or inverted T waves.

Rapid treatment can prevent myocardial necrosis. However, if symptoms persist for more than 6 hours, little can be done to prevent necrosis. That's one of the reasons patients are advised to seek medical attention as soon as symptoms begin.

The telltale Q wave

Q waves can appear hours to days after an MI and signify that an entire thickness of the myocardium has become necrotic. Tall R waves in reciprocal leads may also develop. This type of MI is called a *transmural,* or *Q-wave, MI.*

Back to baseline

Knowing how long such changes last can help you determine how long ago an MI occurred. ST segments return to baseline within a few days to two weeks. Inverted T waves may persist for several months. Although not every patient who has had an MI develops Q waves, those who do may have them on their ECGs indefinitely.

What to do for an MI

The most important step you can take for a patient with an MI is to remain vigilant about detecting changes in his condition and ECG. (See *Monitoring MI patients.*)

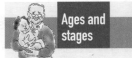

Ages and stages

Q waves in children

Q waves in leads II, III, aV_F, V_5, and V_6 are normal in children. Q waves in other leads suggest cardiac disease, such as an abnormal left coronary artery.

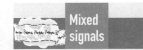

Mixed signals

Monitoring MI patients

Remember that specific leads monitor specific walls of the heart. Here's a quick overview of those leads:

• For an anterior wall myocardial infarction (MI), monitor lead V_1 or MCL_1.

• For a septal wall MI, monitor lead V_1 or MCL_1 to pick up hallmark changes.

• For a lateral wall MI, monitor lead V_6 or MCL_6.

• For an inferior wall MI, monitor lead II.

The primary goal of treatment for an MI is to limit the size of the infarction by increasing oxygen supply to the myocardium and decreasing workload. (See *Improving blood flow.*)

In addition to rest, pain relief, and supplemental oxygen, such medications as nitroglycerin, morphine sulfate, beta-adrenergic blockers, calcium channel blockers, angiotensin-converting enzyme inhibitors, and antiarrhythmics are used. Aspirin or glycoprotein IIb/IIIa inhibitors may be used to reduce platelet aggregation. Thrombolytic therapy may also be prescribed to dissolve a thrombus occluding a coronary artery.

Identifying types of MI

The location of the MI is a critical factor in determining the most appropriate treatment and predicting probable complications. Characteristic ECG changes that occur with each type of MI are localized to the leads overlying the infarction site. (See *Locating myocardial damage.*) Here's a look at characteristic ECG changes that occur with different types of MI.

Anterior wall MI

The left anterior descending artery supplies blood to the anterior portion of the left ventricle. The artery supplies blood to the

Improving blood flow

Increasing the blood supply to the heart of a patient who has had a myocardial infarction can help prevent further damage to his heart. In addition to medications, blood flow to the heart can be improved by:
- intra-aortic balloon pump
- percutaneous transluminal coronary angioplasty
- atherectomy
- laser treatment
- stent placement
- coronary artery bypass graft.

Locating myocardial damage

After you've noted characteristic lead changes of an acute myocardial infarction, use this chart to identify the areas of damage. Match the lead changes in the second column with the affected wall in the first column and the artery involved in the third column. Column four shows reciprocal lead changes.

Wall affected	Leads	Artery involved	Reciprocal changes
Anterior	V_3 to V_4	Left coronary artery, left anterior descending (LAD) artery	II, III, aV_F
Anterolateral	I, aV_L, V_3 to V_6	LAD artery, circumflex artery	II, III, aV_F
Septal	V_1 to V_2	LAD artery	None
Inferior	II, III, aV_F	Right coronary artery	I, aV_L
Lateral	I, aV_L, V_5, V_6	Circumflex artery, branch of left coronary artery	II, III, aV_F
Posterior	V_8, V_9	Right coronary artery, circumflex artery	V_1 to V_4
Right ventricular	V_{4R}, V_{5R}, V_{6R}	Right coronary artery	None

ventricular septum and portions of the right and left bundle-branch systems.

When the anterior descending artery becomes occluded, an anterior wall MI occurs. (See *Recognizing an anterior wall MI.*)

Recognizing an anterior wall MI

This 12-lead ECG shows typical characteristics of an anterior wall myocardial infarction (MI). Note that the R waves don't progress through the precordial leads. Also note the ST-segment elevation in leads V_2 and V_3. As expected, the reciprocal leads II, III, and aV_F show slight ST-segment depression. Axis deviation is normal at +60 degrees.

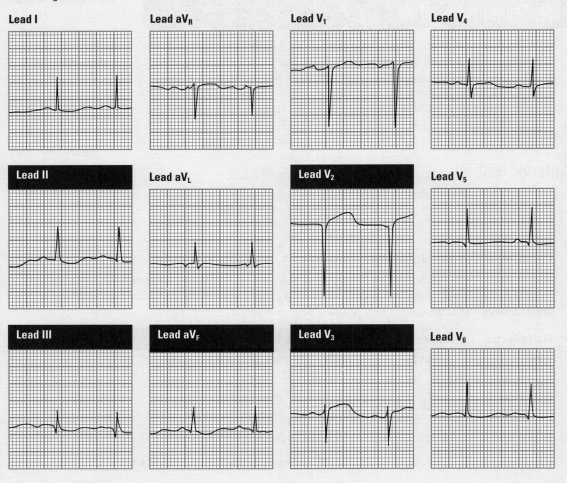

Lead I   Lead aV_R Lead V_1 Lead V_4

Lead II   Lead aV_L Lead V_2 Lead V_5

Lead III   Lead aV_F Lead V_3 Lead V_6

Complications of an anterior wall MI include varying second-degree atrioventricular blocks, bundle-branch blocks, ventricular irritability, and left-sided heart failure.

Changing the leads

An anterior wall MI causes characteristic ECG changes in leads V_3 to V_4. The precordial leads show poor R-wave progression because the left ventricle can't depolarize normally. ST-segment elevation and T-wave inversion are also present.

The reciprocal leads for the anterior wall are the inferior leads II, III, and aV_F. They show tall R waves and depressed ST segments.

Septal wall MI

The patient with a septal wall MI has an increased risk for developing a ventricular septal defect. ECG changes are present in leads V_1 and V_2. In those leads, the R wave disappears, the ST segment rises, and the T wave inverts.

Because the LAD artery also supplies blood to the ventricular septum, a septal wall MI commonly accompanies an anterior wall MI. (See *Recognizing an anteroseptal wall MI*, page 296.)

Lateral wall MI

A lateral wall MI is usually caused by a blockage in the left circumflex artery and shows characteristic changes in the left lateral leads I, aV_L, V_5, and V_6. The reciprocal leads for a lateral wall infarction are leads II, III, and aV_F. (See *Recognizing a lateral wall MI*, page 297.)

This type of infarction typically causes premature ventricular contractions and varying degrees of heart block. A lateral wall MI usually accompanies an anterior or inferior wall MI.

Inferior wall MI

An inferior wall MI is usually caused by occlusion of the right coronary artery and produces characteristic ECG changes in the inferior leads II, III, and aV_F and reciprocal changes in the lateral leads I and aV_L. (See *Recognizing an inferior wall MI*, page 298.) It's also called a *diaphragmatic MI* because the heart's inferior wall lies over the diaphragm.

Patients with inferior wall MI are at risk for developing sinus bradycardia, sinus arrest, heart block, and premature ventricular contractions. This type of MI occurs alone, with a lateral wall MI, or with a right ventricular MI.

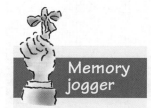

Memory jogger

To remember which leads are critical in diagnosing a lateral wall MI, think of the L's in "lateral MI" and "left lateral leads."

Recognizing an anteroseptal wall MI

This 12-lead ECG shows typical characteristics of an anteroseptal wall myocardial infarction (MI). Note the poor R-wave progression, the elevated ST segments, and the inverted T waves in leads V_1, V_2, and V_3. Reciprocal changes are seen in leads II, III, and aV_F with depressed ST segments and tall, peaked T waves.

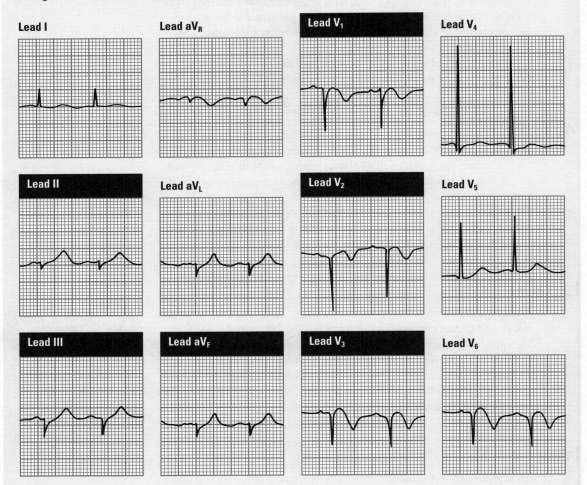

Recognizing a lateral wall MI

This 12-lead ECG shows changes characteristic of a lateral wall myocardial infarction (MI). In leads I, aV$_L$, V$_5$, and V$_6$, note the pathologic Q waves, the ST-segment elevation, and the T-wave inversion.

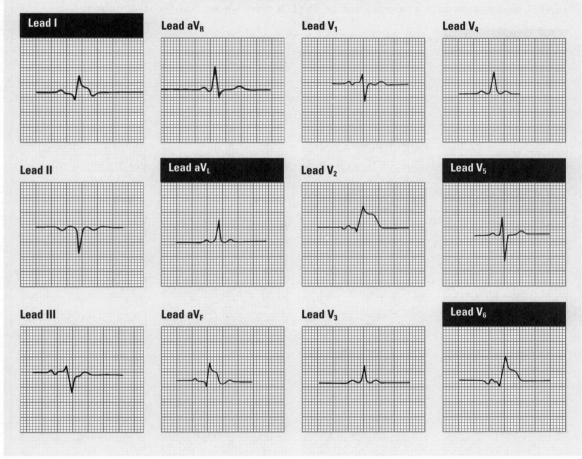

Right ventricular MI

A right ventricular MI usually follows occlusion of the right coronary artery. This type of MI rarely occurs alone. In fact, 40% of all patients with an inferior wall MI also suffer a right ventricular MI.

Recognizing an inferior wall MI

This 12-lead ECG shows the characteristic changes of an inferior wall myocardial infarction (MI). In leads II, III, and aV_F, note the T-wave inversion, ST-segment elevation, and pathologic Q waves. In leads I and aV_L, note the slight ST-segment depression, a reciprocal change. This ECG shows left axis deviation at −60 degrees.

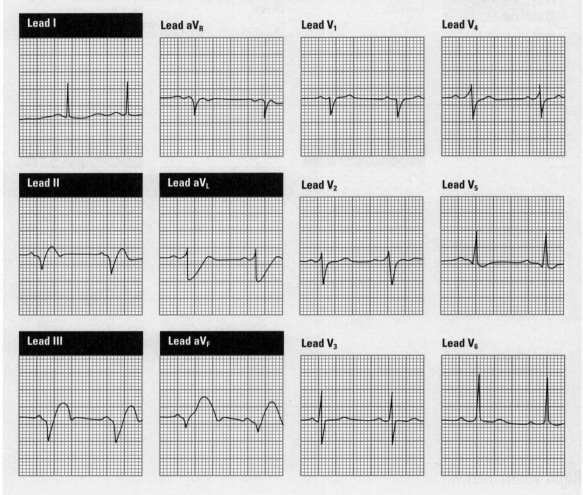

A right ventricular MI can lead to right-sided heart failure or right-sided block. The classic changes are ST-segment elevation, pathologic Q waves, and inverted T waves in the right precordial leads V_{4R} to V_{6R}. (See *Recognizing a right ventricular MI.*)

Recognizing a right ventricular MI

This 12-lead ECG shows typical characteristics of a right ventricular myocardial infarction (MI). Note the T-wave inversion in leads V_{3R}, V_{4R}, V_{5R}, and V_{6R}. Pathologic Q waves and ST-segment elevation are also present.

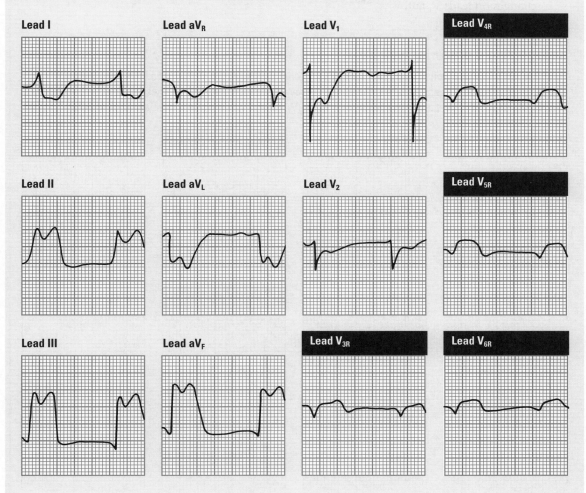

Take the right lead

Identifying a right ventricular MI is difficult without information from the right precordial leads. If these leads aren't available, you can observe leads II, III, and aV_F or watch leads V_1, V_2, and V_3 for ST-segment elevation. If a right ventricular MI has occurred, use lead II to monitor for further damage.

Posterior wall MI

A posterior wall MI is caused by occlusion of either the right coronary artery or the left circumflex arteries. This MI produces reciprocal changes on leads V_1 and V_2.

Recognizing a posterior wall MI

This 12-lead ECG shows typical characteristics of a posterior wall myocardial infarction (MI). Note the tall R waves, the depressed ST segments, and the upright T waves in leads V_1, V_2, and V_3. These are reciprocal changes, because the leads that best monitor a posterior wall MI (V_7, V_8, and V_9) aren't on a standard 12-lead ECG.

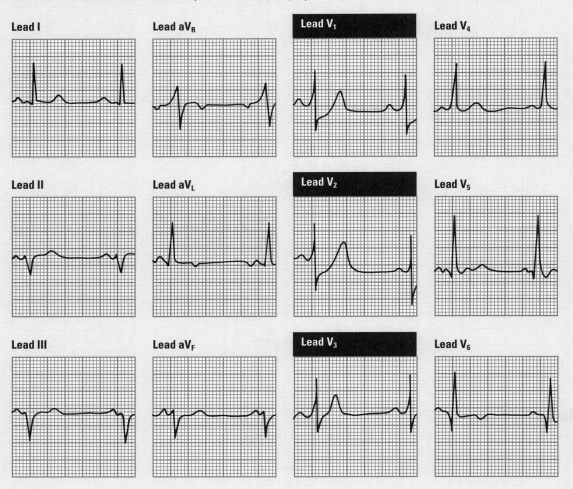

Classic ECG changes in a posterior wall MI include tall R waves, ST-segment depression, and upright T waves. (See *Recognizing a posterior wall MI.*) Posterior infarctions usually accompany inferior infarctions. Information about the posterior wall and pathologic Q waves that might occur can be obtained from leads V_7 to V_9 using a posterior ECG.

Identifying a right ventricular MI is difficult without the right information from the right precordial leads.

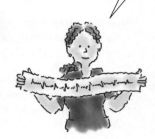

That's a wrap!

12-lead ECG interpretation review

Looking at the waves
- *P waves:* Upright; possibly inverted in lead aV_R or biphasic or inverted in leads III, aV_L, and V_1
- *PR intervals:* Always constant, like QRS-complex durations
- *QRS-complex deflections:* Variable in different leads
- *Q waves:* Possibly pathologic; duration of less than 0.4 second when normal
- *T wave:* Slightly rounded and upright; normal deflection upward in leads I, II, and V_3 through V_6; inverted in leads III, aV_F, aV_R, aV_L, and V_1; shouldn't be tall, peaked, or notched
- *ST segments:* should be isoelectric or have minimal deviation

Electrical axis
- Average direction of the heart's electrical activity during ventricular depolarization

Methods of determining axis
- *Quadrant method:* Determines main deflection of QRS complex in leads I and aV_F
- *Degree method:* Identifies axis by degrees on the hexaxial system

- *Examination of the waveforms from the six frontal leads:* I, II, III, aV_R, aV_L, and aV_F
- *Normal axis:* Between 0 and +90 degrees (−30 to +90 degrees is acceptable)
- *Left axis deviation:* Between 0 and −90 degrees
- *Right axis deviation:* Between +90 and +180 degrees
- *Extreme axis deviation:* Between +180 and −90 degrees

Disorders affecting 12-lead ECGs
Angina
- *Possible ECG changes:* Peaked or flattened T wave, T-wave inversion, and ST-segment depression with or without T-wave inversion

Bundle-branch block
- *QRS complex:* Width increases to greater than 0.12 second with bundle-branch block
- *Lead V_1 (to right of heart) and V_6 (to left of heart):* Used to determine whether block is in right or left bundle
- *RBBB:* QRS complex has rsR′ pattern and T-wave inversion in lead V_1 and widened S wave and upright T wave in lead V_6

(continued)

12-lead ECG interpretation review *(Continued)*

- *LBBB:* Wide S wave (which may be preceded by a Q wave or small R wave) and small positive T wave in lead V_1; tall, notched R wave or slurred R wave and T-wave inversion in lead V_6

Myocardial infarction
- Three pathologic changes on ECG—ischemia, injury, and infarction

Pathologic ECG changes
- *Zone of ischemia:* T-wave inversion
- *Zone of injury:* ST-segment elevation
- *Zone of infarction:* Pathologic Q wave in transmural MI

Locating the MI
- *Anterior wall:* Leads V_3 to V_4; involves LAD artery
- *Septal wall:* V_1 to V_2; involves LAD artery
- *Inferior wall:* Leads II, III, aV_F; involves right coronary artery
- *Lateral wall:* Leads I, aV_L, V_5, V_6; involves left circumflex artery
- *Posterior wall:* Leads V_7, V_8, V_9; involves right coronary or left circumflex arteries
- *Right ventricular wall:* V_{4R}, V_{5R}, V_{6R}; involves right coronary artery

Quick quiz

1. Your patient's ECG shows positively deflected QRS complexes in leads I and aV_F. Using the four-quadrant method for determining the electrical axis, you determine that he has a:
    A. normal axis.
    B. left axis deviation.
    C. right axis deviation.
    D. extreme axis deviation.

Answer: A. If the QRS-complex deflection is positive or upright in both leads, the electrical axis is normal.

2. Your patient's ECG shows a negatively deflected QRS complex in lead I and a positively deflected one in lead aV_F. Using the four-quadrant method for determining electrical axis, you determine that he has a:
    A. normal axis.
    B. left axis deviation.
    C. right axis deviation.
    D. extreme axis deviation.

Answer: C. When lead I points downward and lead aV_F is upright, right axis deviation exists. Both waves pointing down signals indeterminate axis deviation.

3. If your patient has a T-wave inversion, ST-segment elevation, and pathologic Q waves in leads II, III, and aV$_F$, suspect an acute MI in the:
    A. anterior wall.
    B. inferior wall.
    C. lateral wall.
    D. septal wall.

Answer: B. Leads II, III, and aV$_F$ face the inferior wall of the left ventricle, so the ECG changes there are indicative of an acute inferior wall MI.

4. If a patient's QRS complex has an R′ wave in V$_1$, suspect:
    A. right ventricular hypertrophy.
    B. left ventricular hypertrophy.
    C. LBBB.
    D. RBBB.

Answer: D. In RBBB, depolarization of the right ventricle takes longer than normal, thereby creating an R′ wave in lead V$_1$.

5. Myocardial injury is represented on an ECG by the presence of a:
    A. T-wave inversion.
    B. ST-segment elevation.
    C. pathologic Q wave.
    D. ST-segment depression.

Answer: B. ST-segment elevation is the ECG change that corresponds with myocardial injury. It's caused by a prolonged lack of blood supply.

6. On a 12-lead ECG, a posterior wall MI produces:
    A. deep, broad Q waves in leads V$_1$ through V$_4$.
    B. inverse or mirror image changes in V$_1$ and V$_2$.
    C. raised ST segments in all leads.
    D. poor R-wave progression in the precordial leads.

Answer: B. Leads V$_1$ and V$_2$ show reciprocal changes when a posterior wall MI occurs. Look at the mirror images of these leads to determine the presence of a posterior wall MI.

7. An ST segment located 1.5 mm above the baseline is considered:
    A. normal.
    B. slightly depressed.
    C. abnormally elevated.
    D. isoelectric.

Answer: C. ST segments should be isoelectric or have minimal deviation. ST-segment elevation greater than 1 mm above the baseline is considered abnormal.

So far, so good. Now check out the strips on the next page!

Test strips

Okay, it's time to try out a couple of ECG test strips.

8.   In the 12-lead ECG below, you'll see an rsR′ pattern in lead V_1, as well as T-wave inversion. Looking at lead V_6, you'll note a widened S wave and an upright T wave. These changes indicate:

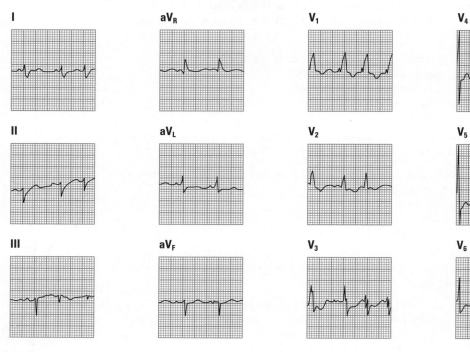

A.   right ventricular MI.
B.   LBBB.
C.   RBBB.
D.   angina.

Answer: C. The rsR′ configuration in lead V_1 and the wide S wave in V_6 indicate RBBB.

9.   Your patient says he thinks he might have had a heart attack about 3 years ago and had never had it checked with his healthcare provider. Looking at his admission ECG, you are certain that he sustained a previous MI based on the presence of a(an):

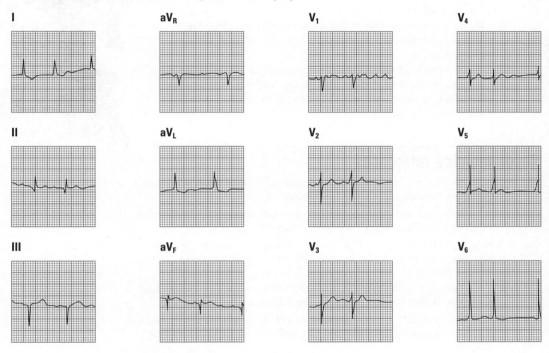

I   aV_R   V_1   V_4

II   aV_L   V_2   V_5

III   aV_F   V_3   V_6

   A.   pathologic Q waves in leads II, III, and aV_F.
   B.   inverted T waves in leads I, aV_L, and V_6.
   C.   depressed ST segments in leads II, aV_L, and V_5.
   D.   axis between 0 and +90 degrees.

Answer: A. Old damage to the myocardium is indicated by the presence of pathologic Q waves, in this case in leads II, III, and aV_F. Those findings lead you to suspect the patient suffered an inferior wall MI at some point.

Scoring

☆☆☆   If you answered all nine questions correctly, wow! You've graduated with honors from the School of 12-Lead ECG Interpretation.

☆☆   If you answered seven or eight questions correctly, super! You're ready to take a graduate course on 12-lead ECG interpretation.

☆   If you answered fewer than seven questions correctly, it takes time to become proficient and you're on your way. You will benefit from further review of your notes from 12-Lead ECG Interpretation 101.

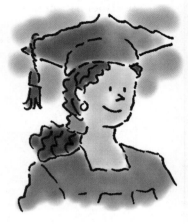

Recommended references

Brown, D. F. M., & Martindale, J. L. (2012). *Rapid interpretation of ECG's in emergency medicine.* Philadelphia, PA: Wolters Kluwer.

Cohen, B. J., & Taylor, J. J. (2013). *Memmler's structure and function of the human body* (10th ed.). Philadelphia, PA: Wolters Kluwer.

García-Niebla, J. (2009). Comparison of P-wave patterns derived from correct and incorrect placement of V1-V2 electrodes. *Journal of Cardiovascular Nursing, 24*(2), 156–161.

Katritsis, D. G., Gersch, B. J., & Camm, A. J. (2013). *Clinical cardiology: Current practice guidelines.* Oxford, United Kingdom: Oxford University Press.

Mann, D. L., Zipes, D. P., Libby, P., & Bonow, R. D. (2014). *Braunwald's heart disease: A textbook of cardiovascular medicine* (10th ed.). St. Louis, MO: Saunders | Elsevier.

McLaughlin, M. A. (clinical ed.) (2014). *Cardiovascular care made incredibly easy* (3rd ed.). Philadelphia, PA: Wolters Kluwer.

Rosen, A. V., Koppikan, S., Shaw, C., & Baranchuk, A. (2014). Common ECG lead placement errors. Part 1: Limb lead reversals. *International Journal of Medical Students, 2*(3), 92–98.

Urden, L., & Stacy, K. (2013). *Critical care nursing* (7th ed.). St Louis, MO: Mosby | Elsevier.

Wagner, G. S., & Strauss, D. G. (2013). *Marriott's practical electrocardiology* (12th ed.). Philadelphia, PA: Wolters Kluwer.

Appendices and index

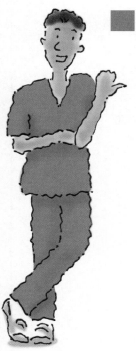

Practice makes perfect

1. You're caring for a patient with a history of mitral valve prolapse. Based on your knowledge of the heart's anatomy, you know that the mitral valve is located:
    A. between the left atrium and left ventricle.
    B. where the left ventricle meets the aorta.
    C. between the right atrium and right ventricle.
    D. between the right ventricle and pulmonary artery.

2. A 45-year-old patient is admitted to your floor for observation after undergoing cardiac catheterization. His test results reveal a blockage in the circumflex artery. The circumflex artery supplies oxygenated blood to which area of the heart?
    A. Anterior wall of the left ventricle
    B. Left atrium
    C. Right bundle branch
    D. Right ventricle

3. Which of the following choices is responsible for slowing heart rate?
    A. Norepinephrine (Levophed)
    B. Vagus nerve
    C. Epinephrine
    D. Isoproterenol (Isuprel)

4. Which cycle describes cardiac cells at rest?
    A. Early repolarization
    B. Polarization
    C. Rapid depolarization
    D. Absolute refractory period

5. A patient admitted with an acute myocardial infarction (MI) complains of chest pain. When you look at his ECG monitor, you note a heart rate of 35 beats/min. Which area of his heart has taken over as the heart's pacemaker?
    A. Sinoatrial (SA) node
    B. Atrioventricular (AV) node
    C. Bundle of His
    D. Purkinje fibers

6. Which lead on a cardiac monitor is equivalent to V_1 on a 12-lead ECG?
    A. Lead I
    B. Lead MCL_6
    C. Lead aV_F
    D. Lead MCL_1

7. A 37-year-old patient comes to the emergency department (ED) complaining of chest pain that began while he was mowing the lawn. You immediately begin cardiac monitoring and administer oxygen. Next you obtain a 12-lead ECG. You know that the six limb leads you apply will give you information about what area of the patient's heart?

    A. The frontal plane   *→ 3rd limb = Six limb = frontal plane*
    B. The horizontal plane
    C. The vertical plane
    D. The posterior plane

8. A patient with heart failure is transferred to your unit from the medical–surgical floor. Before initiating cardiac monitoring you must first:

    A. prepare the skin by rubbing it until it reddens.
    B. press the adhesive edge around the outside of the electrode to the patient's chest.
    C. press one side of the electrode against the patient's skin.
    D. attach the clip-on leadwire to the electrode before placing it on the patient's chest.

9. A 58-year-old patient is admitted with an acute MI. After you begin cardiac monitoring, you note a baseline that's thick and unreadable. How do you interpret this finding?

    A. Electrical interference
    B. Artifact
    C. Wandering baseline
    D. Weak signal

10. What does the horizontal axis of an ECG represent?

    A. Amplitude
    B. Time
    C. Electrical voltage
    D. Heart rate

11. A 65-year-old patient diagnosed with angina is admitted to your telemetry unit. You begin cardiac monitoring and record a rhythm strip. Using the 8-step method of rhythm strip interpretation, what should you do first?

    A. Calculate the heart rate.
    B. Evaluate the P wave.
    C. Check the rhythm.
    D. Measure the PR interval.

12. A 72-year-old patient calls you to his room because he's experiencing substernal chest pain that radiates to his jaw. You record a rhythm strip and monitor his vital signs. Which portion of the patient's ECG complex may become elevated or depressed indicating myocardial damage?
    A. T wave
    B. ST segment
    C. QRS complex
    D. P wave

13. A 76-year-old patient with heart failure is receiving furosemide (Lasix) 40 mg I.V. twice daily. When you look at his rhythm strip, you note prominent U waves. Which condition may have caused U waves to appear on your patient's rhythm strip?
    A. Hypokalemia
    B. Hypocalcemia
    C. Worsening heart failure
    D. Pericarditis

14. An 80-year-old patient with a history of atrial fibrillation is admitted with digoxin toxicity. When you assess his rhythm strip using the 10-times method, you note that his heart rate is 40 beats/min. Based on this finding, you should:
    A. check the patient's pulse and correlate it with the heart rate on the rhythm strip.
    B. recheck the heart rate on the rhythm strip using the sequence method.
    C. record another rhythm strip and reassess the heart rate on the rhythm strip.
    D. recheck the heart rate on the rhythm strip using the 1,500 method.

15. A patient with a history of paroxysmal atrial tachycardia develops digoxin toxicity. Because digoxin toxicity may cause prolongation of the PR interval, you must monitor his rhythm strip closely. What's the duration of a normal PR interval?
    A. 0.06 to 0.10 second
    B. 0.12 to 0.20 second
    C. 0.24 to 0.30 second
    D. 0.36 to 0.44 second

16. A patient is admitted to your telemetry unit with a diagnosis of sick sinus syndrome. Which medication should you keep readily available to treat a symptomatic event?
    A. Isoproterenol (Isuprel)
    B. Verapamil (Calan)
    C. Lidocaine
    D. Atropine

17. A 45-year-old patient is admitted with an acute MI. In the ED, he received nitroglycerin and morphine to treat his chest pain, and he's currently pain-free. His monitor reveals sinus tachycardia at a rate of 123 beats/min. Which statement is true regarding sinus tachycardia after acute MI?

    A. Sinus tachycardia is a normal response that typically abates after the first 24 hours.

    B. Sinus tachycardia is a poor prognostic sign because it may be associated with massive heart damage.

    C. Sinus tachycardia is a typical response to morphine administration.

    D. Sinus tachycardia is a sign that the heart is starting to heal.

18. A patient who has been taking digoxin (Lanoxin) suddenly develops the rhythm shown below. What's your interpretation of the rhythm?

    A. Normal sinus rhythm

    B. Sinus arrhythmia

    C. Sinus bradycardia

    D. Junctional escape rhythm

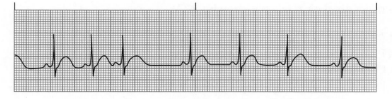

19. A patient develops sinus bradycardia. Which symptoms indicate that his cardiac output is falling?

    A. Hypertension and further drop in heart rate

    B. Hypotension and dizziness

    C. Increased urine output and syncope

    D. Warm, dry skin and hypotension

20. A patient admitted 2 days ago with an acute MI suddenly develops premature atrial contractions (PACs). What's the most likely cause of this arrhythmia in this patient?

    A. Increased caffeine intake

    B. Impending cardiogenic shock

    C. Developing heart failure

    D. Imminent cardiac arrest

21. A patient diagnosed with heart failure is admitted to your telemetry unit. He complains of seeing yellow-green halos around visual images. He also states that he's been nauseated and unable to eat for the past few days. Based on these findings you suspect:
    A.   digoxin toxicity.
    B.   atrial fibrillation.
    C.   worsening heart failure.
    D.   MI.

22. A patient returns to your unit after cardiac surgery in sinus tachycardia. As you perform your assessment of the patient, you note that his cardiac monitor shows a new onset atrial fibrillation at a rate of 160 beats/min. The patient suddenly begins complaining of chest pain. Based on these findings, what's the best treatment?
    A.   Digoxin (Lanoxin) administration
    B.   Defibrillation
    C.   Cardioversion
    D.   Flecainide (Tambocor) administration

23. A 32-year-old patient with a history of Wolff–Parkinson–White (WPW) syndrome is admitted to your floor after gallbladder surgery. Which ECG characteristics are typical in a patient with WPW syndrome?
    A.   Prolonged PR interval and narrowed QRS complex
    B.   Prolonged PR interval and presence of a delta wave
    C.   Shortened PR interval and narrowed QRS complex
    D.   Widened QRS complex and presence of a delta wave

24. A 68-year-old patient with a history of heart failure is receiving digoxin (Lanoxin). At the beginning of your shift, you record the patient's rhythm strip shown below. You interpret this rhythm as:
    A.   junctional tachycardia.
    B.   wandering pacemaker.
    C.   accelerated junctional rhythm.
    D.   sinus tachycardia.

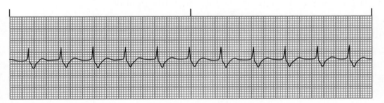

25.   A patient with a history of chronic obstructive pulmonary disease is admitted to your floor with hypoxemia. You begin cardiac monitoring, which reveals the rhythm shown below. You interpret this rhythm as:
   A.   premature junctional contractions.
   B.   wandering pacemaker.
   C.   accelerated junctional rhythm.
   D.   premature atrial contractions.

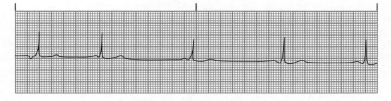

26.   A patient is admitted to your unit with digoxin toxicity. You record a rhythm strip and note that the rhythm is regular, the rate is 80 beats/min, and the P waves are inverted in lead II and occur before each QRS complex. Based on these findings, you interpret the rhythm as:
   A.   accelerated junctional rhythm.
   B.   junctional tachycardia.
   C.   junctional escape rhythm.
   D.   paroxysmal atrial tachycardia.

27.   A patient with an acute MI develops an arrhythmia. You record the rhythm strip shown below and identify the arrhythmia as:
   A.   idioventricular rhythm.
   B.   junctional escape rhythm.
   C.   premature junctional contractions.
   D.   sinus bradycardia.

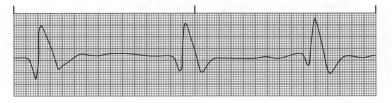

28.   The same patient with the arrhythmia identified in question 27 is hypotensive. You must immediately administer which agent to increase his heart rate?
   A.   Lidocaine
   B.   Isoproterenol (Isuprel)
   C.   Atropine
   D.   Amiodarone (Cordarone)

29.   A patient with a low magnesium level develops an arrhythmia. You record the rhythm strip shown below and identify the arrhythmia as:
   A.   monomorphic ventricular tachycardia.
   B.   ventricular fibrillation.
   C.   paroxysmal supraventricular tachycardia.
   D.   torsades de pointes.

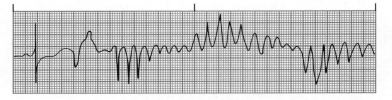

30.   A patient with an acute anterior wall MI develops third-degree heart block. His blood pressure is 78/44 mm Hg, and he's complaining of dizziness. You should immediately administer atropine and:
   A.   follow with a dose of isoproterenol (Isuprel).
   B.   apply a transcutaneous pacemaker.
   C.   place the patient in Trendelenburg position.
   D.   prepare for synchronized cardioversion.

31.   An 86-year-old patient is found in his apartment without heat on a cold winter day. He's admitted to your unit with hypothermia. You begin cardiac monitoring, which displays the rhythm shown below. You document this strip as:
   A.   normal sinus rhythm with first-degree AV block.
   B.   type 1 second-degree AV block.
   C.   sinus tachycardia.
   D.   junctional tachycardia.

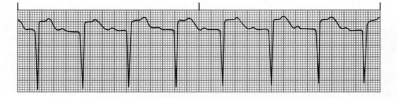

32. You're caring for a patient who developed complications after an acute MI requiring transvenous pacemaker insertion. His monitor alarm sounds and the rhythm strip shown below is recorded. You interpret this rhythm as which type of pacemaker malfunction?
   A. Failure to capture
   B. Failure to pace
   C. Undersensing
   D. Oversensing

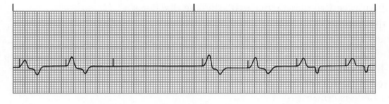

33. A patient admitted to the cardiac care unit with digoxin toxicity required transvenous pacemaker insertion. While assessing the patient, you note the rhythm shown below on the patient's monitor. This rhythm strip displays:
   A. oversensing.
   B. failure to sense.
   C. failure to pace.
   D. undersensing.

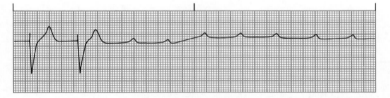

34. Your patient complains that his heart is skipping beats. You immediately record a rhythm strip from his cardiac monitor and take his vital signs. Based on the rhythm strip shown below, you should notify the practitioner of:
   A. failure to sense.
   B. over sensing.
   C. pacemaker-mediated tachycardia.
   D. failure to pace.

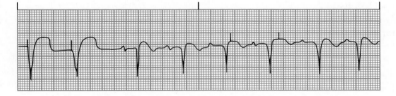

35.   When teaching a patient with a newly inserted permanent pacemaker, you should:

    A.   advise him to avoid computed tomography scans.

    B.   tell him that hiccups are normal for the first few days after pacemaker insertion.

    C.   instruct him to avoid tight clothing.

    D.   explain that magnetic resonance imaging scans are safe.

36.   You're caring for a 75-year-old patient who's receiving oral procainamide to control supraventricular tachycardia. Before discharge, you should instruct the patient:

    A.   to avoid chewing the drug, which may cause him to get too much of the drug at once.

    B.   that lupus-like symptoms are normal and will cease 2 to 3 weeks after initiation of therapy.

    C.   that a bitter taste is common.

    D.   that he may crush the extended-release tablet if it's difficult to swallow.

37.   A patient returns to your floor from the postaesthesia care unit after undergoing a right lower lobectomy. When you begin cardiac monitoring, you note the rhythm strip shown below. Which drug will the practitioner most likely prescribe to rapidly convert this rhythm?

    A.   Propafenone (Rhythmol)

    B.   Digoxin

    C.   Atropine

    D.   Ibutilide (Corvert)

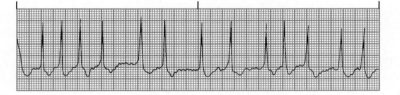

38.   After receiving quinidine, you note that your patient develops a prolonged QT interval on his rhythm strip. You notify the practitioner immediately because you know that prolongation of the QT interval places the patient at risk for what?

    A.   Atrial fibrillation

    B.   Junctional tachycardia

    C.   Polymorphic ventricular tachycardia

    D.   Atrial flutter

39. A 74-year-old patient is admitted to your floor from the ED with syncope. You note the rhythm shown below when you record a rhythm strip from his cardiac monitor. Based on this rhythm strip, you should question an order for which drug on the patient's chart?
   A. Warfarin (Coumadin)
   B. Verapamil (Calan)
   C. Epinephrine
   D. Atropine

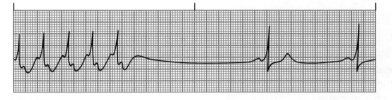

40. A 36-year-old patient with a history of heart transplantation is admitted to your floor for observation after an appendectomy. If the patient develops symptomatic bradycardia, which drug is indicated?
   A. Atropine
   B. Isoproterenol (Isuprel)
   C. Dopamine
   D. Propranolol (Inderal)

41. The surgeon orders a preoperative 12-lead ECG for your patient who's scheduled for a thoracotomy in the morning. Using your knowledge of 12-lead ECGs, which leads are bipolar?
   A. aV_R, aV_L, and aV_F
   B. I, II, and III
   C. V_1, V_2, and V_3
   D. V_4, V_5, and V_6

42. Each of the 12 leads of an ECG views the heart from a different angle. Lead I views which area of the heart?
   A. Inferior wall
   B. Anterior wall
   C. Posterior wall
   D. Lateral wall

43. The practitioner orders a signal-averaged ECG for a patient who sustained an acute MI. Why is this test typically ordered?
   A. To locate posterior wall damage
   B. To identify whether the patient is at risk for sudden death from sustained ventricular tachycardia
   C. To identify whether the patient has suffered damage to his right ventricle
   D. To identify left bundle-branch block in an anterior wall MI

44. You're caring for a patient with a histo[...] you into his room because he's experiencing [...] sion orders included a 12-lead ECG with eac[...] You immediately retrieve the ECG machine. [...] ment, where should you place lead V_1?
   A. Over the fourth intercostal space at t[...]
   B. Over the fourth intercostal space at t[...]
   C. Over the fifth intercostal space at the [...] line
   D. Over the fifth intercostal space at the [...]

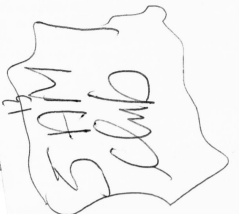

45. A 12-lead ECG is ordered for a 32-year-old[...] to the ED complaining of chest pain. You know [...] necessary to assess conduction of the:
   A. right ventricle.
   B. right and left ventricles.
   C. left ventricle.
   D. right and left atria.

46. You're caring for a 72-year-old patient admitted with unstable angina. He calls you into his room and complains of chest pain that he rates an 8 on a scale of 0 to 10 (10 being the worst). You immediately obtain a 12-lead ECG. Which ECG change would you expect with angina?
   A. Pathologic Q wave
   B. T-wave inversion
   C. Widened QRS complex
   D. Poor R-wave progression

47. A patient's 12-lead ECG reveals left axis deviation. When is left axis deviation considered normal?
   A. In infants
   B. In small children
   C. In pregnant women
   D. In healthy adults

48. A 38-year-old patient is admitted with a diagnosis of unstable angina. Which statement is true about unstable angina?
   A. The pain is typically triggered by exertion or stress.
   B. The pain is typically relieved by rest.
   C. The pain typically lasts less than 2 minutes.
   D. The pain may occur while the patient is sleeping.

49. After experiencing substernal chest pain for about 4 hours, a patient drives himself to the ED. He's triaged immediately and a 12-lead ECG is obtained. Which change on the patient's ECG is associated with myocardial necrosis?
  A. Pathologic Q waves
  B. T-wave inversion
  C. ST-segment elevation
  D. Narrowed QRS complex

50. When examining your patient's 12-lead ECG, you notice a bundle-branch block. Which leads should you check to determine whether the block is in the right or left bundle?
  A. V_1 and V_6
  B. II and aV_F
  C. V_4 and V_5
  D. I and III

51. You obtain a telemetry strip on a patient after coronary artery bypass surgery. After interpreting the rhythm strip shown below, what arrhythmia should you document?
  A. Atrial flutter
  B. Type II second-degree AV block
  C. Sinus arrhythmia
  D. Third-degree AV block

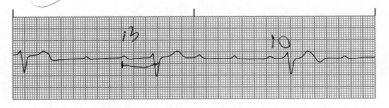

52. You're caring for a patient with an evolving anterolateral wall MI. While examining the patient's 12-lead ECG, you would expect to note changes in which leads? (Select all that apply.)
  A. Lead I
  B. Lead III
  C. Lead aV_F
  D. Lead V_4
  E. Lead V_6

53. As part of a preoperative assessment, you begin preparation for a 12-lead ECG. Using the figure below, identify the area on the patient's chest where you would place lead V_1.

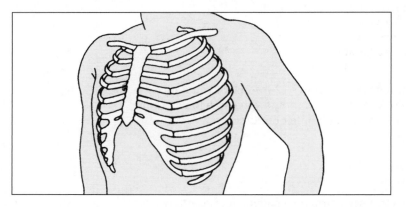

54. While interpreting the rhythm strip shown below for a patient who was just admitted to the telemetry unit, you document the PR interval as how many seconds?

_____ seconds

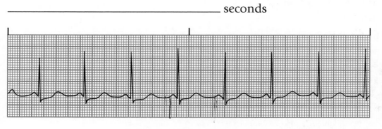

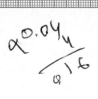

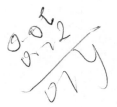

Answers

1.   A. The bicuspid valve, commonly called the mitral valve is located between the left atrium and left ventricle.

2.   B. The circumflex artery supplies oxygenated blood to the lateral walls of the ventricle, the left atrium, and the left posterior fasciculus of the left bundle branch.

3.   B. The vagus nerve carries impulses that slow the heart rate and the conduction of impulses through the AV node and ventricles.

4.   B. Polarization describes cardiac cells at rest.

5.   D. If the Purkinje fibers take over as the heart's pacemaker, impulses are typically discharged at a rate of 20 to 40 beats/min.

6.   D. Lead MCL_1 is the equivalent to V_1 on a 12-lead ECG.

7.   A. The six limb leads—leads I, II, III, aV_R, aV_L, and aV_F—provide information about the heart's frontal plane.

8.   A. Before initiating cardiac monitoring, you must first prepare the patient's skin. Use a special rough patch on the back of the electrode, a dry washcloth, or a gauze pad to briskly rub each site until the skin reddens.

9.   A. Electrical interference appears on the ECG as a baseline that's thick and unreadable. Electrical interference is caused by electrical power leakage. It may also occur due to interference from other equipment in the room or improperly grounded equipment.

10.   B. The horizontal axis of the ECG strip represents time.

11.   C. Using the 8-step method of rhythm strip interpretation, you should check the rhythm first and then calculate the rate. Next, evaluate the P wave, check out the PR interval and the QRS complex, examine the T wave, measure the QT interval and, finally, check for ectopic beats and other abnormalities.

12.   B. A change in the ST segment may indicate myocardial damage. An ST segment may become either elevated or depressed.

13.   A. A U wave isn't present on every rhythm strip. A prominent U wave may be due to hypokalemia, hypercalcemia, or digoxin toxicity.

14.   A. Although you can use the 10-times method, the 1,500 method, or the sequence method to determine heart rate, you shouldn't rely on these methods. Always check a pulse to correlate it with the heart rate on the ECG.

15. B. The normal duration of a PR interval is 0.12 to 0.20 second.

16. D. Atropine or epinephrine may be administered for symptomatic bradycardia that's caused by sick sinus syndrome. Therefore, you should keep these drugs readily available.

17. B. Sinus tachycardia occurs in about 30% of patients after acute MI and is considered a poor prognostic sign because it may be associated with massive heart damage.

18. B. The rhythm strip shows sinus arrhythmia. If sinus arrhythmia develops suddenly in the patient taking digoxin, the patient may be experiencing digoxin toxicity.

19. B. When sinus bradycardia is symptomatic, the resulting drop in cardiac output produces such signs and symptoms as hypotension and dizziness.

20. C. In a patient with an acute MI, PACs can serve as an early sign of heart failure or an electrolyte imbalance.

21. A. The patient with digoxin toxicity may develop arrhythmias, blurred vision, hypotension, increased severity of heart failure, yellow-green halos around visual images, anorexia, nausea, and vomiting.

22. C. If the patient with atrial fibrillation complains of chest pain, emergency measures such as cardioversion are necessary. Digoxin may be used to control the ventricular response in patients with atrial fibrillation who are asymptomatic.

23. D. WPW syndrome causes a shortened PR interval (less than 0.10 second) and a widened QRS complex (greater than 0.10 second). The beginning of the QRS complex may appear slurred. This hallmark sign is referred to as a delta wave.

24. A. The rhythm strip reveals junctional tachycardia. The rhythm is regular, the rate is 110 beats/min, a P wave occurs after each QRS complex, and the PR interval isn't measurable.

25. B. The rhythm strip reveals a wandering pacemaker. The key characteristics are the varying shapes of the P waves.

26. A. Based on these findings, the patient's rhythm strip reveals accelerated junctional rhythm.

27. A. The rhythm strip reveals idioventricular rhythm.

28. C. The agent of choice for treatment of idioventricular rhythm is atropine. A pacemaker may be necessary after atropine administration.

29. D. The rhythm strip shows torsades de pointes.

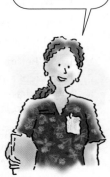

A slurred QRS complex is referred to as a delta wave.

30.   B. If the patient's cardiac output is inadequate (low blood pressure and dizziness), you should immediately administer atropine and apply a transcutaneous pacemaker. The patient may need a transvenous pacemaker until the block resolves. If the block doesn't resolve, he'll need a permanent pacemaker.

31.   A. You should document in your notes that the patient's monitor reveals normal sinus rhythm with first-degree AV block. Hypothermia is one cause of this arrhythmia.

32.   A. The rhythm strip shows the pacemaker's failure to capture. The ECG pacemaker spike isn't followed by a QRS complex.

33.   C. The rhythm strip reveals the pacemaker's failure to pace. After two paced beats, there's no apparent pacemaker activity on the ECG. Begin CPR.

34.   A. The ECG pacemaker spikes fall where they shouldn't, indicating a failure to sense.

35.   C. You should instruct the patient to avoid tight clothing or direct pressure over the pulse generator, to avoid magnetic resonance imaging scans and certain other diagnostic studies, and to notify the practitioner if he feels confused, light-headed, or short of breath. The patient should also notify the practitioner if he has palpitations, hiccups, or a rapid or unusually slow heart rate.

36.   A. Warn the patient taking oral procainamide not to chew it because this might cause him to get too much of the drug at once. Lupus-like symptoms are associated with long-term use of procainamide and may require discontinuation of the drug. A bitter taste is also an adverse effect of procainamide. The extended-release tablet shouldn't be crushed.

37.   D. This rhythm strip reveals atrial fibrillation. Ibutilide is used for rapid conversion of recent-onset atrial fibrillation or flutter to sinus rhythm.

38.   C. Prolongation of the QT interval is a sign that the patient is predisposed to developing polymorphic ventricular tachycardia.

39.   B. The rhythm strip reveals sick sinus syndrome. Verapamil should be avoided in sick sinus syndrome or second- or third-degree AV block without a pacemaker and in atrial fibrillation or flutter due to WPW syndrome.

40.   B. Isoproterenol is the drug of choice for treating symptomatic bradycardia in patients who have undergone heart transplantation. The vagal nerve dissection that occurs during heart transplantation surgery renders atropine ineffective in these patients.

41.   B. The 12 leads include three bipolar limb leads (I, II, and III), three unipolar augmented limb leads (aV_R, aV_L, and aV_F), and six unipolar precordial leads (V_1, V_2, V_3, V_4, V_5, and V_6).

42.   D. Lead I views the lateral wall of the heart.

43.   B. Signal-averaged ECG helps identify patients at risk for sudden death from sustained ventricular tachycardia. The test uses a computer to identify late electrical potentials that can't be detected by a 12-lead ECG.

44.   A. Lead V_1 should be placed over the fourth intercostal space at the right sternal border.

45.   C. A 12-lead ECG is used to assess left ventricular conduction activity. A right-sided ECG is necessary to assess right ventricular conduction activity.

46.   B. Classic ECG changes associated with angina include a peaked T wave, flattened T wave, T-wave inversion, ST-segment depression with T-wave inversion, and ST-segment depression without T-wave inversion.

47.   C. Left axis deviation is a normal finding in pregnant women. Right axis deviation is normal in infants and small children.

48.   D. Unstable angina is more easily provoked and may occur while the patient is sleeping, causing him to awaken. It's also unpredictable and tends to worsen over time. In stable angina, pain is triggered by exertion or stress and is commonly relieved by rest. Each episode follows a similar pattern.

49.   A. The area of myocardial necrosis is called the zone of infarction. The ECG change associated with a necrotic area is a pathologic Q wave. The zone of injury shows up on an ECG as an elevated ST segment. The zone of ischemia is represented by T-wave inversion.

50.   A. After you identify a bundle-branch block, examine lead V_1, which lies to the right of the heart, and lead V_6, which lies to the left of the heart. These leads will tell you if the block is in the right or left bundle.

51.   D. The rhythm strip reveals third-degree AV block. Characteristics of this arrhythmia include a regular atrial rhythm along with a regular but slow ventricular rhythm, an absence of a relationship between P waves and QRS complexes, and P and R waves that march across the strip in rhythm.

52.   A, D, E. In an anterolateral wall MI, ECG changes occur in leads I, aV_L, V_4, V_5, and V_6.

53. Lead V_1 should be placed over the fourth intercostal space at the right sternal border.

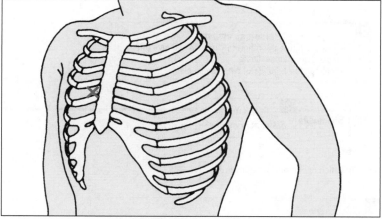

54. 0.14. The PR interval is measured from the beginning of the P wave to the beginning of the QRS complex. The normal duration of the PR interval is 0.12 to 0.20 second.

Pulseless arrest

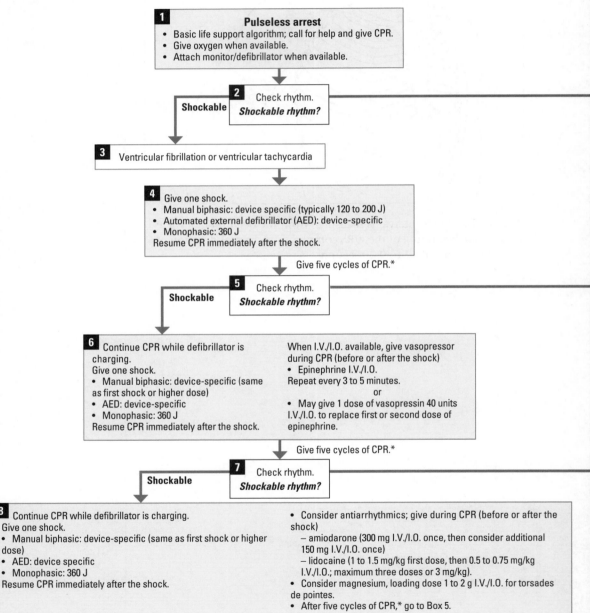

1
Pulseless arrest
- Basic life support algorithm; call for help and give CPR.
- Give oxygen when available.
- Attach monitor/defibrillator when available.

2 Check rhythm.
Shockable rhythm?

Shockable

3 Ventricular fibrillation or ventricular tachycardia

4 Give one shock.
- Manual biphasic: device specific (typically 120 to 200 J)
- Automated external defibrillator (AED): device-specific
- Monophasic: 360 J
Resume CPR immediately after the shock.

Give five cycles of CPR.*

5 Check rhythm.
Shockable rhythm?

Shockable

6 Continue CPR while defibrillator is charging.
Give one shock.
- Manual biphasic: device-specific (same as first shock or higher dose)
- AED: device-specific
- Monophasic: 360 J
Resume CPR immediately after the shock.

When I.V./I.O. available, give vasopressor during CPR (before or after the shock)
- Epinephrine I.V./I.O.
Repeat every 3 to 5 minutes.
or
- May give 1 dose of vasopressin 40 units I.V./I.O. to replace first or second dose of epinephrine.

Give five cycles of CPR.*

7 Check rhythm.
Shockable rhythm?

Shockable

8 Continue CPR while defibrillator is charging.
Give one shock.
- Manual biphasic: device-specific (same as first shock or higher dose)
- AED: device specific
- Monophasic: 360 J
Resume CPR immediately after the shock.

- Consider antiarrhythmics; give during CPR (before or after the shock)
  – amiodarone (300 mg I.V./I.O. once, then consider additional 150 mg I.V./I.O. once)
  – lidocaine (1 to 1.5 mg/kg first dose, then 0.5 to 0.75 mg/kg I.V./I.O.; maximum three doses or 3 mg/kg).
- Consider magnesium, loading dose 1 to 2 g I.V./I.O. for torsades de pointes.
- After five cycles of CPR,* go to Box 5.

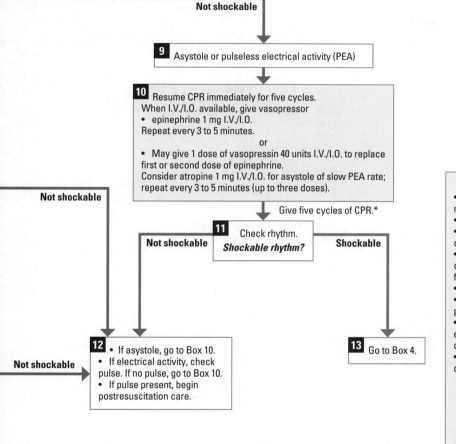

Not shockable

9 Asystole or pulseless electrical activity (PEA)

10 Resume CPR immediately for five cycles.
When I.V./I.O. available, give vasopressor
• epinephrine 1 mg I.V./I.O.
Repeat every 3 to 5 minutes.
        or
• May give 1 dose of vasopressin 40 units I.V./I.O. to replace
first or second dose of epinephrine.
Consider atropine 1 mg I.V./I.O. for asystole of slow PEA rate;
repeat every 3 to 5 minutes (up to three doses).

Not shockable

Give five cycles of CPR.*

11 Check rhythm.
Shockable rhythm?

Not shockable   **Shockable**

Not shockable

12 • If asystole, go to Box 10.
• If electrical activity, check
pulse. If no pulse, go to Box 10.
• If pulse present, begin
postresuscitation care.

Not shockable

13 Go to Box 4.

During CPR
• Push hard and fast (100/
minute).
• Ensure full chest recoil.
• Minimize interruptions in
chest compressions.
• One cycle of CPR: 30
compressions then 2 breaths;
five cycles = 2 minutes.
• Avoid hyperventilation.
• Secure airway and confirm
placement.
• Rotate compressors
every two minutes with rhythm
checks.
• Search for and treat possible
contributing factors, such as:
  – hypovolemia
  – hypoxia
  – hydrogen ion (acidosis)
  – hypokalemia/hyperkalemia
  – hypoglycemia
  – hypothermia
  – toxins
  – tamponade, cardiac
  – tension pneumothorax
  – thrombosis (coronary or
pulmonary)
  – trauma.

* After an advanced airway is placed, rescuers no longer deliver "cycles" of CPR. Give continuous chest
compressions without pauses for breaths. Give 8 to 10 breaths/minute. Check rhythm every 2 minutes.

Bradycardia

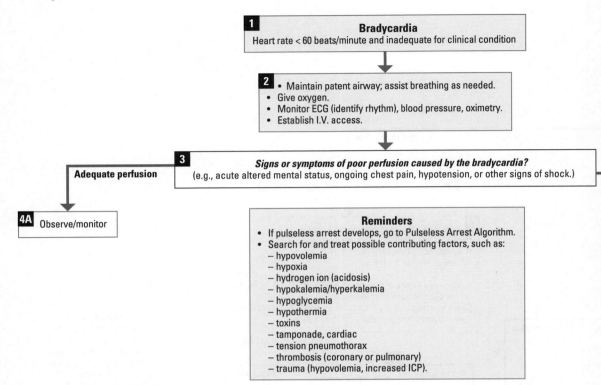

1 **Bradycardia**
Heart rate < 60 beats/minute and inadequate for clinical condition

2
- Maintain patent airway; assist breathing as needed.
- Give oxygen.
- Monitor ECG (identify rhythm), blood pressure, oximetry.
- Establish I.V. access.

3 *Signs or symptoms of poor perfusion caused by the bradycardia?*
(e.g., acute altered mental status, ongoing chest pain, hypotension, or other signs of shock.)

Adequate perfusion

4A Observe/monitor

Reminders
- If pulseless arrest develops, go to Pulseless Arrest Algorithm.
- Search for and treat possible contributing factors, such as:
  - hypovolemia
  - hypoxia
  - hydrogen ion (acidosis)
  - hypokalemia/hyperkalemia
  - hypoglycemia
  - hypothermia
  - toxins
  - tamponade, cardiac
  - tension pneumothorax
  - thrombosis (coronary or pulmonary)
  - trauma (hypovolemia, increased ICP).

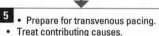

Poor perfusion

4
- Prepare for transcutaneous pacing; use without delay for high-degree block (type II second-degree block or third-degree atrioventricular block).
- Consider atropine 0.5 mg I.V. while awaiting pacer. May repeat to a total dose of 3 mg. If ineffective, begin pacing.
- Consider epinephrine (2 to 10 mcg/minute) or dopamine (2 to 10 mcg/kg/minute) infusion while awaiting pacer or if pacing ineffective.

5
- Prepare for transvenous pacing.
- Treat contributing causes.
- Consider expert consultation.

Reproduced with permission, "2005 American Heart Association Guidelines for Cardiopulmonary Resuscitation and Emergency Cardiovascular Care: Part 7.3-Management of Symptomatic Bradycardia and Tachycardia," *Circulation 2005*: 112(suppl IV): IV–67–IV–77. © 2005, American Heart Association.

Tachycardia

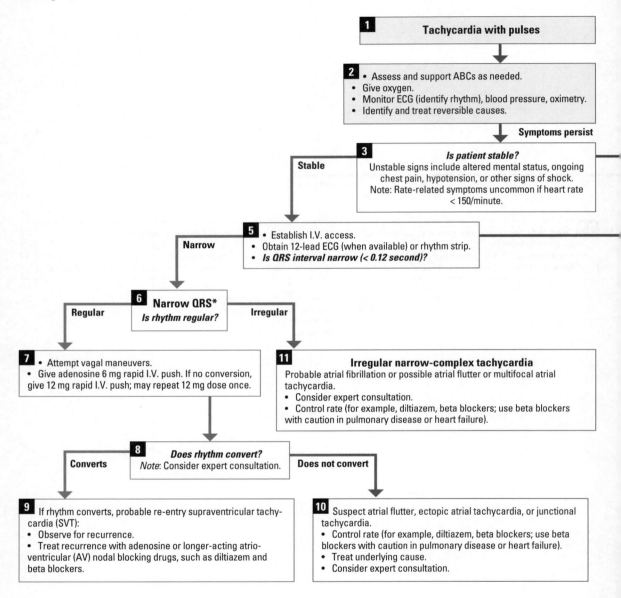

1 **Tachycardia with pulses**

2
- Assess and support ABCs as needed.
- Give oxygen.
- Monitor ECG (identify rhythm), blood pressure, oximetry.
- Identify and treat reversible causes.

Symptoms persist

3 ***Is patient stable?***
Unstable signs include altered mental status, ongoing chest pain, hypotension, or other signs of shock.
Note: Rate-related symptoms uncommon if heart rate < 150/minute.

Stable

5
- Establish I.V. access.
- Obtain 12-lead ECG (when available) or rhythm strip.
- ***Is QRS interval narrow (< 0.12 second)?***

Narrow

6 **Narrow QRS***
Is rhythm regular?

Regular   **Irregular**

7
- Attempt vagal maneuvers.
- Give adenosine 6 mg rapid I.V. push. If no conversion, give 12 mg rapid I.V. push; may repeat 12 mg dose once.

11 **Irregular narrow-complex tachycardia**
Probable atrial fibrillation or possible atrial flutter or multifocal atrial tachycardia.
- Consider expert consultation.
- Control rate (for example, diltiazem, beta blockers; use beta blockers with caution in pulmonary disease or heart failure).

8 ***Does rhythm convert?***
Note: Consider expert consultation.

Converts   **Does not convert**

9 If rhythm converts, probable re-entry supraventricular tachy-cardia (SVT):
- Observe for recurrence.
- Treat recurrence with adenosine or longer-acting atrio-ventricular (AV) nodal blocking drugs, such as diltiazem and beta blockers.

10 Suspect atrial flutter, ectopic atrial tachycardia, or junctional tachycardia.
- Control rate (for example, diltiazem, beta blockers; use beta blockers with caution in pulmonary disease or heart failure).
- Treat underlying cause.
- Consider expert consultation.

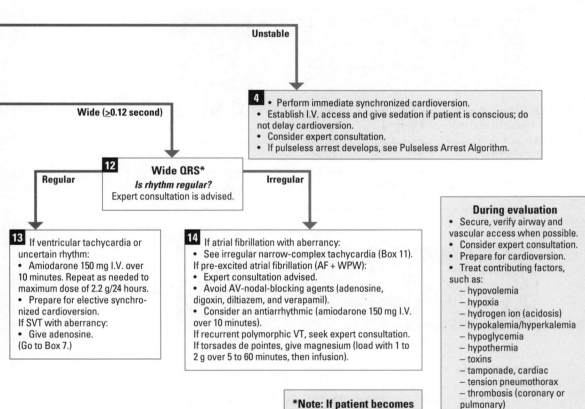

Unstable

4 • Perform immediate synchronized cardioversion.
• Establish I.V. access and give sedation if patient is conscious; do not delay cardioversion.
• Consider expert consultation.
• If pulseless arrest develops, see Pulseless Arrest Algorithm.

Wide (≥0.12 second)

12 **Wide QRS***
Is rhythm regular?
Expert consultation is advised.

Regular   **Irregular**

13 If ventricular tachycardia or uncertain rhythm:
• Amiodarone 150 mg I.V. over 10 minutes. Repeat as needed to maximum dose of 2.2 g/24 hours.
• Prepare for elective synchronized cardioversion.
If SVT with aberrancy:
• Give adenosine.
(Go to Box 7.)

14 If atrial fibrillation with aberrancy:
• See irregular narrow-complex tachycardia (Box 11).
If pre-excited atrial fibrillation (AF + WPW):
• Expert consultation advised.
• Avoid AV-nodal-blocking agents (adenosine, digoxin, diltiazem, and verapamil).
• Consider an antiarrhythmic (amiodarone 150 mg I.V. over 10 minutes).
If recurrent polymorphic VT, seek expert consultation.
If torsades de pointes, give magnesium (load with 1 to 2 g over 5 to 60 minutes, then infusion).

During evaluation
• Secure, verify airway and vascular access when possible.
• Consider expert consultation.
• Prepare for cardioversion.
• Treat contributing factors, such as:
  – hypovolemia
  – hypoxia
  – hydrogen ion (acidosis)
  – hypokalemia/hyperkalemia
  – hypoglycemia
  – hypothermia
  – toxins
  – tamponade, cardiac
  – tension pneumothorax
  – thrombosis (coronary or pulmonary)
  – trauma (hypovolemia).

*Note: If patient becomes unstable, go to Box 4.

Use these sample rhythm strips as a practical way to brush up on your ECG interpretation skills. Record the rhythm, rates, and waveform characteristics in the blank spaces provided, and then compare your findings with the answers beginning on page 351.

1.

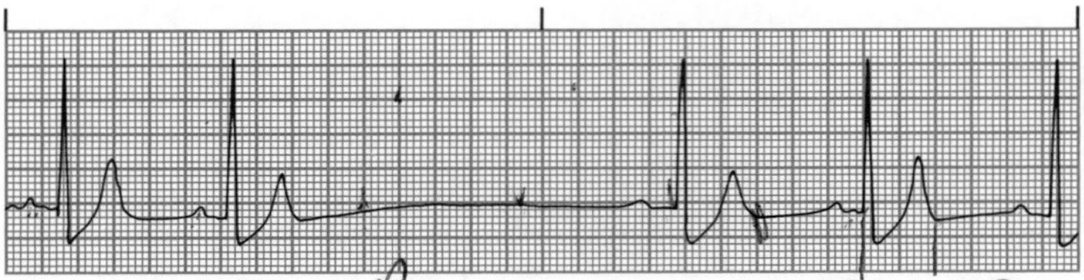

Atrial rhythm: _____ *R*

Ventricular rhythm: _____ irreg

Atrial rate: _____ 70

Ventricular rate: _____ 50

P wave: _____ ✓

PR interval: _____ 0.2, 0.24, 0.62

QRS complex: _____ 0.08

T wave: _____

QT interval: _____

Other: _____

Interpretation: _____

2.

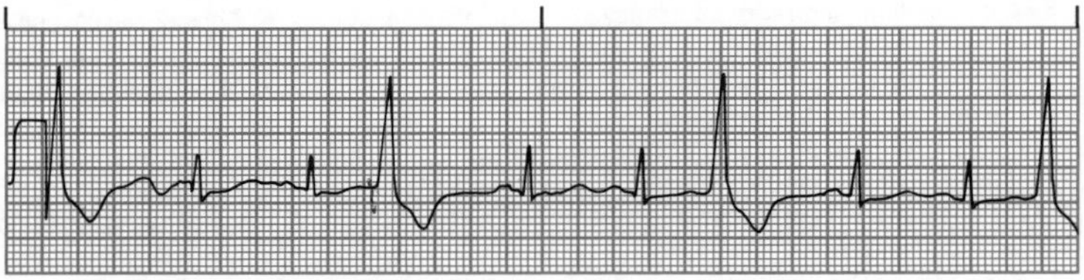

Atrial rhythm: _____

Ventricular rhythm: _____

Atrial rate: _____

Ventricular rate: _____

P wave: _____

PR interval: _____

QRS complex: _____

T wave: _____

QT interval: _____

Other: _____

Interpretation: _____

3.

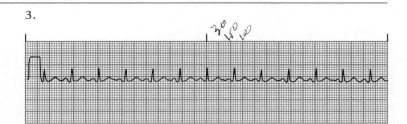

Atrial rhythm: _____   QRS complex: _____
Ventricular rhythm: _____   T wave: _____
Atrial rate: _____   QT interval: _____
Ventricular rate: _____   Other: _____
P wave: _____   Interpretation: _____
PR interval: _____   _____

4.

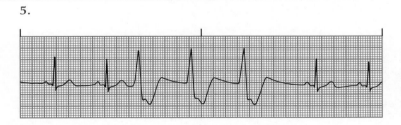

Atrial rhythm: _____   QRS complex: _____
Ventricular rhythm: _____   T wave: _____
Atrial rate: _____   QT interval: _____
Ventricular rate: _____   Other: _____
P wave: _____   Interpretation: _____
PR interval: _____   _____

5.

Atrial rhythm: _____   QRS complex: _____
Ventricular rhythm: _____   T wave: _____
Atrial rate: _____   QT interval: _____
Ventricular rate: _____   Other: _____
P wave: _____   Interpretation: _____
PR interval: _____   _____

6.

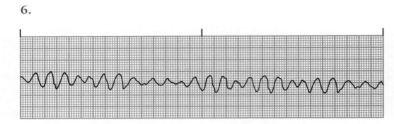

Atrial rhythm: _____
Ventricular rhythm: _____
Atrial rate: _____
Ventricular rate: _____
P wave: _____
PR interval: _____

QRS complex: _____
T wave: _____
QT interval: _____
Other: _____
Interpretation: _____
_____

7.

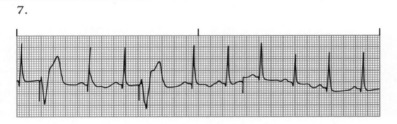

Atrial rhythm: _____
Ventricular rhythm: _____
Atrial rate: _____
Ventricular rate: _____
P wave: _____
PR interval: _____

QRS complex: _____
T wave: _____
QT interval: _____
Other: _____
Interpretation: _____
_____

8.

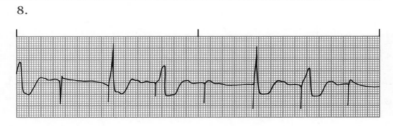

Atrial rhythm: _____
Ventricular rhythm: _____
Atrial rate: _____
Ventricular rate: _____
P wave: _____
PR interval: _____

QRS complex: _____
T wave: _____
QT interval: _____
Other: _____
Interpretation: _____
_____

9.

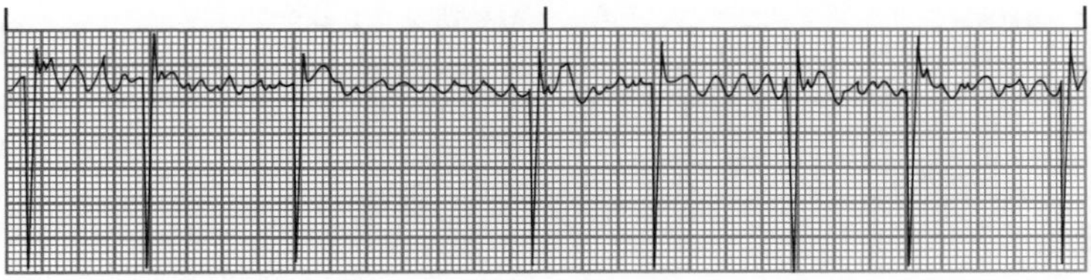

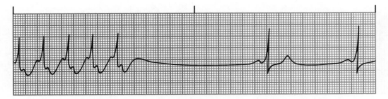

Atrial rhythm: _____ 　 QRS complex: _____
Ventricular rhythm: _____ 　 T wave: _____
Atrial rate: _____ 　 QT interval: _____
Ventricular rate: _____ 　 Other: _____
P wave: _____ 　 Interpretation: _____
PR interval: _____ 　 _____

10.

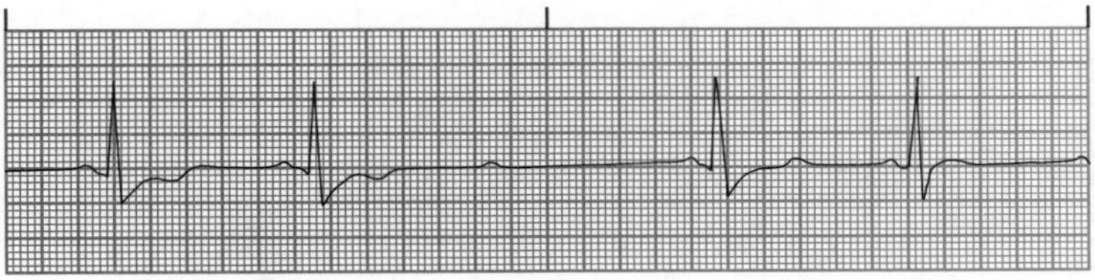

Atrial rhythm: _____ 　 QRS complex: _____
Ventricular rhythm: _____ 　 T wave: _____
Atrial rate: _____ 　 QT interval: _____
Ventricular rate: _____ 　 Other: _____
P wave: _____ 　 Interpretation: _____
PR interval: _____ 　 _____

11.

Atrial rhythm: _____ 　 QRS complex: _____
Ventricular rhythm: _____ 　 T wave: _____
Atrial rate: _____ 　 QT interval: _____
Ventricular rate: _____ 　 Other: _____
P wave: _____ 　 Interpretation: _____
PR interval: _____ 　 _____

12.

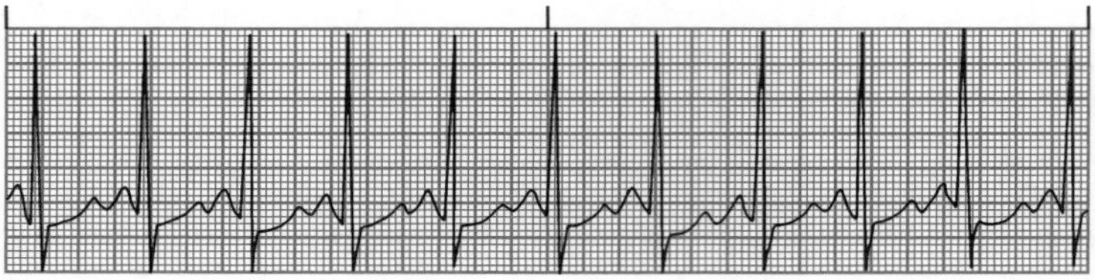

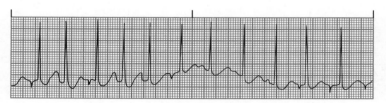

Atrial rhythm: _____   QRS complex: _____
Ventricular rhythm: _____   T wave: _____
Atrial rate: _____   QT interval: _____
Ventricular rate: _____   Other: _____
P wave: _____   Interpretation: _____
PR interval: _____   _____

13.

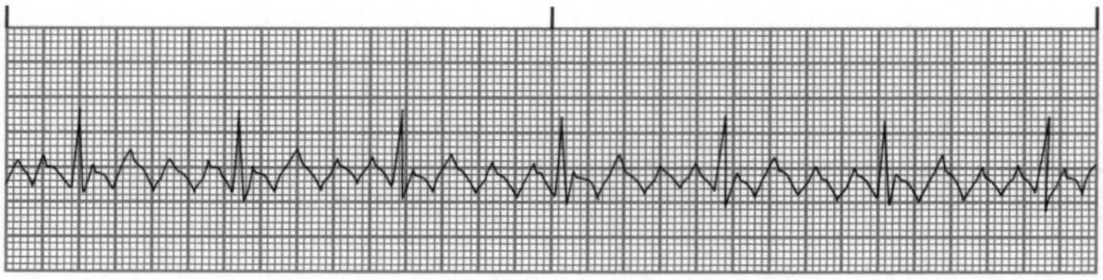

Atrial rhythm: _____   QRS complex: _____
Ventricular rhythm: _____   T wave: _____
Atrial rate: _____   QT interval: _____
Ventricular rate: _____   Other: _____
P wave: _____   Interpretation: _____
PR interval: _____   _____

14.

Atrial rhythm: _____   QRS complex: _____
Ventricular rhythm: _____   T wave: _____
Atrial rate: _____   QT interval: _____
Ventricular rate: _____   Other: _____
P wave: _____   Interpretation: _____
PR interval: _____   _____

15.

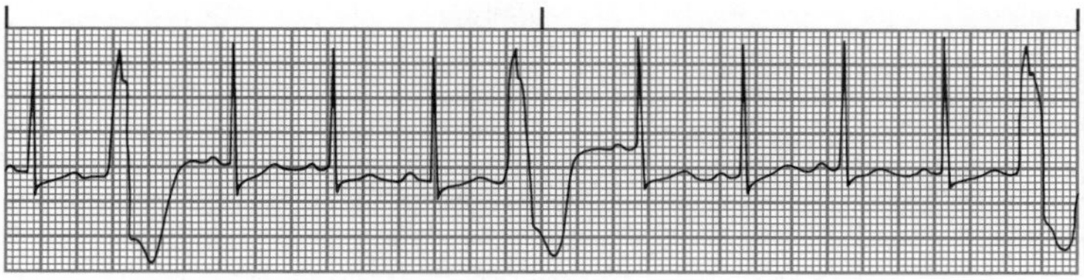

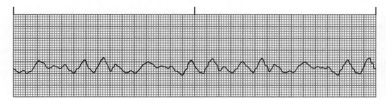

Atrial rhythm: _____   QRS complex: _____
Ventricular rhythm: _____   T wave: _____
Atrial rate: _____   QT interval: _____
Ventricular rate: _____   Other: _____
P wave: _____   Interpretation: _____
PR interval: _____   _____

16.

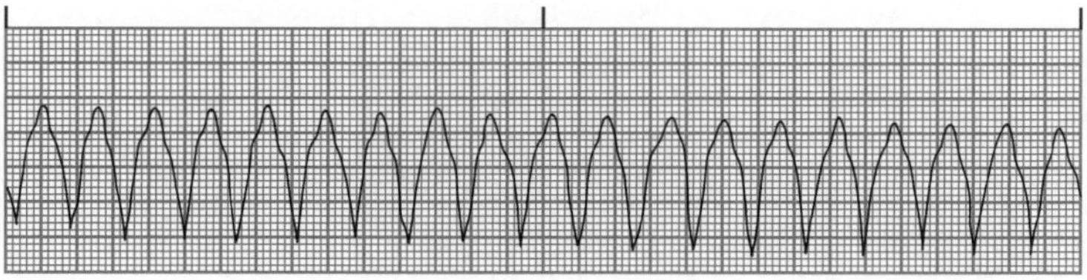

Atrial rhythm: _____   QRS complex: _____
Ventricular rhythm: _____   T wave: _____
Atrial rate: _____   QT interval: _____
Ventricular rate: _____   Other: _____
P wave: _____   Interpretation: _____
PR interval: _____   _____

17.

Atrial rhythm: _____   QRS complex: _____
Ventricular rhythm: _____   T wave: _____
Atrial rate: _____   QT interval: _____
Ventricular rate: _____   Other: _____
P wave: _____   Interpretation: _____
PR interval: _____   _____

18.

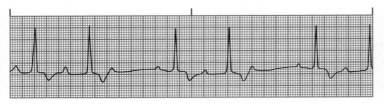

Atrial rhythm: _____   QRS complex: _____

Ventricular rhythm: _____   T wave: _____

Atrial rate: _____   QT interval: _____

Ventricular rate: _____   Other: _____

P wave: _____   Interpretation: _____

PR interval: _____   _____

19.

Atrial rhythm: _____   QRS complex: _____

Ventricular rhythm: _____   T wave: _____

Atrial rate: _____   QT interval: _____

Ventricular rate: _____   Other: _____

P wave: _____   Interpretation: _____

PR interval: _____   _____

20.

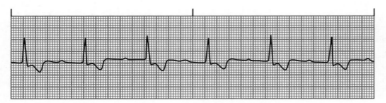

Atrial rhythm: _____   QRS complex: _____

Ventricular rhythm: _____   T wave: _____

Atrial rate: _____   QT interval: _____

Ventricular rate: _____   Other: _____

P wave: _____   Interpretation: _____

PR interval: _____   _____

21.

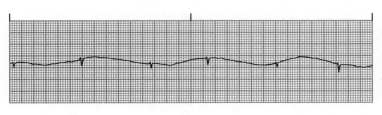

Atrial rhythm: _____ QRS complex: _____
Ventricular rhythm: _____ T wave: _____
Atrial rate: _____ QT interval: _____
Ventricular rate: _____ Other: _____
P wave: _____ Interpretation: _____
PR interval: _____ _____

22.

Atrial rhythm: _____ QRS complex: _____
Ventricular rhythm: _____ T wave: _____
Atrial rate: _____ QT interval: _____
Ventricular rate: _____ Other: _____
P wave: _____ Interpretation: _____
PR interval: _____ _____

23.

Atrial rhythm: _____ QRS complex: _____
Ventricular rhythm: _____ T wave: _____
Atrial rate: _____ QT interval: _____
Ventricular rate: _____ Other: _____
P wave: _____ Interpretation: _____
PR interval: _____ _____

24.

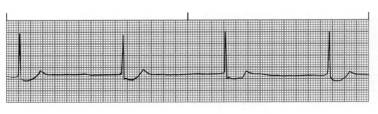

Atrial rhythm: _____   QRS complex: _____

Ventricular rhythm: _____   T wave: _____

Atrial rate: _____   QT interval: _____

Ventricular rate: _____   Other: _____

P wave: _____   Interpretation: _____

PR interval: _____   _____

25.

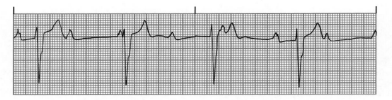

Atrial rhythm: _____   QRS complex: _____

Ventricular rhythm: _____   T wave: _____

Atrial rate: _____   QT interval: _____

Ventricular rate: _____   Other: _____

P wave: _____   Interpretation: _____

PR interval: _____   _____

26.

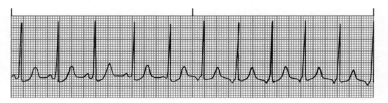

Atrial rhythm: _____   QRS complex: _____

Ventricular rhythm: _____   T wave: _____

Atrial rate: _____   QT interval: _____

Ventricular rate: _____   Other: _____

P wave: _____   Interpretation: _____

PR interval: _____   _____

27.

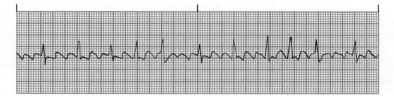

Atrial rhythm: _____ QRS complex: _____
Ventricular rhythm: _____ T wave: _____
Atrial rate: _____ QT interval: _____
Ventricular rate: _____ Other: _____
P wave: _____ Interpretation: _____
PR interval: _____ _____

28.

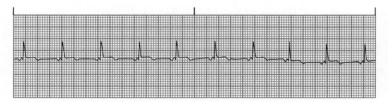

Atrial rhythm: _____ QRS complex: _____
Ventricular rhythm: _____ T wave: _____
Atrial rate: _____ QT interval: _____
Ventricular rate: _____ Other: _____
P wave: _____ Interpretation: _____
PR interval: _____ _____

29.

Atrial rhythm: _____ QRS complex: _____
Ventricular rhythm: _____ T wave: _____
Atrial rate: _____ QT interval: _____
Ventricular rate: _____ Other: _____
P wave: _____ Interpretation: _____
PR interval: _____ _____

30.

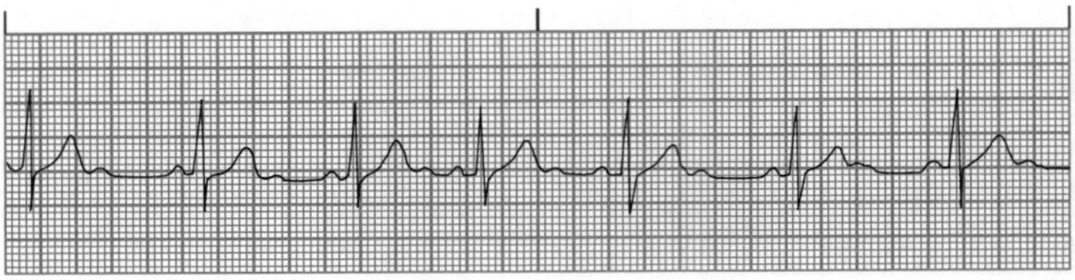

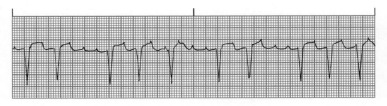

Atrial rhythm: _____   QRS complex: _____
Ventricular rhythm: _____   T wave: _____
Atrial rate: _____   QT interval: _____
Ventricular rate: _____   Other: _____
P wave: _____   Interpretation: _____
PR interval: _____   _____

31.

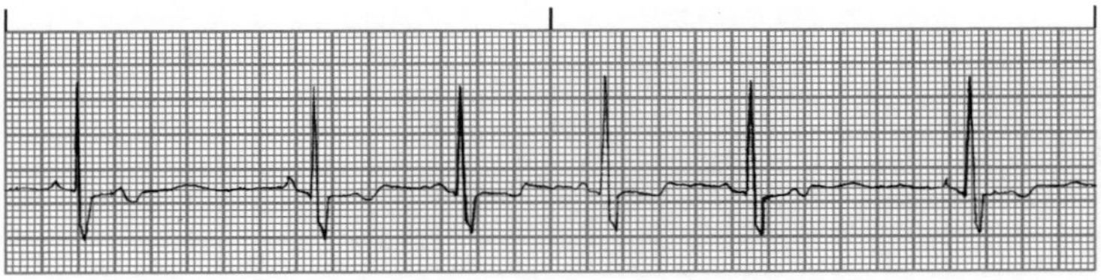

Atrial rhythm: _____   QRS complex: _____
Ventricular rhythm: _____   T wave: _____
Atrial rate: _____   QT interval: _____
Ventricular rate: _____   Other: _____
P wave: _____   Interpretation: _____
PR interval: _____   _____

32.

Atrial rhythm: _____   QRS complex: _____
Ventricular rhythm: _____   T wave: _____
Atrial rate: _____   QT interval: _____
Ventricular rate: _____   Other: _____
P wave: _____   Interpretation: _____
PR interval: _____   _____

33.

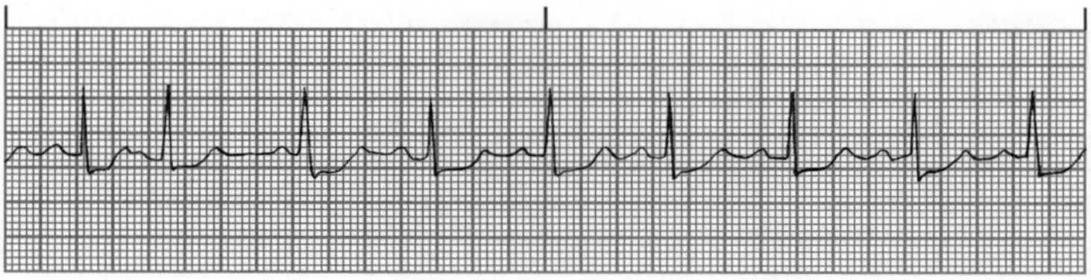

Atrial rhythm: _____   QRS complex: _____

Ventricular rhythm: _____   T wave: _____

Atrial rate: _____   QT interval: _____

Ventricular rate: _____   Other: _____

P wave: _____   Interpretation: _____

PR interval: _____   _____

34.

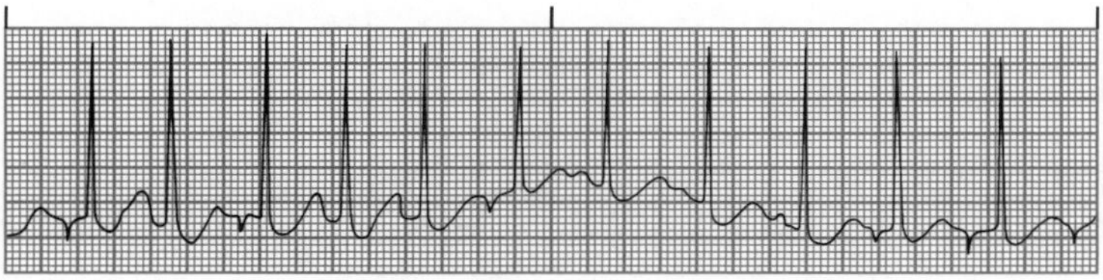

Atrial rhythm: _____   QRS complex: _____

Ventricular rhythm: _____   T wave: _____

Atrial rate: _____   QT interval: _____

Ventricular rate: _____   Other: _____

P wave: _____   Interpretation: _____

PR interval: _____

35.

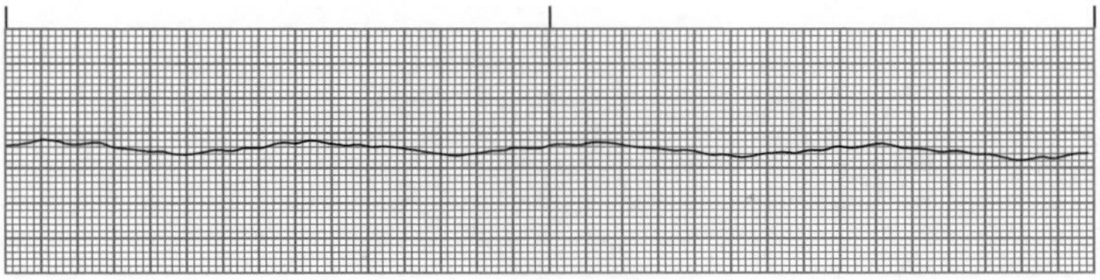

Atrial rhythm: _____   QRS complex: _____

Ventricular rhythm: _____   T wave: _____

Atrial rate: _____   QT interval: _____

Ventricular rate: _____   Other: _____

P wave: _____   Interpretation: _____

PR interval: _____

36.

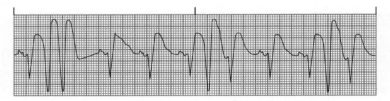

Atrial rhythm: _____   QRS complex: _____
Ventricular rhythm: _____   T wave: _____
Atrial rate: _____   QT interval: _____
Ventricular rate: _____   Other: _____
P wave: _____   Interpretation: _____
PR interval: _____   _____

37.

Atrial rhythm: _____   QRS complex: _____
Ventricular rhythm: _____   T wave: _____
Atrial rate: _____   QT interval: _____
Ventricular rate: _____   Other: _____
P wave: _____   Interpretation: _____
PR interval: _____   _____

38.

Atrial rhythm: _____   QRS complex: _____
Ventricular rhythm: _____   T wave: _____
Atrial rate: _____   QT interval: _____
Ventricular rate: _____   Other: _____
P wave: _____   Interpretation: _____
PR interval: _____   _____

39.

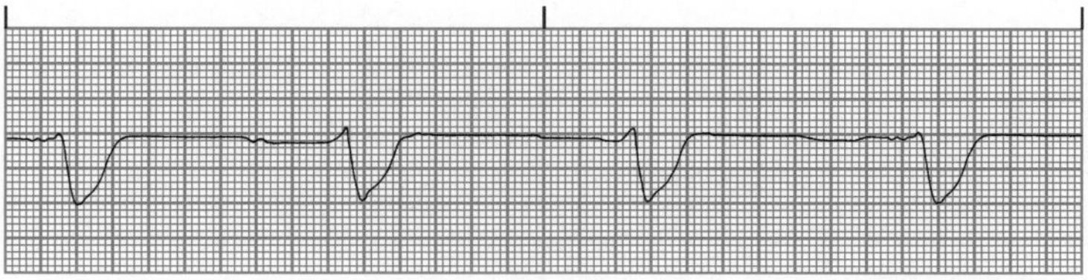

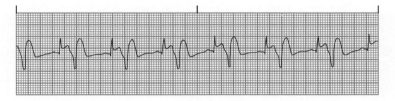

Atrial rhythm: _____   QRS complex: _____
Ventricular rhythm: _____   T wave: _____
Atrial rate: _____   QT interval: _____
Ventricular rate: _____   Other: _____
P wave: _____   Interpretation: _____
PR interval: _____   _____

40.

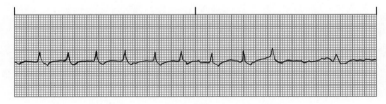

Atrial rhythm: _____   QRS complex: _____
Ventricular rhythm: _____   T wave: _____
Atrial rate: _____   QT interval: _____
Ventricular rate: _____   Other: _____
P wave: _____   Interpretation: _____
PR interval: _____   _____

41.

Atrial rhythm: _____   QRS complex: _____
Ventricular rhythm: _____   T wave: _____
Atrial rate: _____   QT interval: _____
Ventricular rate: _____   Other: _____
P wave: _____   Interpretation: _____
PR interval: _____   _____

42.

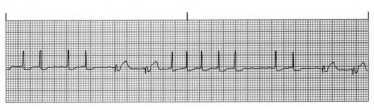

Atrial rhythm: _____   QRS complex: _____
Ventricular rhythm: _____   T wave: _____
Atrial rate: _____   QT interval: _____
Ventricular rate: _____   Other: _____
P wave: _____   Interpretation: _____
PR interval: _____   _____

43.

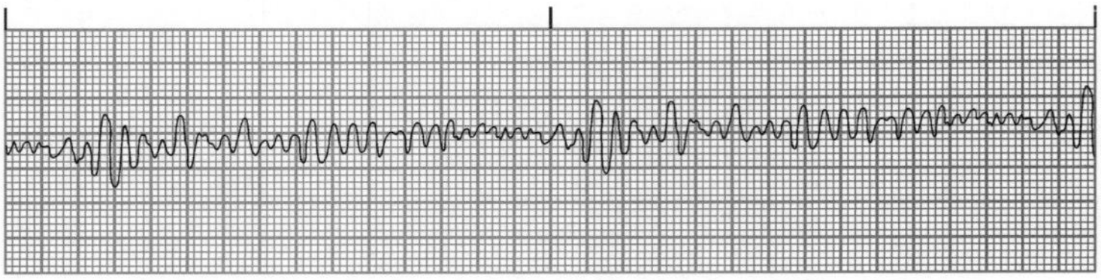

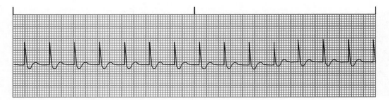

Atrial rhythm: _____   QRS complex: _____
Ventricular rhythm: _____   T wave: _____
Atrial rate: _____   QT interval: _____
Ventricular rate: _____   Other: _____
P wave: _____   Interpretation: _____
PR interval: _____   _____

44.

Atrial rhythm: _____   QRS complex: _____
Ventricular rhythm: _____   T wave: _____
Atrial rate: _____   QT interval: _____
Ventricular rate: _____   Other: _____
P wave: _____   Interpretation: _____
PR interval: _____   _____

45.

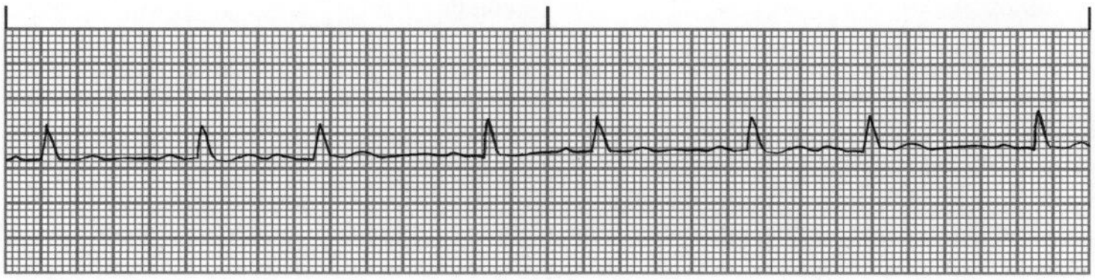

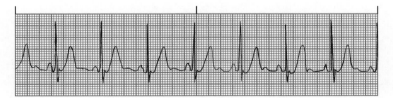

Atrial rhythm: _____   QRS complex: _____

Ventricular rhythm: _____   T wave: _____

Atrial rate: _____   QT interval: _____

Ventricular rate: _____   Other: _____

P wave: _____   Interpretation: _____

PR interval: _____   _____

46.

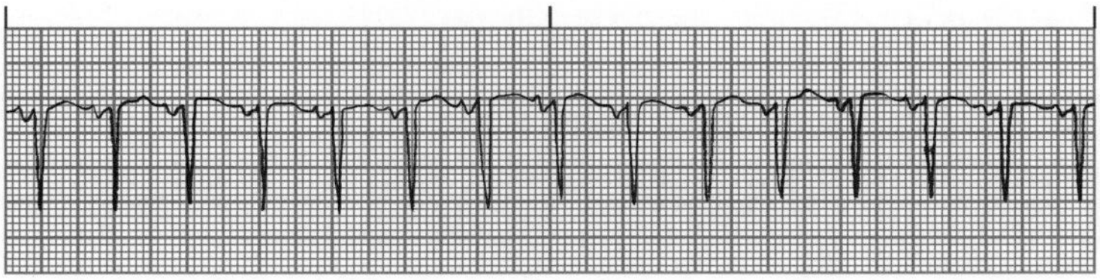

Atrial rhythm: _____   QRS complex: _____

Ventricular rhythm: _____   T wave: _____

Atrial rate: _____   QT interval: _____

Ventricular rate: _____   Other: _____

P wave: _____   Interpretation: _____

PR interval: _____   _____

47.

Atrial rhythm: _____   QRS complex: _____

Ventricular rhythm: _____   T wave: _____

Atrial rate: _____   QT interval: _____

Ventricular rate: _____   Other: _____

P wave: _____   Interpretation: _____

PR interval: _____   _____

48.

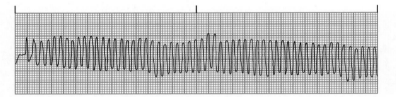

Atrial rhythm: _____   QRS complex: _____
Ventricular rhythm: _____   T wave: _____
Atrial rate: _____   QT interval: _____
Ventricular rate: _____   Other: _____
P wave: _____   Interpretation: _____
PR interval: _____   _____

49.

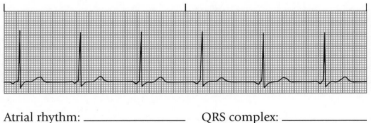

Atrial rhythm: _____   QRS complex: _____
Ventricular rhythm: _____   T wave: _____
Atrial rate: _____   QT interval: _____
Ventricular rate: _____   Other: _____
P wave: _____   Interpretation: _____
PR interval: _____   _____

50.

Atrial rhythm: _____   QRS complex: _____
Ventricular rhythm: _____   T wave: _____
Atrial rate: _____   QT interval: _____
Ventricular rate: _____   Other: _____
P wave: _____   Interpretation: _____
PR interval: _____   _____

51.

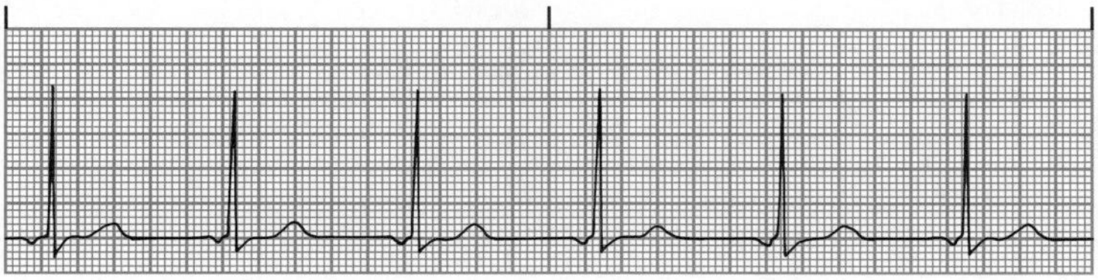

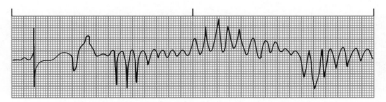

Atrial rhythm: _____   QRS complex: _____
Ventricular rhythm: _____   T wave: _____
Atrial rate: _____   QT interval: _____
Ventricular rate: _____   Other: _____
P wave: _____   Interpretation: _____
PR interval: _____   _____

52.

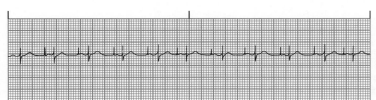

Atrial rhythm: _____   QRS complex: _____
Ventricular rhythm: _____   T wave: _____
Atrial rate: _____   QT interval: _____
Ventricular rate: _____   Other: _____
P wave: _____   Interpretation: _____
PR interval: _____   _____

53.

Atrial rhythm: _____   QRS complex: _____
Ventricular rhythm: _____   T wave: _____
Atrial rate: _____   QT interval: _____
Ventricular rate: _____   Other: _____
P wave: _____   Interpretation: _____
PR interval: _____   _____

54.

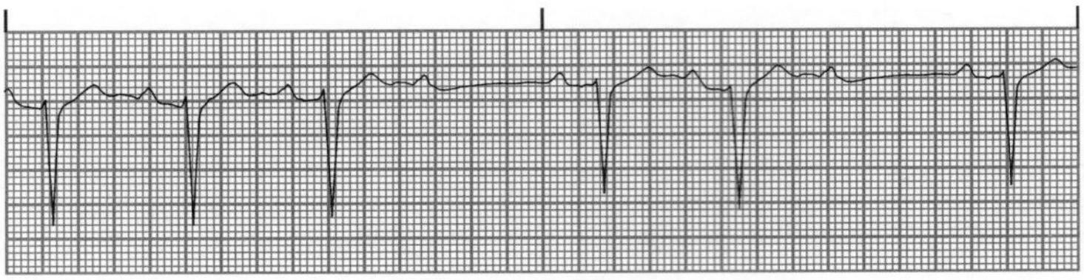

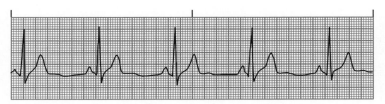

Atrial rhythm: _____   QRS complex: _____
Ventricular rhythm: _____   T wave: _____
Atrial rate: _____   QT interval: _____
Ventricular rate: _____   Other: _____
P wave: _____   Interpretation: _____
PR interval: _____   _____

55.

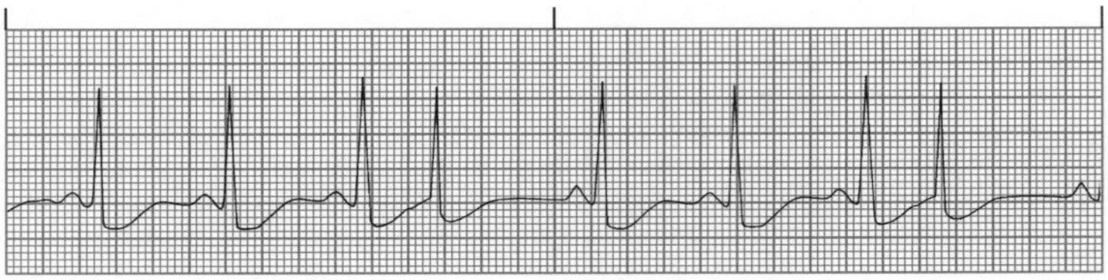

Atrial rhythm: _____   QRS complex: _____
Ventricular rhythm: _____   T wave: _____
Atrial rate: _____   QT interval: _____
Ventricular rate: _____   Other: _____
P wave: _____   Interpretation: _____
PR interval: _____   _____

56.

Atrial rhythm: _____   QRS complex: _____
Ventricular rhythm: _____   T wave: _____
Atrial rate: _____   QT interval: _____
Ventricular rate: _____   Other: _____
P wave: _____   Interpretation: _____
PR interval: _____   _____

Answers

1.
Atrial rhythm: Regular, except for missing PQRST complex
Ventricular rhythm: Regular, except for missing PQRST complex
Atrial rate: 40 beats/min; underlying rate 50 beats/min
Ventricular rate: 40 beats/min
P wave: Normal size and configuration; absent during pause
PR interval: 0.20 second
QRS complex: 0.08 second
T wave: Normal configuration; absent during pause
QT interval: 0.40 second
Other: None
Interpretation: Sinus arrest

2.
Atrial rhythm: Irregular
Ventricular rhythm: Irregular
Atrial rate: 60 beats/min; underlying rate 88 beats/min
Ventricular rate: 90 beats/min
P wave: None with premature ventricular contractions (PVCs);
present with QRS complexes
PR interval: 0.16 second
QRS complex: Underlying rate 0.08 second; 0.16 second with PVCs
T wave: Normal configuration; opposite direction with PVCs
QT interval: 0.42 second
Other: None
Interpretation: Normal sinus rhythm with trigeminal PVCs

3.
Atrial rhythm: Regular
Ventricular rhythm: Regular
Atrial rate: 125 beats/min
Ventricular rate: 125 beats/min
P wave: Normal size and configuration
PR interval: 0.14 second
QRS complex: 0.08 second
T wave: Normal configuration
QT interval: 0.32 second
Other: None
Interpretation: Sinus tachycardia

4.

Atrial rhythm: Irregular
Ventricular rhythm: Irregular
Atrial rate: 60 beats/min; underlying rate 71 beats/min
Ventricular rate: 70 beats/min
P wave: None with PVC; present with QRS complexes
PR interval: 0.16 second
QRS complex: 0.08 second; 0.14 second with PVC
T wave: Normal configuration
QT interval: 0.40 second
Other: None
Interpretation: Normal sinus rhythm with PVC

5.

Atrial rhythm: Irregular
Ventricular rhythm: Irregular
Atrial rate: 40 beats/min; underlying rate 70 beats/min
Ventricular rate: 70 beats/min
P wave: None with PVCs; present with QRS complexes
PR interval: 0.16 second
QRS complex: 0.08 second; 0.16 second with PVCs
T wave: Normal configuration
QT interval: 0.40 second
Other: None
Interpretation: Normal sinus rhythm with run of PVCs

6.

Atrial rhythm: Absent
Ventricular rhythm: Chaotic
Atrial rate: Absent
Ventricular rate: Undetermined
P wave: Absent
PR interval: Unmeasurable
QRS complex: Indiscernible
T wave: Indiscernible
QT interval: Not applicable
Other: None
Interpretation: Ventricular fibrillation

7.
Atrial rhythm: Regular
Ventricular rhythm: Regular
Atrial rate: 90 beats/min; underlying rate 107 beats/min
Ventricular rate: 110 beats/min
P wave: Present in normal QRS complexes
PR interval: 0.16 second
QRS complex: 0.08 second
T wave: Normal configuration
QT interval: 0.32 second
Other: Random pacemaker spikes
Interpretation: Sinus tachycardia with pacemaker failure to sense

8.
Atrial rhythm: Unmeasurable
Ventricular rhythm: Regular
Atrial rate: Unmeasurable
Ventricular rate: Paced rate 40 beats/min; pacer fires at
75 beats/min
P wave: Absent
PR interval: Unmeasurable
QRS complex: Unmeasurable
T wave: Unmeasurable
QT interval: Unmeasurable
Other: None
Interpretation: Paced rhythm with failure to capture

9.
Atrial rhythm: Irregular
Ventricular rhythm: Irregular
Atrial rate: Indiscernible
Ventricular rate: 80 beats/min
P wave: Absent; fine fibrillation waves present
PR interval: Indiscernible
QRS complex: 0.08 second
T wave: Indiscernible
QT interval: Unmeasurable
Other: None
Interpretation: Atrial fibrillation

10.

Atrial rhythm: Regular
Ventricular rhythm: Irregular
Atrial rate: 50 beats/min
Ventricular rate: 40 beats/min
P wave: Normal; some not followed by QRS complexes
PR interval: 0.16 second and constant (may be prolonged)
QRS complex: 0.08 second
T wave: Normal configuration; absent if QRS complexes are absent
QT interval: 0.40 second
Other: None
Interpretation: Type II second-degree atrioventricular (AV) block

11.

Atrial rhythm: Irregular
Ventricular rhythm: Irregular
Atrial rate: 60 beats/min
Ventricular rate: 70 beats/min
P wave: Rate and configuration varies
PR interval: Varies with rhythm
QRS complex: 0.10 second
T wave: Configuration varies
QT interval: Configuration varies
Other: None
Interpretation: Sick sinus syndrome

12.

Atrial rhythm: Regular
Ventricular rhythm: Regular
Atrial rate: 110 beats/min
Ventricular rate: 110 beats/min
P wave: Normal size and configuration
PR interval: 0.16 second
QRS complex: 0.10 second
T wave: Normal configuration
QT interval: 0.36 second
Other: None
Interpretation: Sinus tachycardia

13.

Atrial rhythm: Regular
Ventricular rhythm: Regular
Atrial rate: 270 beats/min
Ventricular rate: 70 beats/min
P wave: Saw-tooth edged
PR interval: Unmeasurable
QRS complex: 0.10 second
T wave: Unidentifiable
QT interval: Unidentifiable
Other: None
Interpretation: Atrial flutter (4:1 block)

14.

Atrial rhythm: Irregular
Ventricular rhythm: Irregular
Atrial rate: About 110 beats/min
Ventricular rate: About 110 beats/min
P wave: Size and configuration vary
PR interval: Rate varies
QRS complex: 0.08 second
T wave: Inverted
QT interval: 0.22 second
Other: None
Interpretation: Multifocal atrial tachycardia

15.

Atrial rhythm: Irregular
Ventricular rhythm: Irregular
Atrial rate: 100 beats/min
Ventricular rate: 100 beats/min
P wave: Normal size and configuration, except during premature beat
PR interval: 0.16 second; unmeasurable for premature beat
QRS complex: 0.06 second
T wave: Normal configuration
QT interval: 0.36 second
Other: None
Interpretation: Sinus tachycardia with PVCs

16.

Atrial rhythm: Unmeasurable
Ventricular rhythm: Regular
Atrial rate: Unmeasurable
Ventricular rate: 187 beats/min
P wave: Absent
PR interval: Unmeasurable
QRS complex: 0.18 second; wide and bizarre
T wave: Opposite direction of QRS complex
QT interval: Unmeasurable
Other: None
Interpretation: Ventricular tachycardia (monomorphic)

17.

Atrial rhythm: Unmeasurable
Ventricular rhythm: Unmeasurable; fibrillatory waves present
Atrial rate: Unmeasurable
Ventricular rate: Unmeasurable
P wave: Absent
PR interval: Absent
QRS complex: Unmeasurable
T wave: Opposite direction of QRS complex
QT interval: Absent
Other: None
Interpretation: Ventricular fibrillation

18.

Atrial rhythm: Regular
Ventricular rhythm: Irregular
Atrial rate: 75 beats/min
Ventricular rate: 50 beats/min
P wave: Normal size and configuration
PR interval: Lengthens with each cycle until dropped
QRS complex: 0.06 second
T wave: Normal configuration
QT interval: 0.38 second
Other: None
Interpretation: Type 1 (Mobitz I or Wenckebach) second-degree
AV block

19.
Atrial rhythm: Regular
Ventricular rhythm: Regular
Atrial rate: 90 beats/min
Ventricular rate: 30 beats/min
P wave: Normal size and configuration, except when hidden within
T wave
PR interval: Rate varies
QRS complex: 0.16 second
T wave: Normal configuration
QT interval: 0.56 second
Other: None
Interpretation: Third-degree AV block

20.
Atrial rhythm: Regular
Ventricular rhythm: Regular
Atrial rate: 60 beats/min
Ventricular rate: 60 beats/min
P wave: Normal size and configuration
PR interval: 0.36 second
QRS complex: 0.08 second
T wave: Normal configuration
QT interval: 0.40 second
Other: None
Interpretation: Normal sinus rhythm with first-degree AV block

21.
Atrial rhythm: Regular
Ventricular rhythm: Regular
Atrial rate: 35 beats/min
Ventricular rate: 35 beats/min
P wave: Normal configuration
PR interval: 0.18 second
QRS complex: 0.12 second
T wave: Normal configuration
QT interval: 0.44 second
Other: None
Interpretation: Sinus bradycardia

22.

Atrial rhythm: Irregular
Ventricular rhythm: Irregular
Atrial rate: 50 beats/min
Ventricular rate: 50 beats/min
P wave: Normal configuration
PR interval: 0.20 second
QRS complex: 0.08 second
T wave: Normal configuration
QT interval: 0.52 second
Other: None
Interpretation: Sinus bradycardia with premature atrial contraction (PAC)

23.

Atrial rhythm: Irregular
Ventricular rhythm: Irregular
Atrial rate: Unmeasurable
Ventricular rate: 60 beats/min
P wave: Not present
PR interval: Unmeasurable
QRS complex: 0.06 second
T wave: Flattened
QT interval: Unmeasurable
Other: None
Interpretation: Junctional escape rhythm

24.

Atrial rhythm: Regular
Ventricular rhythm: Regular
Atrial rate: Unmeasurable
Ventricular rate: 38 beats/min
P wave: Absent
PR interval: Unmeasurable
QRS complex: 0.04 second
T wave: Normal configuration
QT interval: 0.44 second
Other: None
Interpretation: Junctional rhythm

25.
Atrial rhythm: Regular
Ventricular rhythm: Regular
Atrial rate: 68 beats/min
Ventricular rate: 43 beats/min
P wave: Normal configuration
PR interval: Unmeasurable
QRS complex: 0.12 second
T wave: Normal configuration
QT interval: Unmeasurable
Other: P wave no correlation with QRS complex
Interpretation: Third-degree AV block

26.
Atrial rhythm: Regular
Ventricular rhythm: Regular
Atrial rate: 100 beats/min
Ventricular rate: 100 beats/min
P wave: Normal initially, then becomes inverted with shortened PR interval
PR interval: 0.14 second initially, then unmeasurable
QRS complex: 0.08 second
T wave: Normal configuration
QT interval: 0.36 second
Other: None
Interpretation: Sinus tachycardia leading to junctional tachycardia

27.
Atrial rhythm: Not present
Ventricular rhythm: Regular
Atrial rate: Not present
Ventricular rate: 30 beats/min
P wave: Absent
PR interval: Unmeasurable
QRS complex: Abnormal
T wave: Abnormal configuration
QT interval: Unmeasurable
Other: None
Interpretation: Idioventricular rhythm

28.

Atrial rhythm: Irregular
Ventricular rhythm: Irregular
Atrial rate: 280 beats/min
Ventricular rate: 110 beats/min
P wave: Flutter waves
PR interval: Unmeasurable
QRS complex: 0.08 second
T wave: Indiscernible
QT interval: Unmeasurable
Other: None
Interpretation: Atrial flutter with variable block

29.

Atrial rhythm: Regular
Ventricular rhythm: Regular
Atrial rate: 94 beats/min
Ventricular rate: 94 beats/min
P wave: Inverted
PR interval: 0.12 second
QRS complex: 0.08 second
T wave: Inverted
QT interval: 0.30 second
Other: None
Interpretation: Accelerated junctional rhythm

30.

Atrial rhythm: Irregular
Ventricular rhythm: Irregular
Atrial rate: 70 beats/min
Ventricular rate: 70 beats/min
P wave: Normal
PR interval: 0.16 second
QRS complex: 0.10 second
T wave: Biphasic
QT interval: 0.38 second
Other: None
Interpretation: Sinus arrhythmia

31.
Atrial rhythm: Irregular
Ventricular rhythm: Irregular
Atrial rate: 60 beats/min
Ventricular rate: 60 beats/min
P wave: Variable configurations
PR interval: 0.16 second
QRS complex: 0.10 second
T wave: Inverted
QT interval: 0.36 second
Other: None
Interpretation: Wandering pacemaker

32.
Atrial rhythm: Irregular
Ventricular rhythm: Irregular
Atrial rate: 180 beats/min
Ventricular rate: 100 beats/min
P wave: Abnormal; slight saw-tooth appearance
PR interval: Unmeasurable
QRS complex: 0.10 second
T wave: Abnormal configuration
QT interval: Unmeasurable
Other: None
Interpretation: Atrial flutter with varying conduction ratios

33.
Atrial rhythm: Irregular
Ventricular rhythm: Irregular
Atrial rate: 88 beats/min
Ventricular rate: 88 beats/min
P wave: Normal
PR interval: 0.16 second
QRS complex: 0.08 second
T wave: Normal
QT interval: 0.40 second
Other: ST-segment depression
Interpretation: Normal sinus rhythm with PACs

34.

Atrial rhythm: Slightly irregular
Ventricular rhythm: Slightly irregular
Atrial rate: 110 beats/min
Ventricular rate: 110 beats/min
P wave: P-wave shape different for multiple P waves
PR interval: Unmeasurable
QRS complex: 0.08 second
T wave: Indiscernible
QT interval: Unmeasurable
Other: None
Interpretation: Multifocal atrial tachycardia

35.

Atrial rhythm: Absent
Ventricular rhythm: Absent
Atrial rate: Absent
Ventricular rate: Absent
P wave: Absent
PR interval: Unmeasurable
QRS complex: Absent
T wave: Absent
QT interval: Unmeasurable
Other: None
Interpretation: Asystole

36.

Atrial rhythm: Regular
Ventricular rhythm: Irregular
Atrial rate: 80 beats/min
Ventricular rate: 60 beats/min
P wave: Biphasic
PR interval: 0.12 second
QRS complex: 0.12 second
T wave: Normal
QT interval: 0.34 second
Other: Two P waves without QRS complex
Interpretation: Second-degree AV block type II

37.
Atrial rhythm: Absent
Ventricular rhythm: Absent
Atrial rate: Absent
Ventricular rate: Absent
P wave: Absent
PR interval: Unmeasurable
QRS complex: Absent
T wave: Absent
QT interval: Unmeasurable
Other: None
Interpretation: Asystole

38.
Atrial rhythm: Irregular
Ventricular rhythm: Irregular
Atrial rate: 60 beats/min
Ventricular rate: 120 beats/min
P wave: Biphasic when present
PR interval: 0.16 second
QRS complex: 0.10 second
T wave: Elevated
QT interval: 0.40 second when measurable
Other: None
Interpretation: Normal sinus rhythm with PVCs

39.
Atrial rhythm: Indiscernible
Ventricular rhythm: Regular
Atrial rate: Indiscernible
Ventricular rate: 38 beats/min
P wave: Indiscernible
PR interval: Unmeasurable
QRS complex: 0.36 second
T wave: Indiscernible
QT interval: Unmeasurable
Other: None
Interpretation: Idioventricular rhythm

40.
Atrial rhythm: Regular
Ventricular rhythm: Irregular
Atrial rate: 70 beats/min
Ventricular rate: 140 beats/min
P wave: Normal with sinus beats
PR interval: 0.14 second
QRS complex: 0.08 second
T wave: Distorted
QT interval: Unmeasurable
Other: None
Interpretation: Normal sinus rhythm with PVCs (bigeminy)

41.
Atrial rhythm: Irregular
Ventricular rhythm: Irregular
Atrial rate: Indiscernible
Ventricular rate: 100 beats/min
P wave: Indiscernible
PR interval: Unmeasurable
QRS complex: 0.08 second
T wave: Flattened
QT interval: Unmeasurable
Other: None
Interpretation: Atrial fibrillation

42.
Atrial rhythm: Irregular
Ventricular rhythm: Irregular
Atrial rate: Indiscernible
Ventricular rate: 150 beats/min
P wave: None
PR interval: Unmeasurable
QRS complex: 0.04 second in nonpaced beats
T wave: Flattened
QT interval: Unmeasurable
Other: ST-segment depression
Interpretation: Atrial fibrillation with ventricular pacing

43.
Atrial rhythm: None
Ventricular rhythm: Chaotic
Atrial rate: None
Ventricular rate: Unmeasurable
P wave: Indiscernible
PR interval: Unmeasurable
QRS complex: Unmeasurable
T wave: Indiscernible
QT interval: Unmeasurable
Other: None
Interpretation: Ventricular fibrillation

44.
Atrial rhythm: Not visible
Ventricular rhythm: Regular
Atrial rate: Indiscernible
Ventricular rate: 150 beats/min
P wave: Not visible
PR interval: Unmeasurable
QRS complex: 0.12 second
T wave: Normal
QT interval: 0.24 second
Other: None
Interpretation: Junctional tachycardia

45.
Atrial rhythm: Irregular
Ventricular rhythm: Irregular
Atrial rate: 80 beats/min
Ventricular rate: 80 beats/min
P wave: Normal configuration
PR interval: 0.22 second
QRS complex: 0.10 second
T wave: Normal configuration
QT interval: 0.38 second
Other: None
Interpretation: First-degree AV block with bigeminal PACs

46.

Atrial rhythm: Regular
Ventricular rhythm: Regular
Atrial rate: 150 beats/min
Ventricular rate: 150 beats/min
P wave: Peaked
PR interval: 0.12 second
QRS complex: 0.08 second
T wave: Flattened
QT interval: 0.24 second
Other: None
Interpretation: Atrial tachycardia

47.

Atrial rhythm: Regular
Ventricular rhythm: Regular
Atrial rate: 79 beats/min
Ventricular rate: 79 beats/min
P wave: Normal configuration
PR interval: 0.16 second
QRS complex: 0.08 second
T wave: Normal configuration
QT interval: 0.40 second
Other: None
Interpretation: Normal sinus rhythm

48.

Atrial rhythm: None
Ventricular rhythm: Regular
Atrial rate: Indiscernible
Ventricular rate: 60 beats/min
P wave: Not present
PR interval: Unmeasurable
QRS complex: 0.06 second
T wave: Normal configuration
QT interval: 0.32 second
Other: None
Interpretation: Junctional escape rhythm

49.

Atrial rhythm: Indiscernible
Ventricular rhythm: Chaotic
Atrial rate: Unmeasurable
Ventricular rate: Greater than 300 beats/min
P wave: Indiscernible
PR interval: Unmeasurable
QRS complex: Abnormal
T wave: Indiscernible
QT interval: Unmeasurable
Other: None
Interpretation: Ventricular tachycardia

50.

Atrial rhythm: Slightly irregular
Ventricular rhythm: Slightly irregular
Atrial rate: 70 beats/min
Ventricular rate: 70 beats/min
P wave: Normal configuration
PR interval: 0.20 second
QRS complex: 0.08 second
T wave: Normal configuration
QT interval: 0.36 second
Other: Phasic slowing and quickening
Interpretation: Sinus arrhythmia

51.

Atrial rhythm: Regular
Ventricular rhythm: Regular
Atrial rate: 60 beats/min
Ventricular rate: 60 beats/min
P wave: Inverted
PR interval: 0.08 second
QRS complex: 0.12 second
T wave: Normal configuration
QT interval: 0.44 second
Other: None
Interpretation: Junctional escape rhythm

52.

Atrial rhythm: Unmeasurable
Ventricular rhythm: Irregular
Atrial rate: Unmeasurable
Ventricular rate: Unmeasurable
P wave: Absent
PR interval: Absent
QRS complex: Unmeasurable
T wave: Indiscernible
QT interval: Unmeasurable
Other: Continuous switching of ventricular rhythm between positive and negative directions
Interpretation: Torsades de pointes

53.

Atrial rhythm: Regular
Ventricular rhythm: Regular
Atrial rate: 107 beats/min; pacemaker generated
Ventricular rate: 107 beats/min; pacemaker generated
P wave: Follows pacer spike
PR interval: 0.12 second
QRS complex: 0.06 second
T wave: Normal configuration
QT interval: 0.28 second
Other: Pacemaker spikes
Interpretation: AV pacing

54.

Atrial rhythm: Regular
Ventricular rhythm: Irregular
Atrial rate: 80 beats/min
Ventricular rate: 60 beats/min
P wave: Normal configuration
PR interval: 0.24 second
QRS complex: 0.12 second
T wave: Normal configuration
QT interval: 0.38 second
Other: Dropped ventricular beats
Interpretation: Normal sinus rhythm with Type II second-degree AV block

55.

Atrial rhythm: Irregular
Ventricular rhythm: Irregular
Atrial rate: 70 beats/min
Ventricular rate: 80 beats/min
P wave: Normal configuration but absent on premature beats
PR interval: 0.20 second
QRS complex: 0.08 second
T wave: Flattened
QT interval: Unmeasurable
Other: None
Interpretation: Normal sinus rhythm with premature junctional complexes

56.

Atrial rhythm: Regular
Ventricular rhythm: Regular
Atrial rate: 50 beats/min
Ventricular rate: 50 beats/min
P wave: Normal configuration
PR interval: 0.16 second
QRS complex: 0.12 second
T wave: Normal configuration
QT interval: 0.44 second
Other: None
Interpretation: Sinus bradycardia

Differentiating ECG rhythm strips can often be a tricky proposition, especially when waveform patterns appear strikingly similar. These pairs of rhythm strips are among the most challenging to interpret. Test your knowledge and skill by correctly identifying each rhythm strip; answers begin on page 374.

1.

Rhythm strip A

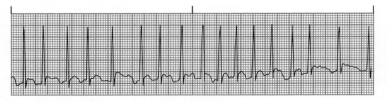

Rhythm strip A is: _____

Rhythm strip B

Rhythm strip B is: _____

2.

Rhythm strip A

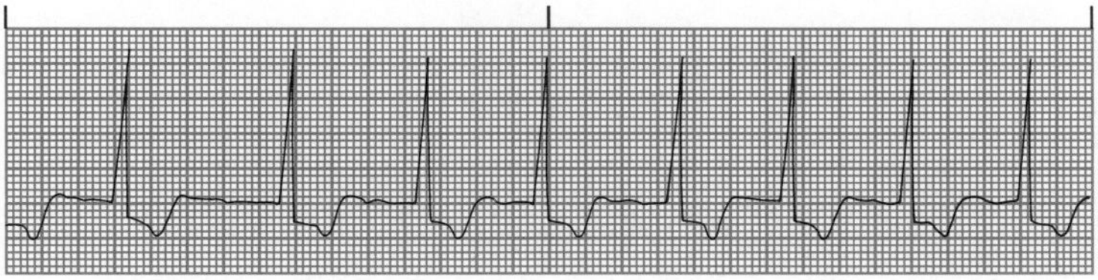

Rhythm strip A is: _____

Rhythm strip B

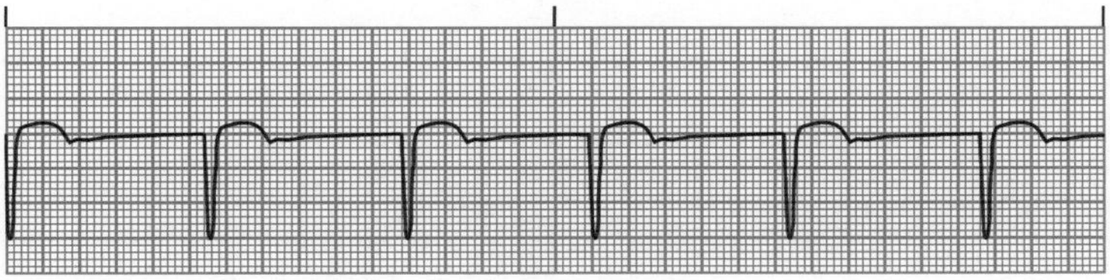

Rhythm strip B is: _____

3.

Rhythm strip A

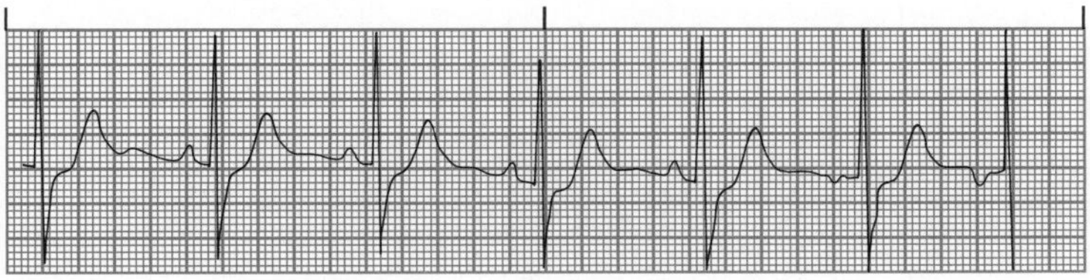

Rhythm strip A is: _____

Rhythm strip B

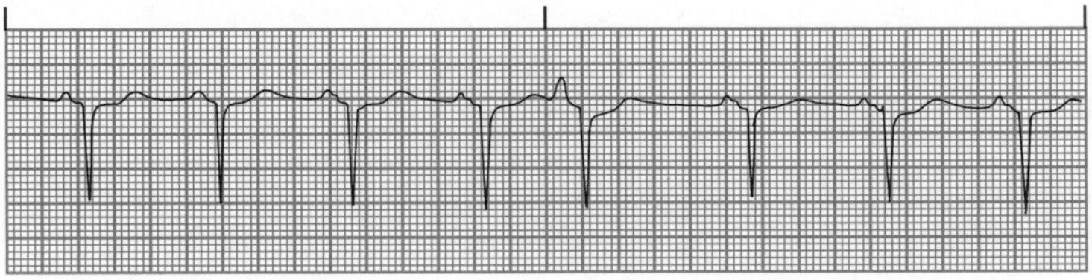

Rhythm strip B is: _____

4.

Rhythm strip A

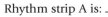

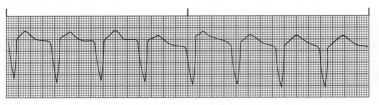

Rhythm strip A is: _____

Rhythm strip B

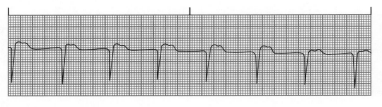

Rhythm strip B is: _____

5.

Rhythm strip A

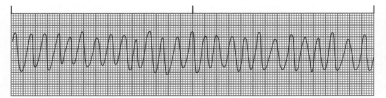

Rhythm strip A is: _____

Rhythm strip B

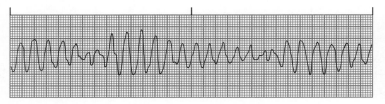

Rhythm strip B is: _____

6.

Rhythm strip A

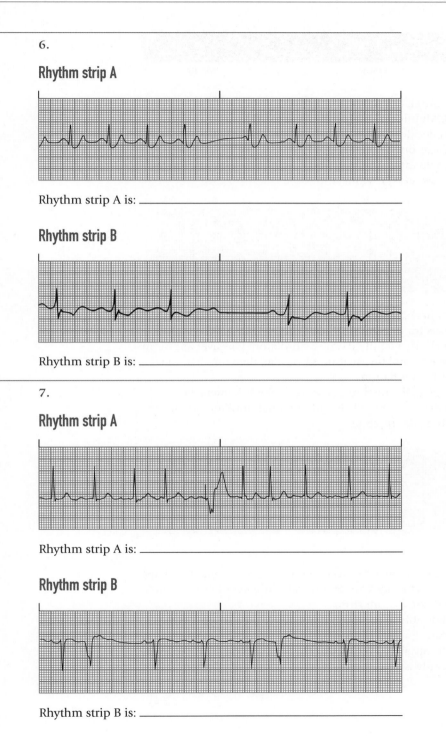

Rhythm strip A is: _____

Rhythm strip B

Rhythm strip B is: _____

7.

Rhythm strip A

Rhythm strip A is: _____

Rhythm strip B

Rhythm strip B is: _____

Answers

1.

Rhythm strip A: Atrial fibrillation
Rhythm strip B: Multifocal atrial tachycardia (MAT)

To help you decide whether a rhythm is atrial fibrillation or the similar MAT, focus on the presence of P waves as well as the atrial and ventricular rhythms. You may find it helpful to look at a longer (greater than 6 seconds) rhythm strip.

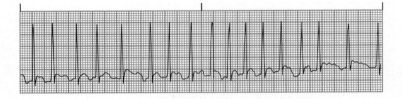

Atrial fibrillation
- Carefully look for discernible P waves before each QRS complex.
- If you can't clearly identify P waves, fibrillatory (f) waves appear in place of P waves, and the rhythm is irregular, then the rhythm is probably atrial fibrillation.
- Carefully look at the rhythm, focusing on the R-R intervals. Remember that one of the hallmarks of atrial fibrillation is an irregularly irregular rhythm.

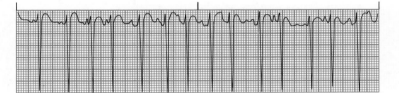

MAT
- P waves are present in MAT. Keep in mind, however, that the shape of the P waves will vary, with at least three different P wave shapes visible in a single rhythm strip.
- You should be able to see most, if not all, of the various P wave shapes repeat.
- Although the atrial and ventricular rhythms are irregular, the irregularity generally isn't as pronounced as in atrial fibrillation.

2.

Rhythm strip A: Atrial fibrillation
Rhythm strip B: Junctional rhythm

At times, it can be easy to mistake atrial fibrillation for junctional rhythm. Here's how to tell the two apart.

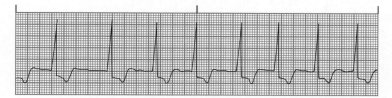

Atrial fibrillation

- Examine lead II, which provides a clear view of atrial activity. Look for fibrillatory (f) waves, which appear as a wavy line. These waves indicate atrial fibrillation. The rhythm is irregular with atrial fibrillation.
- Chronic atrial fibrillation tends to have fine or small f waves and a controlled ventricular rate (less than 100 beats/min).

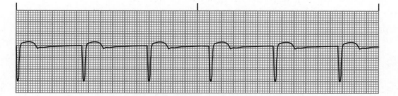

Junctional rhythm

- Junctional rhythm is always regular.
- Examine lead II. The P wave may occur before, be hidden in, or occur after the QRS complex (see shaded areas above). If visible, the P wave is inverted; if the P wave is before the QRS complex, the PR interval is less than 0.12 second.

3.

Rhythm strip A: Wandering pacemaker

Rhythm strip B: Premature atrial contraction (PAC)

Because PACs are commonly encountered, it's possible to mistake wandering pacemaker for PACs unless the rhythm strip is carefully examined. In such cases, you may find it helpful to look at a longer (greater than 6 seconds) rhythm strip.

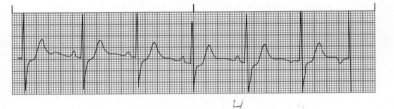

Wandering pacemaker

- Carefully examine the P waves. You must be able to identify at least three different shapes of P waves (see shaded areas above) in wandering pacemaker.
- Atrial rhythm varies slightly, with an irregular P-P interval. Ventricular rhythm also varies slightly, with an irregular R-R interval. These slight variations in rhythm result from the changing site of impulse formation.

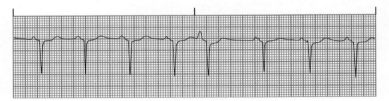

PAC

- The PAC occurs earlier than the sinus P wave, with an abnormal configuration when compared with a sinus P wave (see shaded area above). It's possible, but rare, to see multifocal PACs, which originate from multiple ectopic pacemaker sites in the atria. In this setting, the P waves have different shapes.
- With the exception of the irregular atrial and ventricular rhythms that result from the PAC, the underlying rhythm is usually regular.

4.

Rhythm strip A: Accelerated idioventricular rhythm
Rhythm strip B: Accelerated junctional rhythm

Idioventricular rhythm and junctional rhythm appear similar but have different causes. To distinguish between the two, closely examine the duration of the QRS complex and then look for P waves.

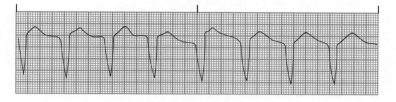

Accelerated idioventricular rhythm

- The QRS duration will be greater than 0.12 second.
- The QRS complex will have a wide and bizarre configuration.
- P waves are usually absent.
- The ventricular rate is generally between 40 and 100 beats/min.

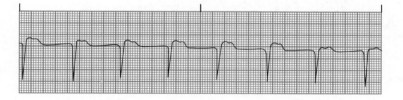

Accelerated junctional rhythm

- The QRS duration and configuration are usually normal.
- Inverted P waves generally occur before or after the QRS complex (see shaded area above). However, remember that P waves may also be buried within QRS complexes.
- The ventricular rate is typically between 60 and 100 beats/min.

5.

Rhythm strip A: Ventricular flutter
Rhythm strip B: Torsades de pointes

Torsades de pointes is a variant form of ventricular tachycardia, with a rapid ventricular rate that varies between 250 and 350 beats/min. It's characterized by QRS complexes that gradually change back and forth, with the amplitude of each successive complex gradually increasing then decreasing. This results in an overall outline of the rhythm commonly described as *spindle-shaped.*

Ventricular flutter, although rarely recognized, results from the rapid, regular, repetitive beating of the ventricles. It's produced by a single ventricular focus firing at a rapid rate of 250 to 350 beats/min. The hallmark of this arrhythmia is its smooth sine-wave appearance.

The illustrations shown here highlight key differences in the two arrhythmias.

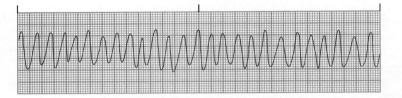

Ventricular flutter
• Smooth sine-wave appearance

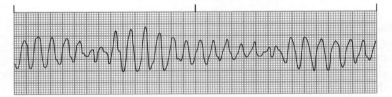

Torsades de pointes
• Spindle-shaped appearance

6.

Rhythm strip A: Nonconducted PAC

Rhythm strip B: Type II second-degree atrioventricular (AV) block

An isolated P wave that doesn't conduct through to the ventricle (P wave without a QRS complex following it; see shaded areas in both illustrations below) may occur with either a nonconducted PAC or type II second-degree AV block. To differentiate the two, look for constancy of the P-P interval. Be aware that mistakenly identifying AV block as nonconducted PACs may have serious consequences. The latter is generally benign, whereas the former can be life-threatening.

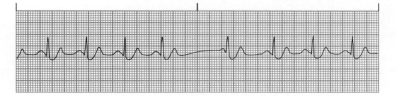

Nonconducted PAC

- If the P-P interval, including the extra P wave, isn't constant, it's a nonconducted PAC.

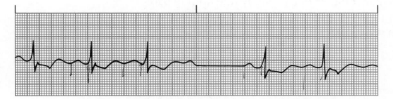

Type II second-degree AV block

- If the P-P interval is constant, including the extra P wave, it's type II second-degree AV block.

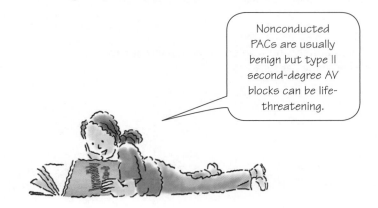

Nonconducted PACs are usually benign but type II second-degree AV blocks can be life-threatening.

7.
Rhythm strip A: Intermittent ventricular pacing
Rhythm strip B: Premature ventricular contraction (PVC)

Knowing whether your patient has an artificial pacemaker will help you avoid mistaking a ventricular paced beat for a PVC. If your facility uses a monitoring system that eliminates artifact, make sure the monitor is set up correctly for a patient with a pacemaker. Otherwise, the pacemaker spikes may be eliminated as well.

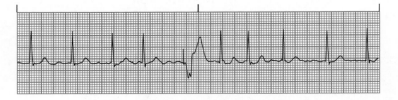

Intermittent ventricular pacing

- The paced ventricular complex will have a pacemaker spike preceding it (see pacemaker spike before the down sloping ventricular beat in the strip above). You may need to look in different leads for a bipolar pacemaker spike because it's small and may be difficult to see.
- The paced ventricular complex of a properly functioning pacemaker won't occur early or prematurely. It will occur only when the patient's own ventricular rate falls below the rate set for the pacemaker.

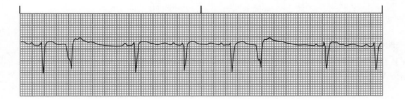

PVC

- PVCs will occur prematurely and won't have pacemaker spikes preceding them (see shaded areas above).

Quick guide to arrhythmias

Sinus arrhythmia

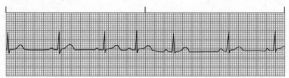

Features
- Rhythm irregular; varies with respiratory cycle
- P and R-R intervals shorter during inspiration, longer during expiration
- Normal P wave preceding each QRS complex

Treatment
- Typically no treatment necessary; possible correction of underlying cause

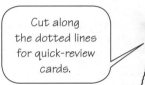

Cut along the dotted lines for quick-review cards.

Sinus bradycardia

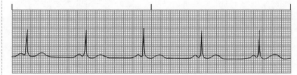

Features
- Rhythm regular
- Rate < 60 beats/min
- Normal P wave preceding each QRS complex
- Normal QRS complex
- QT interval may be prolonged

Treatment
- No treatment needed if patient is asymptomatic; if drugs are cause, possibly discontinuation of use
- For low cardiac output, dizziness, weakness, altered level of consciousness, or low blood pressure, consider temporary or permanent pacemaker and atropine, dopamine, or epinephrine

Sinus tachycardia

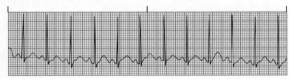

Features
- Rhythm regular
- Atrial and ventricular rates > 100 beats/min
- Normal P wave preceding each QRS complex
- Normal QRS complex
- QT interval commonly shortened

Treatment
- No treatment necessary if patient is asymptomatic
- Correction of underlying cause
- Beta-adrenergic blocker or calcium channel blocker administration, if cardiac ischemia occurs

Sinus arrest

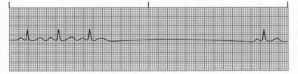

Features
- Rhythm normal, except for missing PQRST complexes
- P wave is periodically absent with entire PQRST complexes missing; when present, normal P wave precedes each QRS complex

Treatment
- No treatment needed if patient is asymptomatic
- For mild symptoms, possible discontinuation of drugs that contribute to arrhythmia
- Atropine administration if patient is symptomatic
- Temporary or permanent pacemaker for repeated episodes

Premature atrial contractions (PACs)

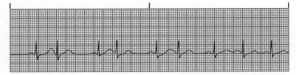

Features
- Premature, abnormal P waves (differ in configuration from normal P waves)
- QRS complexes after P waves, except in blocked PACs
- P wave often buried or identified in preceding T wave

Treatment
- No treatment needed if patient is asymptomatic
- Beta-adrenergic blockers or calcium channel blockers, if PACs occur frequently
- Treatment of underlying cause; avoidance of triggers (caffeine or smoking) and use of stress-reduction measures

Atrial tachycardia

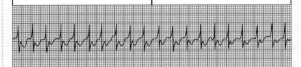

Features
- Rhythm regular if block is constant; irregular if not
- Rate 150 to 250 beats/min
- P waves regular but hidden in preceding T wave; precede QRS complexes
- Usually has sudden onset and termination

Treatment
- Vagal stimulation and adenosine administration
- Calcium channel blocker, beta-adrenergic blocker, amiodarone, procainamide, sotalol, or digoxin administration; cardioversion
- Atrial overdrive pacing
- If other treatment fails, synchronized cardioversion may be considered

Atrial flutter

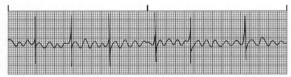

Features
- Atrial rhythm regular; ventricular rhythm variable
- Atrial rate 250 to 400 beats/min; ventricular rate depends on degree of AV block
- Sawtooth P-wave configuration (F waves)

Treatment
- Calcium channel blockers or beta-adrenergic blockers if patient is stable and heart function is normal
- Amiodarone, ibutilide, flecainide, propafenone, or procainamide if arrhythmia is present for less than 48 hours
- Synchronized cardioversion immediately if patient is unstable
- Anticoagulation before cardioversion if rhythm is present for more than 48 hours

Atrial fibrillation

Features
- Atrial and ventricular rhythms grossly irregular
- Atrial rate > 400 beats/min; ventricular rate varies
- No P waves; replaced by fine fibrillatory waves

Treatment
- Calcium channel blockers or beta-adrenergic blockers if patient is stable
- Amiodarone, ibutilide, flecainide, propafenone, or procainamide if arrhythmia is present for less than 48 hours
- Synchronized cardioversion immediately if patient is unstable
- Anticoagulation before cardioversion if rhythm is present for more than 48 hours

Wandering pacemaker

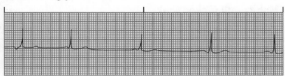

Features
- Rhythm irregular
- PR interval varies
- P waves change in configuration, indicating origin in sinoatrial node, atria, or AV junction (*Hallmark:* At least three different P-wave configurations)

Treatment
- No treatment if patient is asymptomatic
- Treatment of underlying cause if patient is symptomatic

Premature junctional contractions

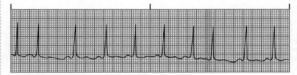

Features
- Rhythm irregular
- P waves before, hidden in, or after QRS complexes; inverted if visible
- PR interval < 0.12 second, if P wave precedes QRS complex
- QRS configuration and duration normal

Treatment
- No treatment if patient is asymptomatic
- Correction of underlying cause
- Discontinuation of digoxin, if appropriate
- Possible elimination of caffeine

Junctional tachycardia

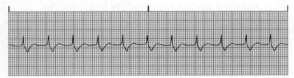

Features
- Rhythm regular
- Rate 100 to 200 beats/min
- P waves before, hidden in, or after QRS complexes; inverted if visible

Treatment
- Correction of underlying cause
- Discontinuation of digoxin, if appropriate
- Vagal maneuvers, adenosine, amiodarone, beta-adrenergic blockers, or calcium channel blockers to slow rate
- Possible pacemaker insertion
- Ablation therapy, if recurrent

Junctional escape rhythm

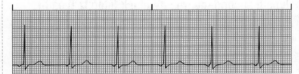

Features
- Rhythm regular
- Rate 40 to 60 beats/min
- P waves before, hidden in, or after QRS complexes; inverted if visible
- PR interval < 0.12 second (measurable only if P wave appears before QRS complex)

Treatment
- Treatment of underlying cause
- Atropine administration for symptomatic slow rate
- Pacemaker insertion if refractory to drugs
- Discontinuation of digoxin, if appropriate

First-degree AV block

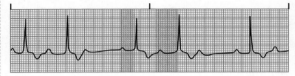

Features
- Rhythm regular
- PR interval > 0.20 second
- P wave preceding each QRS complex; QRS complex normal

Treatment
- Cautious use of digoxin, calcium channel blockers, and beta-adrenergic blockers
- Correction of underlying cause

Type I second-degree AV block (Mobitz I, Wenckebach)

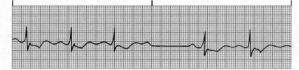

Features
- Atrial rhythm regular
- Ventricular rhythm irregular
- Atrial rate exceeds ventricular rate
- PR interval progressively, but only slightly, longer with each cycle until a P wave appears without a QRS complex (dropped beat)

Treatment
- Treatment of underlying cause
- Atropine administration or temporary pacemaker, for symptomatic bradycardia
- Discontinuation of digoxin, if appropriate

Type II second-degree AV block (Mobitz Type II)

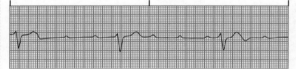

Features
- Atrial rhythm regular
- Ventricular rhythm possibly irregular, varying with degree of block
- QRS complexes periodically absent

Treatment
- Treatment of underlying cause
- Atropine, dopamine, or epinephrine administration, for symptomatic bradycardia (Atropine may worsen ischemia with MI.)
- Temporary or permanent pacemaker
- Discontinuation of digoxin, if appropriate

Third-degree AV block (complete heart block)

Features
- Atrial and ventricular rhythms regular
- Ventricular rate is 40 to 60 beats/min (AV node origin); <40 beats/min (Purkinje system origin)
- No relationship between P waves and QRS complexes
- QRS complex normal (originating in AV node) or wide and bizarre (originating in Purkinje system)

Treatment
- Treatment of underlying cause
- Atropine, dopamine, or epinephrine for symptomatic bradycardia (Don't use atropine with wide QRS complexes.)
- Temporary or permanent pacemaker

Premature ventricular contractions (PVCs)

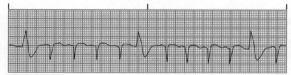

Features

- Underlying rhythm regular; P wave absent with PVCs
- Ventricular rhythm irregular during PVC
- QRS premature, usually followed by compensatory pause
- QRS complex wide and bizarre, duration > 0.12 second
- Premature QRS complexes occurring singly, in pairs, or in threes; possibly unifocal or multifocal
- Most ominous when clustered, multifocal, and with R wave on T pattern

Treatment

- If warranted, procainamide, lidocaine, or amiodarone administration
- Treatment of underlying cause
- Potassium chloride I.V. if induced by hypokalemia

Ventricular tachycardia

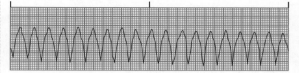

Features

- Ventricular rate 100 to 250 beats/min
- QRS complexes wide and bizarre; duration > 0.12 second
- P waves indiscernible

Treatment

- Monomorphic VT with pulse: Give amiodarone, using Advanced Cardiac Life Support (ACLS) protocol; if unsuccessful, synchronized cardioversion
- Polymorphic VT with normal QT interval: Amiodarone or sotalol using ACLS protocol; if unsuccessful, synchronized cardioversion
- Polymorphic ventricular tachycardia with prolonged QT interval: Stop drugs that may prolong QT interval and treat electrolyte imbalances
- Pulselessness: Initiate cardiopulmonary resuscitation (CPR) and follow treatment for ventricular fibrillation

Ventricular fibrillation

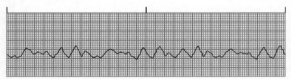

Features

- Ventricular rhythm rapid and chaotic
- QRS wide and irregular; no visible P waves

Treatment

- Defibrillation and CPR
- Epinephrine or vasopressin, amiodarone or lidocaine; if ineffective, magnesium sulfate or procainamide
- Endotracheal intubation
- Implanted cardioverter-defibrillator if at risk for recurrent ventricular fibrillation

Asystole

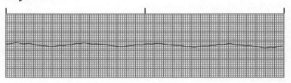

Features

- No atrial or ventricular rate or rhythm
- No discernible P waves, QRS complexes, or T waves

Treatment

- CPR, following ACLS protocol
- Endotracheal intubation
- Transcutaneous pacemaker
- Treatment of underlying cause
- Repeated doses of epinephrine and atropine, as ordered

Glossary

aberrant conduction: abnormal pathway of an impulse traveling through the heart's conduction system

ablation: surgical or radio-frequency removal of an irritable focus in the heart; used to prevent tachyarrhythmias

afterload: resistance that the left ventricle must work against to pump blood through the aorta

amplitude: height of a waveform

arrhythmia: disturbance of the normal cardiac rhythm from the abnormal origin, discharge, or conduction of electrical impulses

artifact: waveform interference in an ECG tracing that results from patient movement or poorly placed or poorly functioning equipment

atrial kick: amount of blood pumped into the ventricles as a result of atrial contraction; contributes approximately 30% of total cardiac output

automaticity: ability of a cardiac cell to initiate an impulse on its own

bigeminy: premature beat occurring every other beat; alternates with normal QRS complexes

biotransformation: series of chemical changes of a substance as a result of enzyme activity; end result of drug biotransformation may be active or inactive metabolites

biphasic: complex containing both an upward and a downward deflection; usually seen when the electrical current is perpendicular to the observed lead

bundle-branch block: slowing or blocking of an impulse as it travels through one of the bundle branches

capture: successful pacing of the heart, represented on the ECG tracing by a pacemaker spike followed by a P wave or QRS complex

cardiac output: amount of blood ejected from the left ventricle per minute; normal value is 4 to 8 L/min

cardioversion: restoration of normal rhythm by electric shock or drug therapy

carotid sinus massage: manual pressure applied to the carotid sinus to slow the heart rate

circus re-entry: delayed impulse in a one-way conduction path in which the impulse remains active and re-enters the surrounding tissues to produce another impulse

compensatory pause: period following a premature contraction during which the heart regulates itself, allowing the sinoatrial node to resume normal conduction

conduction: transmission of electrical impulses through the myocardium

conductivity: ability of one cardiac cell to transmit an electrical impulse to another cell

contractility: ability of a cardiac cell to contract after receiving an impulse

couplet: pair of premature beats occurring together

defibrillation: termination of fibrillation by electrical shock

deflection: direction of a waveform, based on the direction of a current

depolarization: response of a myocardial cell to an electrical impulse that causes movement of ions across the cell membrane, which triggers myocardial contraction

diastole: phase of the cardiac cycle when both atria (atrial diastole) or both ventricles (ventricular diastole) are at rest and filling with blood

ECG complex: waveform representing electrical events of one cardiac cycle; consists of five main waveforms (labeled P, Q, R, S, and T), a sixth waveform (labeled U) that occurs under certain conditions, the PR and QT intervals, and the ST segment

ectopic beat: contraction that occurs as a result of an impulse generated from a site other than the sinoatrial node

electrical axis: direction of the depolarization waveform as seen in the frontal leads

enhanced automaticity: condition in which pacemaker cells increase the firing rate above their inherent rate

excitability: ability of a cardiac cell to respond to an electrical stimulus

extrinsic: not inherently part of the cardiac electrical system

indicative leads: leads that have a direct view of an infarcted area of the heart

intrinsic: naturally occurring electrical stimulus from within the heart's conduction system

inverted: negative or downward deflection on an ECG

late electrical potentials: cardiac electrical activity that occurs after depolarization; predisposes the patient to ventricular tachycardia

lead: perspective of the electrical activity in a particular area of the heart through the placement of electrodes on the chest wall

monomorphic: form of ventricular tachycardia in which the QRS complexes have a uniform appearance from beat to beat

multiform or multifocal: type of premature ventricular contractions that have differing QRS configurations as a result of their originating from different irritable sites in the ventricle

nonsustained ventricular tachycardia: ventricular tachycardia that lasts less than 30 seconds

pacemaker: group of cells that generates impulses to the heart muscle or a battery-powered device that delivers an electrical stimulus to the heart to cause myocardial depolarization

paroxysmal: episode of an arrhythmia that starts and stops suddenly

polymorphic: type of ventricular tachycardia in which the QRS complexes change from beat to beat

preload: stretching force exerted on the ventricular muscle by the blood it contains at the end of diastole

proarrhythmia: rhythm disturbance caused or made worse by drugs or other therapy

quadrigeminy: premature beat occurring every fourth beat that alternates with three normal QRS complexes

reciprocal leads: leads that take a view of an infarcted area of the heart opposite that taken by indicative leads

re-entry mechanism: failure of a cardiac impulse to follow the normal conduction pathway; instead, it follows a circular path

refractory: type of arrhythmia that doesn't respond to usual treatment measures

refractory period: brief period during which excitability in a myocardial cell is depressed

repolarization: recovery of the myocardial cells after depolarization during which the cell membrane returns to its resting potential

retrograde depolarization: depolarization that occurs backward toward the atrium instead of downward toward the ventricles; results in an inverted P wave

rhythm strip: length of ECG paper that shows multiple ECG complexes representing a picture of the heart's electrical activity in a specific lead

Stokes-Adams attack: sudden episode of light-headedness or loss of consciousness caused by an abrupt slowing or stopping of the heartbeat

sustained ventricular tachycardia: type of ventricular tachycardia that lasts longer than 30 seconds

systole: phase of the cardiac cycle when both of the atria (atrial systole) or the ventricles (ventricular systole) are contracting

trigeminy: premature beat occurring every third beat that alternates with two normal QRS complexes

triplet: three premature beats occurring together

uniform or unifocal: type of premature ventricular contraction that has the same or similar QRS configuration and that originates from the same irritable site in the ventricle

vagal stimulation: pharmacologic or manual stimulation of the vagus nerve to slow the heart rate

Valsalva's maneuver: technique of forceful expiration against a closed glottis; used to slow the heart rate

Index

i refers to an illustration; t refers to a table.

to → 5.00 – 5:20   exercise

20 → Review goals   520 – 540

20 –   5:40 → 6⁰⁰